Threat Intelligence and Cloud Trust Models for Healthcare Security

Chin-Shiuh Shieh
National Kaohsiung University of Science and Technology, Taiwan

Pawan Kumar Goel
Raj Kumar Goel Institute of Technology, India

Mong-Fong Horng
National Kaohsiung University of Science and Technology, Taiwan

Hari Mohan Pandey
Bournemouth University, UK

IGI Global
Scientific Publishing
Publishing Tomorrow's Research Today

Vice President of Editorial	Melissa Wagner
Director of Acquisitions	Mikaela Felty
Director of Book Development	Jocelynn Hessler
Production Manager	Mike Brehm
Cover Design	Jose Rosado

Published in the United States of America by
IGI Global Scientific Publishing
701 East Chocolate Avenue
Hershey, PA, 17033, USA
Tel: 717-533-8845 | Fax: 717-533-7115
Website: https://www.igi-global.com E-mail: cust@igi-global.com

Library of Congress Cataloging-in-Publication Data

Names: Shieh, Chin Shiuh, 1965- editor | Goel, Pawan (Pawan Kumar), 1983- editor | Horng, Mong-Fong editor | Pandey, Hari (Hari Mohan), 1982- editor
Title: Threat intelligence and cloud trust models for healthcare security / edited by: Chin-Shiuh Shieh, Pawan Kumar Goel, Mong-Fong Horng, Hari Mohan Pandey.
Description: Hershey PA : IGI Global Scientific Publishing, [2026] | Includes bibliographical references. | Summary: "This book explores and addresses the critical challenges surrounding the security and trustworthiness of healthcare systems empowered by IoT and cloud technologies"-- Provided by publisher.
Identifiers: LCCN 2025029846 (print) | LCCN 2025029847 (ebook) | ISBN 9798337349183 hardcover | ISBN 9798337349190 paperback | ISBN 9798337349206 ebook
Subjects: LCSH: Medical informatics--Security measures | Cloud computing--Security measures | Internet of things--Security measures
Classification: LCC R859.7.S43 T47 2026 (print) | LCC R859.7.S43 (ebook)
LC record available at https://lccn.loc.gov/2025029846
LC ebook record available at https://lccn.loc.gov/2025029847

British Cataloguing in Publication Data
A Cataloguing in Publication record for this book is available from the British Library.

Table of Contents

Detailed Table of Contents

The synthesis of the Internet of Things (IoT) systems and cloud computing in the healthcare sphere created the opportunity to monitor, provide diagnostic support, and predictively analyse the data in real time. However, through this development, extremely crucial problems related to privacy, data integrity, and regulatory compliance have cropped up. This chapter addresses the challenge of reaching cloud-based healthcare systems. It examines the current trust models, including reputation, policy, behavioural and hybrid and draws attention to the constraints of these models in the medical care contexts, where they fail to achieve the high-quality requirements in compliance and dealing with life-sensitive data. The gaps that may arise due to this can be addressed with a holistic cloud trust model proposed in the chapter involving identity and access control, data-centric security, a zero-trust architecture, cryptographic attestation, and enriched by real-time threat intelligence. Lastly, the chapter argues that technological advancement is the key to the sustainability of healthcare IoT

The healthcare sector is increasingly vulnerable to cybersecurity threats, particularly from insider threats and social engineering attacks that target sensitive patient data. Insider threats, originating from individuals with authorized access, can result in data theft and unauthorized access to electronic health records (EHRs). Social engineering tactics exploit trust to manipulate personnel into disclosing protected health information. While cloud trust models enhance security in interconnected environments, challenges remain in balancing security with privacy rights and regulatory compliance. Future directions include the use of artificial intelligence for predictive threat analysis, with careful consideration of ethical implications. The evolving nature of attack tactics necessitates adaptive defense mechanisms. Collaboration among stakeholders is crucial to establish frameworks and promote resilience. A comprehensive approach that integrates technology, training, and policy is essential to safeguard patient data and ensure operational continuity.

Digital technologies in healthcare have created connected health ecosystems using IoT devices and cloud computing. While enabling real-time monitoring and personalized care, these systems raise data privacy challenges. This chapter examines health information protection in interconnected environments. Electronic records, wearable data, and genomic information face risks of breaches and unauthorized access. The chapter explores consequences of data exposure, including identity theft and legal issues, along with patient consent and bias concerns. It analyzes medical device threats from ransomware and weak security, discussing data lifecycle management. Regulatory frameworks like HIPAA and GDPR are reviewed, alongside cloud trust models and privacy-preserving techniques. The chapter examines emerging solutions like post-quantum cryptography and self-sovereign identity, emphasizing stakeholder collaboration for data security in connected health ecosystems.

The expeditious digitization of healthcare has intended to enhance service delivery, operational efficacy, and patient involvement. Also, it suffers from unprecedented cybersecurity limitations. Data breaches in healthcare industry are considered to be regulatory indicators of insufficient knowledge, systematic inadequacies, and developing threat landscapes. This chapter explores real-time data breaches from a multidisciplinary lens, emphasizing institutional education, digital ethics, and policy reform. Under the application of six intensive case studies from Anthem to Medibankit examines how breaches evolved, what went wrong, and how they can be prevented. As a result, a brief resilience framework has been developed, helping healthcare firms towards a human-based digital ecosystem. Recommendations are deployed for providers, policymakers, technical developers, and scholars to arrange cyber-security principle with patient security, belief, and dignity.

The convergence of digital healthcare and electric vehicles (EVs) helps in reshaping the delivery of medical services, by enabling mobile diagnostics, emergency care and health outreach specifically in underserved areas. This integration leads to complex cybersecurity and data discretion due to its reliance on cloud infrastructures and real-time communication. This chapter describes a novel cybersecure healthcare intersection within electric mobility network which emphasizes the role of adaptive cloud trust models and threat intelligence. This study discusses emerging use cases such as smart ambulances by analyzing the evolving cyber threat landscape and proposing a layered architectural framework that controls real-time encrypted data exchange mechanisms . The practical application of these concepts has been discussed using real-world case study of an EV-based smart ambulance system. The chapter concludes by delineating regulatory consideration and technical challenges which aimed at fostering secure, scalable and resilient mobile healthcare systems in electric mobility.

The development of quantum computing systems functions as the leader in creating technological advancements that will transform healthcare delivery. Quantum computing systems have substantial potential for healthcare facilities as the worldwide market will grow to $8.45 billion by 2027. The chapter assesses the advancement of quantum healthcare science through innovation, system challenges, and ethical limitations. It illustrates how quantum computing networks with cryptography combine to form a system that enhances healthcare through fast operations, precise medical research, drug creation, and robust data security. Two key barriers exist for quantum healthcare transformation due to resource allocation and security verification. The implementation meets substantial hurdles because data protection requirements, consent, and accessibility need proper handling. The advantages of quantum healthcare systems depend on stakeholders' ethical guidelines, multi-disciplinary partnerships, and planned investments to maintain patient equity and safety while developing systems.

Preface

The transformation of healthcare through digital innovation has been one of the defining advancements of the 21st century. The convergence of cloud computing, the Internet of Things (IoT), artificial intelligence (AI), blockchain, and quantum technologies has redefined how healthcare organizations store, process, and utilize sensitive patient data. As hospitals, clinics, and public health institutions adopt intelligent cloud-based systems for diagnostics, treatment, and analytics, the need to ensure data security, privacy, and trust has become an urgent global concern.

In recent years, healthcare data breaches, ransomware attacks, and insider threats have exposed the sector's vulnerabilities. Patient data is not merely informational—it represents personal identity, medical history, and even life-critical information. A single cyberattack can compromise medical devices, disrupt emergency care, and undermine public confidence in healthcare institutions. Consequently, threat intelligence and trust-based cloud models have emerged as critical mechanisms for building resilient and reliable healthcare infrastructures.

This book, *Threat Intelligence and Cloud Trust Models for Healthcare Security*, presents a comprehensive overview of the strategies, architectures, and technologies essential for securing modern healthcare systems. It is designed to bridge the gap between theoretical research and practical implementation by combining insights from multiple disciplines—cybersecurity, cloud computing, artificial intelligence, cryptography, and healthcare management.

Purpose and Rationale

Healthcare organizations today rely heavily on cloud-enabled IoT systems for real-time monitoring, telemedicine, electronic health record management, and clinical data analytics. However, this growing dependence on connected technologies introduces challenges related to data integrity, access control, and regulatory compliance.

Traditional security frameworks are no longer sufficient to combat sophisticated and adaptive cyber threats targeting healthcare environments.

The aim of this book is to provide a structured and holistic framework that integrates:

- **Threat Intelligence:** to anticipate, detect, and mitigate emerging threats before they disrupt healthcare operations.
- **Cloud Trust Models:** to ensure transparency, accountability, and reliability in cloud-based healthcare ecosystems.
- **Privacy and Compliance Mechanisms:** to align digital innovation with ethical and regulatory obligations under frameworks like HIPAA and GDPR.
- **Emerging Technologies:** such as blockchain, federated learning, and quantum cryptography, to redefine security for next-generation healthcare systems.

By addressing these dimensions, this book serves as a comprehensive guide for researchers, practitioners, and policymakers aiming to design secure and trustworthy healthcare infrastructures.

Organization of the Book

The book is composed of eight interrelated chapters, each offering a distinct yet interconnected perspective on strengthening cybersecurity and trust in healthcare.

Chapter 1. Cloud Trust Models for Secure Healthcare IoT: Ensuring Privacy, Integrity, and Compliance
Introduces the integration of IoT and cloud computing in healthcare and explores various trust models, including policy-based and behavior-based frameworks. It proposes a holistic cloud trust model incorporating identity management, zero-trust architecture, and real-time threat intelligence.

Chapter 2. Insider Threats and Social Engineering in Healthcare
Examines how insider misuse and social engineering tactics exploit human vulnerabilities within healthcare environments. The chapter underscores the importance of AI-assisted predictive threat analysis and adaptive defense strategies.

Chapter 3. Data Sensitivity and Privacy in Connected Health Ecosystems
Discusses the challenges of protecting sensitive health data across wearable devices, cloud servers, and EHR systems. It introduces privacy-preserving frameworks and regulatory models, emphasizing post-quantum cryptography and self-sovereign identity for secure data exchange.

Chapter 4. Lessons from Real-World Data Breaches in Healthcare: Toward Stronger Digital Safeguards
Presents an analytical study of major healthcare data breaches such as Anthem and Medibank, identifying systemic weaknesses and providing a resilience framework for healthcare organizations.
Chapter 5. Cybersecure Healthcare in Electric Mobility
Explores the emerging field of digital healthcare in electric mobility, such as smart ambulances and mobile diagnostics. It presents a layered security architecture that integrates threat intelligence for safe, encrypted, and real-time data communication in mobile health environments.
Chapter 6. Quantum Healthcare Innovations, Challenges, and Ethical Frontiers
Highlights the transformative potential of quantum computing in healthcare research, data processing, and cryptography. It also addresses ethical considerations including patient equity, consent, and data ownership.
Chapter 7. Cloud Security for Healthcare: Threat Intelligence and Risk Management
Focuses on implementing threat intelligence and risk management strategies in cloud infrastructures. The chapter emphasizes aligning best practices with compliance standards and emerging healthcare security frameworks.
Chapter 8. Blockchain-Based Trust and Data Integrity Models for Healthcare Security
Demonstrates how blockchain can enhance data transparency, integrity, and interoperability across healthcare systems. It examines smart contracts and consensus mechanisms that eliminate single points of failure and improve data trustworthiness.

Together, these chapters create a cohesive narrative that reflects the synergy between advanced technologies and secure healthcare delivery systems.

Intended Audience

This book is designed for a diverse audience, including:

- **Researchers and academicians** exploring innovative frameworks for healthcare data protection.
- **IT and cybersecurity professionals** responsible for securing healthcare cloud infrastructures and IoT networks.
- **Healthcare administrators and policymakers** seeking to implement regulatory-compliant security frameworks.

- **Students and scholars** pursuing advanced studies in cybersecurity, AI, and healthcare technology.

By blending theory, real-world case studies, and practical frameworks, the book aims to serve as both an academic reference and a professional guide.

Conclusion and Acknowledgment

Threat Intelligence and Cloud Trust Models for Healthcare Security represents more than a compilation of research chapters—it is a roadmap toward building resilient, privacy-conscious, and ethically sound digital healthcare ecosystems. The book emphasizes that true security in healthcare is achieved not only through technology but also through informed policy, organizational culture, and continuous innovation.

We extend our heartfelt gratitude to all contributors for their scholarly dedication and to the reviewers and editorial team at IGI Global for their invaluable support throughout the publication process. It is our sincere hope that this book will inspire continued research, foster collaboration, and strengthen the global pursuit of secure and trustworthy healthcare systems.

Chin-Shiuh Shieh
National Kaohsiung University of Science and Technology, Taiwan

Pawan Kumar Goel
Raj Kumar Goel Institute of Technology, India

Mong-Fong Horng
National Kaohsiung University of Science and Technology, Taiwan

Hari Mohan Pandey
Bournemouth University, UK

Chapter 1
Cloud Trust Models for Secure Healthcare IoT:
Ensuring Privacy, Integrity, and Compliance

Nathaniel Adeniyi Akande
https://orcid.org/0009-0001-5930-3116
University of Bradford, UK

ABSTRACT

The synthesis of the Internet of Things (IoT) systems and cloud computing in the healthcare sphere created the opportunity to monitor, provide diagnostic support, and predictively analyse the data in real time. However, through this development, extremely crucial problems related to privacy, data integrity, and regulatory compliance have cropped up. This chapter addresses the challenge of reaching cloud-based healthcare systems. It examines the current trust models, including reputation, policy, behavioural and hybrid and draws attention to the constraints of these models in the medical care contexts, where they fail to achieve the high-quality requirements in compliance and dealing with life-sensitive data. The gaps that may arise due to this can be addressed with a holistic cloud trust model proposed in the chapter involving identity and access control, data-centric security, a zero-trust architecture, cryptographic attestation, and enriched by real-time threat intelligence. Lastly, the chapter argues that technological advancement is the key to the sustainability of healthcare IoT

DOI: 10.4018/979-8-3373-4918-3.ch001

1.0. INTRODUCTION

It was more than a data stream; the beat that superimposed itself rhythmically in the long-distance monitor was the promise of modern medicine. Mr. Patient Evans was a heart disease patient, but fitted with an IoT-enabled pacemaker transmitting some much-needed telemetry magic to the dashboard of his cardiologist, who happened to be in a cloud environment. This distant control that allowed him to be treated and the absence of disruptions are pillars of the proactive care system that provided freedom and clinicians with insights unheard of. But here, another incident occurred in the hospital, i.e. there was a complex ransomware attack that happened without any warning to encrypt a significant fraction of the network, thereby paralysing the ability to plan the schedules of patients, among other outcomes, causing access blockers of the electronic health record (EHRs). This difference of contrast between evolution and the system's weakness provokes an analytical question: Did the data still come out in the pacemaker of Mr. Evans, who is now bleeding onto the private, untested cloud system? The worst and the worst, think to yourself that the machine, already at this distance, is somehow to be governed? The situation preconditions the ambisomeness of the Internet of Things (IoT) that manifests itself in healthcare. A ubiquitous device, such as implanted glucose sensors and infusion pumps, alters patient results and operational effectiveness and establishes the order of concentrate treatment. The driver of change, which is irreplaceable, is the cloud, which unites and analyses big data and processes it to create life-saving knowledge (Zeydan et al., 2024). However, that physical, digital, and biological interlacement provides a limitlessly compounding expanded attack space. The very relationship that makes forward flow possible has terrific vulnerabilities, supplies a triad of archetypal issues, and involves the obvious challenge of healthcare cybersecurity protection, Privacy of highly sensitive protected health information (PHI), achieving Integrity of life-critical data and commands, and achieving Compliance when among heavy loads of regulations and bypass of HIPAA and GDPR. As a result, the cloud cannot be considered a panacea but a powerful and versatile partner. The authority to believe that it is irrevocably united with its utility. This chapter implies that this trust-building exercise constitutes an architectural project more than a performance. Its role is to investigate and articulate the artistic relevance of Cloud Trust Models, as the foundational model of healthcare IoT security. These models furnish the posts and procedures by which the challenges mentioned above are addressed, such that the cloud would have a security vulnerability that can be transformed into an asset of security that can be leveraged to protect patients and not hinder responsible innovation. The chapter will then establish a distinctive security issue of the Internet of healthcare security and reverse engineer the fundamentals of a working reparation framework, before summarising an overall plan of execution, and, ultimately, present the vision of remaking the healthcare future of trust.

2.0. WHY HEALTHCARE IOT IS A UNIQUE SECURITY CHALLENGE

Healthcare Internet of Things (HIoT) 's power is so substantial that it is a transformative force, combined with structural dangerousness as an attack surface, that it is on the scale and harm that no single plan or project has ever posed. To estimate the testament of resilience cloud trust models preliminarily, one must analytically assess the characteristic hostile ground characterising this degree of security leap. They are not necessarily technical nuisances, but essential attributes and risks that can recalibrate the previously upheld paradigms of cybersecurity into irrelevance and render a platform upon which cyber vulnerability can translate into immediate physical consequences.

2.1. The Expanding and Heterogeneous Attack Surface

The primary threat of the Healthcare Internet of Things (HIoT) systems is preconditioned by its character and its bans (or absence of these) of operation. The heterogeneous nature is very high in the HIoT environment, though, these devices are only characteristic of the environment though exceptionally unlike other traditional enterprise IT infrastructures; patient monitors and magnet resonance imaging devices and implantable cardiac pacemakers and wearable self-control devices are varied in nature in terms of type and heterogeneity of device hardware, operating systems, and communications protocols (Habibzadeh et al., 2019). This diversity poses a monumental challenge to realising integrative security reforms (Bollineni et al., 2025). Most such devices are mainly clinical equipment. Thus, manufacturers aim at performance and safety, overlooking security, which leads to a lack of computing power, information memory and battery capacity. Such constraints are obstacles in embedding secure encryption or advanced intrusion-detection software that leaves open the gadgets as the targets of attack (Abomhara & Køien, 2015).

Besides this, human beings possess millennium-long technological medical equipment. This means that, at the expiry of its operating system, or the software that enables it to operate, i.e. it will never be given the eye cover up, installing appropriate security patches (Montesinos, et. al. 2024). This creates a backlog of unaddressed vulnerabilities that persist and occur in practices within clinical settings. Physical accessibility is also discussed, last but not least. Unlike the servers installed in unobtrusive data centres, many IoT gadgets are deployed in hospitals' open or semi-hospitable spaces or even in a patient's residence (Yogi et al., 2025). By their open posture, they are open to handling, theft or installation of rogue hardware exploits that can serve as a base point upon which long-distance network hacking can be committed.

2.2. The Trinity of Existential Risks

There are grave dangers in exploiting the exposed surface of an attack. The institution's reputation and patient safety make IoT security an urgent question instead of a technical issue because three existential threats exist beyond a technical problem.

Privacy Breaches: Invasion of privacy threatens the confidentiality of the highly sensitive Protected Health Information (PHI). Smooth IoT devices generate volumes of data on a vast scale, and they face high sensitivity, including real-time physiological telemetry, detailed medical history and ID (Srivastava et al., 2025). This is not only a breach of financial and reputational damage but also a legal violation that will lead to the loss of money and harm to patient autonomy and trust. Disclosure of such information can bring about discrimination, social vices and medical malpractice. Meanwhile, the regulatory systems, e.g., HIPAA and GDPR, impose individual fines of up to a few million dollars, and the human and ethical price is even harder to quantify.

Integrity Compromises: As the shift from visual threat to physical threat, the latter's intensity goes through the roof because it is not defined by the loss of information but only the real damage (Nadji, 2024). Imagine there is a rogue hacker that hacks/intercepts the transmission of a blood-glucose monitor - now a physician can make a life-or-death decision based on false data. The fact that the attacker is in control of the basic workings of the device is even more detestable; the effects may be catastrophic. Gollakata et al. (2011) also disclosed that insulin pump-induced enjoyment of the victim. On the other hand, Fu and Blum (2013) demonstrated the subvertability of even implants that belong to others, such as anaesthesia. These scenarios weaponise medical equipment, and integrity becomes not only the most essential safety concern, but also one of the points in the security checklist.

Compliance Failure Risk: The laws of health data do not stagnate. The HIPAA and HITECH laws include several laws to protect personal health data in the US (Kaplan, 2020), and the HIPAA had a regulatory framework on data-management responsibilities and data-breach requirements in the European Union (GDPR) (Voss, 2019). At the same time, the U.S. Food and Drug Administration (FDA) offers advisory services on medical devices both before and after market, paying more attention to cybersecurity (Stern et al.,

2019). The cloud-based analytics and IoT devices, as the very instruments of providing the existence of the modern health care, will also require message sharing and storage every day, and the tension is quite acutely felt and becomes apparent. These technologies must be integrated into a patchwork of compromising and, in fact, contradictory regulations. Otherwise, the consequences of such negligence can be grievous in terms of fines and publicity, and his life-saving technology might even need to be, in reality, removed from the market.

2.3. The Legacy and Modernity Divide

The biggest obstacle is the distance separating old-fashioned infrastructure from the modern cloud-based technical platform. Hospitals are not a green field, as they are complex organisms with dozens of technologies. The combination of these old systems and new cloud-based Healthcare Internet of Things (HIoT) systems, including traditional Hospital Information Systems (HIS), or older Picture Archiving and Communication Systems (PACS), is one type of security gap, as dangerous in its own right. The problem with these antique systems is that they do not challenge the Web and can be tested against an array of cloud services. This forces the administrators to devise workarounds that are both insecure and violate the principle of having the net opened to interoperability, and that this would have an impact on a network perimeter riddled with some holes that would allow data to reach the cloud and, in the process, expose the system to severe clinical outcomes to external threats (Chin et al, 2025).

It also makes management a nightmare and a form of division between the old and the new. Security agents must lock down a network with an ultra-modern cloud service next to a Windows XP-powered patient monitor. The perimeter is very sensitive, weak, and permeable since the device can not be patched or dismantled without disrupting the central care processes.

In simple terms, the crossing of a naturally hostile environment, the life and demise of data welfare and the emergence of disorder of controls and heritage constraints announce the end of the archetypal perimeter defence model. There is no surety in relying on the internal network to be secure, especially when a hacked insulin pump, with a hacked hospital Wi-Fi network, leaves an intrusion point into the entire organisation. These facts cannot be overstated: the new paradigm is required and works on Zero trust, where nothing can be trusted by default. All operations pass through the authentication and are secured by the cryptographic measures. A current cloud trust design is founded on that.

3.0. DECONSTRUCTING CLOUD TRUST MODELS

The healthcare sector must seek an alternative solution to the familiar vulnerability, risk, and legacy systems. A single tool is not the solution, but merely a collection of principles and architectural design and construction structures that can create resiliency onboard at the very start. These are the main characters in this story, Cloud Trust Models. They leave the outmoded idea of a single and porous set of perimeters, and establish a world in which security is designed, continuous and perceived to be present. Moving ahead, we deconstruct such models by offering abstract concepts of the substantia nesia upon which sound and inventive IoT in healthcare (HIoT) can likely be administered.

3.1. The Concept of Computational Trust

The element of trust makes it immaterial that individuals would want to examine and assign to one another without an analogous favourable outcome. It is not until a person has experienced several successful mutually beneficial interactions with someone that the individual can earn a reputation of trustworthiness (Gunia, 2023). Being the central element of the widely recognised computational Healthcare IoT (HIoT), however, trust does not mediate need-based, but grounded-based as a solvable, left-of-the-art notion where there is an audit reality bearing tangible evidence and cryptographic authentication (Rauf et al., 2022). A trust model in this sense can be described as a formal system architecture of construction, measuring and contextualising trust in both the structures of the system and the agents acting within it, in both the humans and the non-human mechanisms other than humans, including the medical machines. It transpires through regular assessment and confirmation (Mayer and Mayer, 2024). This re-imagining requires a sceptical twist: the old saying, trust but verify, has been substituted by never trust, always verify. This model aims to support accurate, contextual and risk-based security decisions. An example of this is the authorization to a sensitive real-time feed of patient data will require the dynamic analysis of an impossible number of prioritised factors: who is using and to what extent the use of the data, what machine is accessed and what special device ident identifying which machine is being accessed, demonstrated integrity of the software of that machine, the high sensitivity of the data being accessed, the larger modern threat environment. The strict evidence-based architecture of trust is the deterministic foundation of any other forms of security, which are more predictable and defensive, and audit, a rock-solid bedrock of inherently turbulent digital space clinical operations.

3.2. The Four Pillars of a Healthcare IoT Trust Model

To provide a cloud trust model that can handle the healthcare IoT in singular ways, the model must combine four pillars that depend on each other.

1. **Identity and Access Management (IAM):** The most significant one is IAM since it guarantees that all data entities, human ones and machine users, can be uniquely identified and authenticated before interaction between each other and data or systems (Anand and Khemchandani, 2019). In HIoT, this does not end at a surface level with usernames and passwords. A given device, like a bedside monitor or implantable sensor, should have a cryptographically strong and unique machine identity (e.g., a digital certificate) that is verified before accessing a network (Rose et al., 2020). This can permit fine-grained access control policies. In the classical Role-Based Access Control (RBAC), a user is granted permissions based on a user role: cardiologist, nurse, etc. (Alturi and Ferraiolo, 2025). A more liberal and powerful alternative is the attribute-based access control (ABAC). The decision of ABAC is founded on real-time analysis based on a few distinctive features: user role, device health condition, patient authorisation and access time, and even the device's whereabouts (Atlam and Yang, 2025). One such case is that a surgeon is restricted to working with specialised work equipment, working within the framework of the hospital, when he has a set procedure. Multi-Factor Authentication (MFA) is another mechanism that human subjects need to protect against error.
2. **Data-Centric Security:** The data that may be stored is the centre of data-centric security, where IAM guards the boundaries that define entry. It already recognises the violation of boundaries and awareness of access failure, so the information has to be secured because it is needed on every level. This is ensured by pervasive encryption as the data rests in the cloud or waits in different positions along the network. Above all, caution is given when the data in question is being actively used in the cloud memory, which belongs to the most crucial subfield of the Internet of Things. The less invasive mechanisms, such as Confidential Computing, which relies on a trusted execution environment (TEE) as hardware, provide the prospects of processing data without leaving it decrypted even in the absence of the cloud running administrators (Zobaed, 2025). Workflows that integrate sensitive PHI with synthetic or non-sensitive tokens can allow analytics and testing without real patient data, drastically reducing the likelihood of patient privacy breach (Jain & Puri, 2020).
3. **Zero Trust Architecture (ZTA):** Zero Trust is the general strategic concept of the pillars. It was first given the name of Forerester; it was formalised by NIST in SP 800-207. Zero Trust Architecture (ZTA) is premised on a never trust, al-

ways verify doctrine (Mensah, 2024) and rooted in the idea that a breach is on its way- there is no quietly trusted internal network. Health-IoT (HIoT) is prone to this change (transformative). Install a smart inhaler at home that supports Wi-Fi: it has always had to prove its right to use the resources of the hospitals, and cannot be given a blanket trust. One of the most critical technical supports of ZTA is the micro-segmentation. It also ensures that communication between and among the used impressions of IoT devices is blocked, and access to the most significant flows in the network is prohibited (Al-Ofeishat & Alshorman, 2023). Had an insulin pump been dreaded, the micro-segmentation policies must ensure that the attacker cannot lateralize to the EHR database or infuse bad-codes to other tools, and essentially end the blast radius of the attack and protect the underlying clinical systems.

4. **Attestation and Integrity Verification:** Device compromise is the most significant risk to Health IoT (HIoT). This is not simply a question of identification of the kind of device--we must know at which mode it occurs at any given moment. The attestation is the cryptographic protection which guarantees that. In effect, the machine can perform a self-signing operation in which it can show that its hardware and software are honest with itself to an external authority, such as a cloud service. This verification is carried out through attestation, which requires verification of the bootloader, operating system, and firmware against a known (XML) image called a gold image (Hardjono and Smith, 2021). The diagnostic imaging machine will need a signed report if a study is uploaded to the cloud. The report testified that the machine has executed a signed and unaltered software, including all the requisite security updates. Failing to detect any parts beyond the trusted baseline- an indication of malware or interference- the mechanism puts the machine under quarantine. It prevents entries to the network until the situation is amended. The ability is an overwhelming means of ensuring the reliability of the same device and data it produces in guaranteeing the absence of the disintegrating risks of deployments of HIoT.

3.3. The Role of Threat Intelligence

A model of trust that relies on the immutable set of policies is a precarious impediment, with weaknesses in the duration that cannot predict emerging or constructed ways of attack, since it is people-based. This is a risky susceptibility of this kind of environment, as the dynamic health care environment, where new threats emerge regularly. In this instance, however, the central knowledge in this book, Threat Intelligence (TI), finally gets pushed to a sidefeed to become the aversion voice of the trust model, in a word. The real-world advances by TI are long overdue to move from a reactive and incident-responsible methodology to a proactive and predictive scope of operation of cybersecurity (Sarker, 2024). It is an unending illusion of evidence-based knowledge concerning existing and possible hostile challenges, possibilities, infrastructure, motivation, and most importantly, their own dry by wire technologies, techniques and processes (TTPs) (Skopik and Pahi, 2020). This intelligence introduces a very critical situation awareness in the security ecosystem.

The trust model parameters offer the exosystem, in direct, dynamic, information-furnished form in TA; attributing it to HGV theory requires additional clarification of the spatiality of the appended comity (Tahmasebi, 2024). Opening an example, one may see a TI alert about a campaign targeting a popular infusion pump model and a well-known vulnerability being attacked. Once this intelligence is incorporated into the trust model, it can switch computationally. IAM policies may be strengthened to cause a more robust authentication of that specific device, and attestation and integrity checking can be escalated on the identifiers linked to the potentially malicious identity being suspected (IoCs). A risk-based adjustment like that cannot be regarded as an adaptive trust model. It stays up-to-date with the suggestions of the new threat and answers the fundamental question of what to keep track of and who to guard. As a result, there is always an update of the checks and balances that support the model's core to resolve the most significant risks and offer a stable and thoughtful security posture (Feng et al., 2024). It is a vital synergy needed to secure critical health infrastructures.

These heroes-IAM, data-centric security, Zero Trust, attestation and threat intelligence are not in a vacuum. They form a synergistic structure with strong identity, allowing appropriate access control that secures the intrinsically meaningless data throughout, and the repressive presumption of Zero Trust, with the well-being of devices ongoing and the health of the system in totality dynamic with real-world threat intelligence. The pairing will provide a robust, verifiable, and responsive cloud environment in which the full potential of the Healthcare IoT will finally be realised, and patient safety, privacy, and compliance will not be compromised.

4.0. IMPLEMENTING A HOLISTIC TRUST FRAMEWORK

The theoretical breakdown offered by the model of the cloud trust provides the playbook. Still, it is exclusively by applying it that the protagonist, the healthcare organisation, becomes involved in the conflict. The idea of a two-step process, translating the concept into undertaken and second planned initiatives, is key in transforming the Forces of ZeroTrust and verifiable security into the genome of the conceptualised healthcare IoT (HIoT) ecosystem. It is not a single time implementing initiative but creating a dynamic, ongoing process that makes security into a cost-effective, enabling and value creation process.

4.1. Architectural Blueprint

Even a vertically integrated trust structure does not provide a bolt-on that can be assembled but must be structurally embedded. This also includes distinctive upgrading of a flat network to a custom layered topology to decentralise security services to the entire information pathway, starting with a patient at one end and the cloud dashboard at the other.

The Device Layer: Weak devices are notorious so that they can be the first line of defence of an IoT ecosystem. This vulnerability implies that security has to begin at the hardware level. One of the most critical aspects of this method is the Secure Boot software, which enables a device to execute only cryptographically signed firmware by the manufacturer. Consequently, these unauthorised or malicious code passes are obstructed at the first boot (Rashmi and Karthikeyan, 2018). Secure Boot introduces a Hardware-Rooted Trust (HRT) option, five a tamper-resistant microcontroller that generates and secures the cryptographic keys. The keys are attached to devices, tying the devices with individual X.509-style identity certificates during the factory. The certificate offers a cryptographically secure, non-repudiable, and non-retractable identity that easily replaces weak default passwords, and such a certificate is the foundation of all future signing processes. This certificate is presented when a device tries to connect to a network, and will authenticate its appearance before sending any data (Kagita et al., 2022). In such a way, all IoT units will become verifiable and identifiable participants that can be recognised only by authorised staff.

The Gateway Layer: A sophisticated security agent cannot be encrypted by a multinational since the poor quarters of most medical devices lack the means. Such a job is assigned to an active gateway, which is the hardware or software appliance, and it is there that the local devices' data is amalgamated. The gateway is a gateway to the enforcement of such critical activities and is also termed the front line of defence. It offers local filtering and collects and presents up-to-date traffic data on apparent anomalies or protocols targeting attacks before they can even be extrapolated to the remainder of the network. It is also used to perform protocol translation, which is the translation of older or proprietary comorbid medical device protocols (e.g. DICOM, HL7) into standard web protocols (e.g. HTTPS, MQTT), which may be securely loaded in the cloud. More importantly, the network gateway can employ micro-segmentation to isolate a compromised device at each of the wards or departments to restrict the horizontal movement, which is one of the principal ideals of Zero Trust Architecture.

The Cloud Layer: At the central part of the nervous system, the interactions among the policy, intelligence, and analytics are consolidated into the cloud platform. The Identity and Access Management (IAM) system is hosted at this level, where the point of truth lies in authenticating all creatures, humans and machines, and enforcing the ABAC policy on the entire ecosystem. It involves data at rest on an encryption management service, with keys held in a hard disc security module (HSM), FIPS 140- 2. It also collects all logs, such as the result of a device attestation, a traversed gateway, a user attempt, and system events on behalf of another app, Security Information and Event Management (SIEM). The Threat Intelligence-driven SIEM is engaged in correlation analysis to detect the incidences of multi-stage attacks because sophisticated multi-stage attacks have stages in one form or another, ignoring that aspect at any of the stages (Skopik and Pahi, 2020). Lastly, auditing logs are an immutable, tamper-resistant history of anything that has happened, which is the root of conformity and forensic analysis.

4.2. The Continuous Cycle of Trust

Threats are not in a standard pattern, so a tight architecture fails to keep up. Rivalry, verification or earned trust should be distributed and maintained by an automated and iterative cycle.

1. **Establish:** The cycle starts with secure device onboarding. The device offers self-authentication through its embedded certificate with the cloud IAM system (Maksuti et al., 2021). After confirmation of the initial attestation report, access policies are dynamically issued by the system according to the type and group of the organisation. The enrollment is fully computerised and human error has been removed, hence only authorised devices are allowed in the network.
2. **Measure:** Credibility is unrelated to one award; after a device has been onboarded, the position must be repeatedly proven. Constant monitoring also ensures that the health of the device being utilised and its behaviour is monitored. This involves regular remote attestation to identify infections caused or unusual behaviour, and analytics that would be used to determine a benchmark of expected behaviour- such as the normal frequency and transmission volume. The system reacts individually to anomalies that could present a translation of compromise (Fournaris et al., 2020). In the meantime, the security information and event management (SIEM) engine performs continuous multi-level logging to detect an advanced warning of an attack.
3. **Maintain:** The use of information in the Measure phase dictates the relevant maintenance action for the future. Dynamic responses (automated policy en-

gines) are temporary access permissions to devices exhibiting erratic behaviour. Credential and certificate lifecycles are managed. Computer-assisted and roll-over jobs are managed to maintain the service disruption. The vulnerabilities are patched considering the urgency, and the updates are securely signed with cryptography and transmitted on the management plane.

4. **Revoke:** And finally, a revocable trust should exist. Unplanned loss of attestation of a board, malignant conduct or decommissioning should be terminated automatically and on the spot. The IAM system withdraws its credentials, and the local gateway gives it a command to isolate the device at the network level. It is a real-time automated revocation, which has exerted threat moves in real-time to render accessibility by the attackers perpetual.

4.3. Automating Compliance

The immense advantages of the applied framework are that compliance became a manual dated liability to a continuous and integration-less security engagement product. These are rules such as HIPAA, GDPR, and HITECH, but are not necessarily just a checklist since, in fact, they have already codified a body of supporting checks and balances that data privacy, integrity and availability have masqueraded as being (Isibor, 2024). These regulatory controls may form part and parcel of a good design trust model, which will be modelled with zero-trust principles, to which regulation is designed into its own designs, and can be realised. In the example, HIPAA 164.312(A) of Access Control Requirements, the attribute-based controls access of train dynamic HIPAA policies out of hap to (train)s) hold via a centralised IAM system (Oluoha et al., 2022). These policies effectively purport to the principle of least privilege. Only an immutable audit log can be employed by someone who cannot in any manner challenge real-time evidence of who has accessed what data and when. Likewise, the cryptographic attestation mechanism (which phases out the state of the software of the device and cryptographic message-digest mixtures) that creates integrity of the data in motion and rest (Nadji, 2024) is enforced on the integrity Controls (irq164.312(c)). Since this is done, it is possible that the evidence that led to this finding has not been compromised, with the systems and information being above board. In addition, the Audit Controls requirement (SSC164.312(b)) is fulfilled, but even surpassed by SIEM and centralised logging infrastructure (McCallen et al., 2022), as it would offer an end-to-end, tamper-proof account of the entire system activity.

As a result, rather than the classic and historically valuable reaction, rushing to the end of the year during the construction of the audit, an effort-consuming physical evidence gathering operation by accessing a large number of systems that, as often, were separated historically, a read-only access to automated compliance dashboards can be offered to compliance officers and external auditors. Such a dashboard alive displays would give one a glass, which would already display live reports on the state of the health of the data encryption, user access review, device health attestation and security incident response, and would become an objectifiable and testable product of a sound, Polarsit generate position good, Baroque of security, in its essence. However, an automated system does more than reduce the overheads of working and increase the organisation's credibility to the regulators since easily understandable and ready-to-grasp evidence of due care is available (Imoize et al., 2023).

To sum up, the holistic trust framework is the plot twist that can not make the healthcare organisation a victim but a catalyst for change. The introduction of the layered defence architecture, where the continuity cycle of trust is realised through its automation to form compliance, enables the organisation to develop a strong, innovative, and ultimately reliable world of trust. Precisely, the promise made by the trust paradigm heroes who fit into the practice contributes to the possibility of creating contemporary healthcare delivery in a non-compliant and safe way.

5.0. ACHIEVING RESILIENCE AND FUTURE-PROOFING

This direction of the state of vulnerability, a reactionary situation to the state of confident security, results in a fundamental alteration of the working relations of the healthcare organisation. An introduction of an integrated cloud trust model is not merely the solution to the risks being reduced, but a complete solution to the conflict inherent in the initial stages of this story, because of the tendency of the care delivery to occur within a climate of resiliency in which the Hazard is a permanent challenge. The behaviour analysis in such a resolution would be most characterised by reentry of our original vignette re-engineered on cultivated security posture.

Remember Mr. Evans, the heart disease patient and the ransomware invasion that happened in tandem in a manner that felled the traditional IT architecture at the plant. This mature form does not result in a clinical disaster following a disruptive attack on administrative activity. The sensitive data stream Mr. Evans' pacemaker is transmitting is a secure, authenticated transaction. That is how a cryptogram based on a hardware root of trust and a determining identity certificate has been built into the device, which is then cryptographically measured with respect to the health of a device locally in contact with the cloud gateway over which an assuring channel is subsequently formed. Even though it has obtained the key to the network's components, the ransomware cannot spy on this communication, as it not only does not have the required cryptography keys, but it also eavesdrops or spoofs not even the device in its fortified state.

Moreover, attribute-based access control (ABAC) policies in real-time control Mr. Evans' access to real-time physiological data. A clinician's request to access such data will only be granted under stringent conditions, in the clinician's functions, location, and the device's accessing time and security posture. Any attempt to access the data using an unfamiliar device or address would automatically be barred, even when the attacker had stolen the credentials of a clinician. The SIEM would elevate the correlated query into threat intelligence feeds since it would have been included in the ironing-out process of the event. Even without a permeable perimeter, the safety of the patient and even data integrity are facilitated in part due to the endogenous security inherent in all layers of the architecture. It also has the capability or capacity to be struck by a cyber shock that affects its strategic and central mission operations (Linkov and Kott, 2019).

The positive merits of this perseverance materialise, which justifies construction investing. The first value, patient safety, is influenced positively since now, the data property is a defined line of data between the medical device and the clinician; as a result, all diagnostic and curative decisions are performed based on the originally unchanged information. The position of maximum utility makes cybersecurity a core, not a cost centre of activities, in patient safety (Williams and Woodward, 2015). In the meantime, simple encryption with several layers and Data-centric security will continue to keep the patient privacy intact, addressing the ethical implications this claims and creating the required patient-nurse trust.

Operationally, the framework streamlines compliance. The requirement to cause two items of regulation audit by imposing such a burden on the base of regulation, the requirement to design lets go of the need to create as a mandatory enhancement, and the post-event-let go concern as an evident and transparent task are made apparent by the fact that the trust model is evidence generating and creates irrevocable logs of access, a result of attestation and policy decisions. This compliance is a product of the daily security activities, which can, in practice, be proven to have succeeded instead of being a goal (Memon et al., 2014). This pivot of safety, privacy, and compliance is the mark of which, in a particular position, ultimately leads to the most desirable feature: the ability to invent freely. When a deep base is established, healthcare organisations are ready to install and embrace new, radical technologies, either of which is driven by default diagnostics through artificial intelligence or by high-resolution surgical technology, as they are assured that the trusted paradigm will be in a position to proliferate in their favour.

However, this resolution is not the predetermined goal. This transformation of the protagonist may be called the realisation that trust is neither a state nor a process but a practice that needs to be cultivated. The environment of threats is not simply standing still; the vulnerabilities are constantly discovered, and the strategy of the enemy changes. In that regard, the established measure, maintenance, and revoke mission cycle must be vertically supplied as regular observation and threat intelligence are provided and responding to the alterations. In its turn, the ability to learn and develop out of that is not resilience but the absence of attacks (Linkov and Kott, 2019). Security posture within organisations should be dynamic, tested under various stress levels, and matured into dynamic intelligence and technology. In summation, the healthcare IoT security dilemma cannot be resolved as a tool but rather as the philosophical and architectural adherence to a verifiable and zero-trust solution. With the opportunity to make this model successful, the healthcare organisation is no longer the attack target. It is fortified, a data structure that can ensure the safety of its patients and even the safest numbers, even in the realm of cyber propaganda. The last solution is such a demanding strength because it gives the firm the basis within which medicine would be established in the future, with a sense of confidence and with assurance of innovation and care for the patient.

6.0. FUTURE OUTLOOK: EVOLVING TRUST MODELS IN HEALTHCARE SECURITY

Establishing the modernised frameworks of cloud confidence is among the decisive achievements in the healthcare sector of IoT safety. But this is only a stepping-stone, not a finished product. These models do not travel over a blank mantle but over the extensphere burnt by the retrenchless technology. What is required in the future should be resilient trust structures, anticipatory, adaptive, and, most critically, intelligent.

6.1. The Cognitive Layer

The future of the trust models lies in their evolution, which could be defined as no longer being a rule-based system but more of a cognition-based one. AI and ML will no longer place themselves on the sacrificial altar as aids, but as children of safety operations (Goel et al., 2023). Its existing models are also very effective in implementing pre-set policies and checking the state, but are mainly focused on the reactionary. The second is predictive analytics, which can look at the difference in the looming threats in advance and assume the form of violations. To identify ultra-fine baselines of normality, the ML software will follow the immense volumes of machine-generated data in attestation logs, network traffic, and user action to determine the utilisation of the device (Lin et al., 2022). Through it, they will get conversant with detecting the slightest, out-of-shape patterns, which implies a complex, low and slow assault that will never be identified using the customary signature-based solution. Then it will be possible to transcend not believing in becoming independent and tested, predict risks, and respond to them beforehand. More so is the fact that AIs will enable automation in ensuring that the entire continuous cycle of trust is involved in dynamically adjusted access in real-time, in terms of the perceived threat and incident response orchestration, leveraging the issue of scale that human teams will be limited to.

6.2. The Quantum Conundrum

The other paradigm that is soon changing in the world is the arrival of quantum computing. This technology is up-and-coming in the health sector with several implications for drug discovery, but a death threat to the cryptographical secrecy of the modern reliability models of trust. Existing asymmetric encryption protocols, including RSA and ECC, to authenticate devices, verify connections, and send encrypted data streams, are at risk due to running the Shor algorithm on a quantum computer with adequate power to do so (LaPierre, 2021). It should be a deplorable revelation that not only will a prospective quantum opponent essentially control to devalue messages of medical data in reality conveying trusting-being in beneficial in a nonsensical seeking will also gravitate that it intends to procure the detectability of a genuine revelation dispatched during the next decade, decoding information detached from the validating keying incorporations. This necessitates an active paradigm shift to post-quantum cryptography (PQC). The cryptographic computation algorithms, which are resistant against the attacks of classical and quantum computation, are to be utilised to construct our model of trust to be applied in the future. When companies, such as the NIST, actively experiment with and distinguish in the implementation of the PQC standards, into the hardware of the device, into the clouds, into the communication network, it is no longer an imaginary research question, but an operating demand (Alagic et al., 2022). The multifaceted decades-long process of backwards compatibility and international standardisation is in the varied interest of any healthcare organisation to ensure the security of its data for decades and to affect it in the early stages.

6.3. The Expanding Battlefield

It is a drama of toppling insecurity whose mandate is becoming an issue. The emergence of cross-border telemedicine and global fields of research results in the delocalisation of healthcare, but the future disruption of technological benefits is attached to the imminent 6G networks implementation. This enlarged storey brings in new storey faces. Some laws will be antagonistic, like data sovereignty (e.g. GDPR over national laws), and the trust model will have to recognise dynamic dependence on physical location and data jurisdiction. This 6G level of hyper-connectedness index with extremely low latencies will bring the use of artificial intelligence (AI) and the internet of things (IoT) closer to the current reality and reveal the surface of attacks that is far larger and significantly quicker (Giordani et al., 2020). And this led to the closing and a general cliffhanger. The price of a security breach that will escalate to data breaches is increasingly risking service discontinuity nationwide as the sphere of health care gets increasingly smarter, and therefore mandated and interconnected. Such adversaries, be it cybercriminals or nation-state hacktivists, will consider AI and automation to coordinate more precise and destructive campaigns against them. The central question, which will define the next decade, is not whether we can develop models of trust but instead whether our models of trust can develop quickly enough to be present amid expensive enemies. It will be an answer to the capability of the healthcare profession to internalise the culture of constantly changing, and that safety would be an inseparable element of the system and not a separately provisioned item that would be added on the end. The race has already begun.

7.0. CONCLUSION

The chapter presents the essential changes needed to bring the healthcare organisation to the pinnacle of acute vulnerability defence and resilience achievement. This started with establishing how the healthcare internet of things infrastructure has distinctive vulnerabilities: the sheer scale of attack, the stakes of life and health, the integrity of the information, and the growing disparity between the outdated technology and the current cloud service. In response to all these threats, we have tapped into all the facets of a good cloud model- verifiable identity, data-centric security, ZTP, and it must be guaranteed that we present it on a standby basis. The second was applying these pillars to a multi-layered architecture and automated trust life cycle to make compliance the natural outcome of savings. The net effect is a safe, regulatory ecosystem in which patient safety, privacy, and innovation can all co-exist and thrive assuredly.

As soon as the ever-constructed force of personality has taken its reality and becomes a fact, it introduces a new stage of troubles; faith in self begins a world-long probation. Even the information based on cryptographic principles ensuring the basis of security procedures in the machines and confidential information nowadays are exposed even before quantum computers get highly Ubiquitous, along with the coexisting development of a new form of dynamic malware and social-engineering arms and weapons capable simultaneously of being, similarly to and as and when needed, scaled and paced like criminals, rogue AI is also producing a new breed of even smarter malware and social-engineering arms. That pessimistic fact is a reminder that no trust model can be such. The strength we constantly strengthen ourselves now must be strong enough to meet future challenges.

That imminent evolution preconditions the following chapter. The actual game-changers can be the provision of the trust models' footprint, threat-intelligence platforms on the augmenting level, and tools that utilise AI to manage security operations. Think of an artificial intelligence immune system, anticipating attacks, rebuffing AI risks, and AI continuing to solidify the trust structure it contains, i.e., thus, that will be the next step of healthcare protection. We have found ourselves at this junction and are doing our level best to assist in forming an impregnable circle around tomorrow regarding the security of the medical cyber-ecosystem.

Another motivating factor is healthcare security, which is based on a more ethically sound prerogative than any other industry, where financial or reputational losses usually accompany breaches. A compromise is one of the possible catastrophes in this case, and it threatens people's health. It prospers on the sacrosanctness of the medical system, and the digital tools that we are integrating into a medical system must have earned, or will need to earn, that trust. It is not just a matter of technique, but of morality, an unstoppable obligation to design and maintain an effective and safe order to stabilise life and the pulse of modern medicine.

REFERENCES

Abomhara, M., & Køien, G. M. (2015). Cyber security and the internet of things: Vulnerabilities, threats, intruders and attacks. *Journal of Cyber Security and Mobility*, *4*(1), 65–88. DOI: 10.13052/jcsm2245-1439.414

Al-Ofeishat, H. A., & Alshorman, R. (2023). Build a secure network using segmentation and micro-segmentation techniques. *International Journal of Computing and Digital Systems*, *14*(1), 1–16.

Alagic, G., Alagic, G., Apon, D., Cooper, D., Dang, Q., Dang, T., Kelsey, J., Lichtinger, J., Liu, Y.K., Miller, C. and Moody, D. (2022). Status report on the third round of the NIST post-quantum cryptography standardization process.

Alturi, V., & Ferraiolo, D. (2025). Role-based access control. In *Encyclopedia of Cryptography, Security and Privacy* (pp. 2124–2127). Springer Nature Switzerland. DOI: 10.1007/978-3-030-71522-9_829

Anand, D., & Khemchandani, V. (2019). Identity and access management systems. *Security and Privacy of Electronic Healthcare Records: Concepts, Paradigms and Solutions*, 61.

Atlam, H. F., & Yang, Y. (2025). Enhancing Healthcare Security: A Unified RBAC and ABAC Risk-Aware Access Control Approach. *Future Internet*, *17*(6), 262. DOI: 10.3390/fi17060262

Bollineni, C., Sharma, M., Hazra, A., Kumari, P., Manipriya, S., & Tomar, A. (2025). IoT for Next-Generation Smart Healthcare: A Comprehensive Survey. *IEEE Internet of Things Journal*, *12*(16), 32616–32639. DOI: 10.1109/JIOT.2025.3570188

Chin, M. H., Bruch, J. D., Grogan, C. M., Huang, E. S., Kandula, N. R., Kim, D. D., Peek, M. E., & Pollack, H. A. (2025). How to Fix a Broken Health Care System: Pathways to Maximize Health and Well-being for All. *Diabetes Care*, •••, dci250001. DOI: 10.2337/dci25-0001 PMID: 40542616

Feng, D., Qin, Y., Feng, W., Li, W., Shang, K., & Ma, H. (2024). Survey of research on confidential computing. *IET Communications*, *18*(9), 535–556. DOI: 10.1049/cmu2.12759

Fournaris, A. P., Dimopoulos, C., Lampropoulos, K., & Koufopavlou, O. (2020). Anomaly detection trusted hardware sensors for critical infrastructure legacy devices. *Sensors (Basel)*, *20*(11), 3092. DOI: 10.3390/s20113092 PMID: 32486125

Fu, K., & Blum, J. (2013). Controlling for cybersecurity risks of medical device software. *Communications of the ACM*, *56*(10), 35–37. DOI: 10.1145/2508701

Giordani, M., Polese, M., Mezzavilla, M., Rangan, S., & Zorzi, M. (2020). Toward 6G networks: Use cases and technologies. *IEEE Communications Magazine*, *58*(3), 55–61. DOI: 10.1109/MCOM.001.1900411

Goel, A., Goel, A. K., & Kumar, A. (2023). The role of artificial neural network and machine learning in utilizing spatial information. *Spatial Information Research*, *31*(3), 275–285. DOI: 10.1007/s41324-022-00494-x

Gunia, A. (2023). The role of trust in human-machine interaction: Cognitive science perspective. In *Artificial Intelligence, Management and Trust* (pp. 85-126). Routledge.

Habibzadeh, H., Dinesh, K., Shishvan, O. R., Boggio-Dandry, A., Sharma, G., & Soyata, T. (2019). A survey of healthcare Internet of Things (HIoT): A clinical perspective. *IEEE Internet of Things Journal*, *7*(1), 53–71. DOI: 10.1109/JIOT.2019.2946359 PMID: 33748312

Hardjono, T., & Smith, N. (2021). Towards an attestation architecture for blockchain networks. *World Wide Web (Bussum)*, *24*(5), 1587–1615. DOI: 10.1007/s11280-021-00869-4

Imoize, A. L., Balas, V. E., Solanki, V. K., Lee, C. C., & Obaidat, M. S. (Eds.). (2023). *Handbook of Security and Privacy of AI-Enabled Healthcare Systems and Internet of Medical Things* (pp. 1–460). CRC press.

Isibor, E. (2024). Regulation of healthcare data security: Legal obligations in a digital age. *Available at SSRN* 4957244. DOI: 10.2139/ssrn.4957244

Jain, R. B., & Puri, M. (2020). An approach towards the development of scalable data masking for preserving privacy of sensitive business data. In *Artificial Intelligence and Evolutionary Computations in Engineering Systems* (pp. 733–743). Springer Singapore. DOI: 10.1007/978-981-15-0199-9_63

Kagita, M. K., Thilakarathne, N., Gadekallu, T. R., & Maddikunta, P. K. R. (2022). A review on security and privacy of internet of medical things. *Intelligent internet of things for healthcare and industry*, 171-187.

Kaplan, B. (2020). Phi protection under hipaa: An overall analysis. *Kaplan, B.(with appendix by Monteiro, APL)," PHI Protection under HIPAA: An Overall Analysis," LGPD na Saúde (LGPD Applicable to Health), Dallari, AB, Monaco, GFC, ed., São Paulo: Editora Revista dos Tribunais (Thomsom Reuters), 2021*, 61-88.

LaPierre, R. (2021). *Introduction to quantum computing*. Springer Nature. DOI: 10.1007/978-3-030-69318-3

Lin, Y. D., Wang, Z. Y., Lin, P. C., Nguyen, V. L., Hwang, R. H., & Lai, Y. C. (2022). Multi-datasource machine learning in intrusion detection: Packet flows, system logs and host statistics. *Journal of Information Security and Applications*, *68*, 103248. DOI: 10.1016/j.jisa.2022.103248

Linkov, I., & Kott, A. (2019). Fundamental concepts of cyber resilience: Introduction and overview. In *Cyber resilience of systems and networks* (pp. 1–25). Springer. DOI: 10.1007/978-3-319-77492-3_1

Maksuti, S., Bicaku, A., Zsilak, M., Ivkic, I., Péceli, B., Singler, G., Kovács, K., Tauber, M., & Delsing, J. (2021). Automated and secure onboarding for system of systems. *IEEE Access : Practical Innovations, Open Solutions*, *9*, 111095–111113. DOI: 10.1109/ACCESS.2021.3102280

Mayer, R. C., & Mayer, B. M. (2024). Towards interdisciplinary scholarship in trust: the needs, some leads, and a seed. In *A Research Agenda for Trust* (pp. 1–10). Edward Elgar Publishing. DOI: 10.4337/9781802200942.00008

McCallen, J., Schmardebeck, R., Shipman, J. E., & Whited, R. L. (2022). Evidence on the 2020 exemption of low-revenue issuers from the internal control audit requirement. *Available at SSRN* 3420787.

Memon, M., Wagner, S. R., Pedersen, C. F., Beevi, F. H. A., & Hansen, F. O. (2014). Ambient assisted living healthcare frameworks, platforms, standards, and quality attributes. *Sensors (Basel)*, *14*(3), 4312–4341. DOI: 10.3390/s140304312 PMID: 24599192

Mensah, F. (2024). Zero trust architecture: A comprehensive review of principles, implementation strategies, and future directions in enterprise cybersecurity. [IJAIRI]. *International Journal of Academic and Industrial Research Innovations*, *10*, 339–346.

Montesinos, L., Checa Rifá, P., Rifá Fabregat, M., Maldonado-Romo, J., Capacci, S., Maccaro, A., & Piaggio, D. (2024). Sustainability across the medical device lifecycle: A scoping review. *Sustainability (Basel)*, *16*(4), 1433. DOI: 10.3390/su16041433

Nadji, B. (2024). Data security, integrity, and protection. In *Data, Security, and Trust in Smart Cities* (pp. 59–83). Springer Nature Switzerland. DOI: 10.1007/978-3-031-61117-9_4

Oluoha, O. M., Odeshina, A., Reis, O., Okpeke, F., Attipoe, V., & Orieno, O. H. (2022). A Unified Framework for Risk-Based Access Control and Identity Management in Compliance-Critical Environments.

Rashmi, R. V., & Karthikeyan, A. (2018, March). Secure boot of embedded applications-a review. In *2018 Second International Conference on Electronics, Communication and Aerospace Technology (ICECA)* (pp. 291-298). IEEE.

Rauf, A., Shaikh, R. A., & Shah, A. (2022). Trust Modelling and management for IoT healthcare. *International Journal of Wireless and Microwave Technologies, 12*(5), 21–35. DOI: 10.5815/ijwmt.2022.05.03

Rose, S., Borchert, O., Mitchell, S., & Connelly, S. (2020). *Zero Trust Architecture. National Institute of Standards and Technology (NIST), Special Publication 800-207.*

Sarker, I. H. (2024). Introduction to AI-driven cybersecurity and threat intelligence. In *AI-driven cybersecurity and threat intelligence: Cyber automation, intelligent decision-making and explainability* (pp. 3–19). Springer Nature Switzerland. DOI: 10.1007/978-3-031-54497-2_1

Skopik, F., & Pahi, T. (2020). Under false flag: Using technical artifacts for cyber attack attribution. *Cybersecurity, 3*(1), 8. DOI: 10.1186/s42400-020-00048-4

Srivastava, D., Budhiraja, V., Srivastava, A., & Verma, M. (2025). A systematic review of applications, challenges, data collection and academic research in healthcare using IoT. *Transforming Healthcare: Mode, Technologies, and Implementation*, 181.

Stern, A. D., Gordon, W. J., Landman, A. B., & Kramer, D. B. (2019). Cybersecurity features of digital medical devices: An analysis of FDA product summaries. *BMJ Open, 9*(6), e025374. DOI: 10.1136/bmjopen-2018-025374 PMID: 31256020

Tahmasebi, M. (2024). Beyond defense: Proactive approaches to disaster recovery and threat intelligence in modern enterprises. *Journal of Information Security, 15*(2), 106–133. DOI: 10.4236/jis.2024.152008

Voss, W. G. (2019). Cross-border data flows, the GDPR, and data governance. *Wash. Int'l LJ, 29*, 485.

Williams, P. A., & Woodward, A. J. (2015). Cybersecurity vulnerabilities in medical devices: a complex environment and multifaceted problem. *Medical Devices: Evidence and Research*, 305-316.

Yogi, M. K., MangaDevi, A., & Mundru, Y. (2025). Heartbeat Hackers: Protecting Privacy in the IoMT Age. *Convergence of Internet of Medical Things (IoMT) and Generative AI*, 133-170.

Zeydan, E., Arslan, S. S., & Liyanage, M. (2024). Managing distributed machine learning lifecycle for healthcare data in the cloud. *IEEE Access : Practical Innovations, Open Solutions, 12*, 115750–115774. DOI: 10.1109/ACCESS.2024.3443520

Zobaed, S. M., & Amini Salehi, M. (2025). Confidential Computing Across Edge-To-Cloud for Machine Learning: A Survey Study. *Software, Practice & Experience*, *55*(5), 896–924. DOI: 10.1002/spe.3398

Chapter 2

Insider Threats and Social Engineering in Healthcare

Olatunde Ayomide Olasehan
https://orcid.org/0009-0004-3069-7168
GOSH, UK

ABSTRACT

The healthcare sector is increasingly vulnerable to cybersecurity threats, particularly from insider threats and social engineering attacks that target sensitive patient data. Insider threats, originating from individuals with authorized access, can result in data theft and unauthorized access to electronic health records (EHRs). Social engineering tactics exploit trust to manipulate personnel into disclosing protected health information. While cloud trust models enhance security in interconnected environments, challenges remain in balancing security with privacy rights and regulatory compliance. Future directions include the use of artificial intelligence for predictive threat analysis, with careful consideration of ethical implications. The evolving nature of attack tactics necessitates adaptive defense mechanisms. Collaboration among stakeholders is crucial to establish frameworks and promote resilience. A comprehensive approach that integrates technology, training, and policy is essential to safeguard patient data and ensure operational continuity.

1.0. INTRODUCTION

The healthcare sector, increasingly dependent on digital technologies for patient care and data management, is confronted with escalating cybersecurity risks originating from both internal and external sources. This chapter explores insider threats and social engineering attacks, which exploit human and systemic vulnerabilities to compromise sensitive information and critical operations. By integrating insights

DOI: 10.4018/979-8-3373-4918-3.ch002

from established research, it underscores the unique challenges in healthcare, where breaches can directly endanger lives, and proposes advanced mitigation strategies to enhance resilience in this vital domain (Wasserman & Wasserman, 2022).

1.1. Overview of Insider Threats and Social Engineering in Healthcare

Definition of Insider Threats and Social Engineering in the Healthcare Context

Insider threats within the healthcare sector pertain to risks associated with individuals who possess authorized access to organizational systems, such as employees, contractors, and partners. These individuals may engage in malicious activities, including data theft, unauthorized access to electronic health records (EHRs), or the sabotage of medical devices, often exploiting their comprehensive understanding of internal vulnerabilities (Alsowail & Al-Shehari, 2022). Such threats encompass both deliberate misconduct, such as the deployment of ransomware or data exfiltration for personal benefit, and negligent actions that inadvertently compromise security protocols. In contrast, social engineering involves psychological manipulation techniques, such as phishing, pretexting, or baiting, designed to deceive healthcare personnel into disclosing protected health information (PHI) or granting unauthorized access, thereby exploiting trust-based relationships in high-pressure clinical settings (Hijji & Alam, 2021).

Importance of Addressing These Issues in the Increasingly Digital Healthcare Landscape

The digitization of healthcare, encompassing the extensive adoption of Electronic Health Records (EHRs), interconnected medical devices, and cloud-based systems, has significantly expanded the attack surface. This expansion renders insider threats and social engineering particularly potent, given the sensitive nature of patient data and the potential for direct harm to patient safety (Wasserman & Wasserman, 2022). With over 60% of organizations reporting insider incidents annually and breaches incurring an average global cost of $4.88 million, these threats extend beyond financial losses to include reputational damage, regulatory penalties under frameworks such as the General Data Protection Regulation (GDPR) and the Health Insurance Portability and Accountability Act (HIPAA), and risks to operational continuity. This underscores the urgent need for proactive defenses in a sector where 73% of privacy incidents involve electronic data (Cui & Song, 2025).

Brief Overview of the Chapter's Structure and Objectives

This chapter is organized to offer a thorough analysis, commencing with a detailed examination of insider threats in Section 2.0, encompassing their nature, characteristics, types, and impacts on healthcare. Section 3.0 addresses social engineering tactics, vulnerabilities, and notable incidents, while Section 4.0 explores threat intelligence frameworks and behavioral analytics for detection. Section 5.0 investigates cloud-based trust models and zero-trust architectures as mitigation strategies. The objectives are to elucidate current risks, evaluate preventive measures, and propose forward-looking solutions to strengthen healthcare cybersecurity against evolving threats (Garbis & Chapman, 2021).

1.2. Mission Statement

The primary objective of this chapter is to provide a comprehensive understanding of insider threats and social engineering by distinguishing between malicious and negligent behaviors. It explores motivations such as financial gain or extortion and analyzes their implications for patient care, data integrity, and institutional stability, drawing on empirical evidence from healthcare-specific studies.

Emphasis is placed on current challenges, such as the detection difficulties arising from insiders' legitimate access and the exploitation of human factors through social engineering. Additionally, future trends like AI-enhanced attacks and the integration of IoT devices are highlighted. To address these evolving risks, advanced solutions are advocated, including real-time monitoring, anomaly detection algorithms, and privacy-preserving technologies.

The primary emphasis is on threat intelligence frameworks for proactive risk assessment and their integration into security operations. This is enhanced by cloud-based trust models that incorporate multi-factor authentication, blockchain for secure identity management, and zero-trust principles to mitigate vulnerabilities in distributed healthcare environments.

2.0. INSIDER THREATS IN HEALTHCARE

This section examines the complex nature of insider threats within the healthcare sector, distinguishing between malicious and negligent actions. It further investigates the motivations underlying these behaviors and their specific effects on patient care, data integrity, and operational continuity. Comprehending these intricacies is essential for formulating effective mitigation strategies that address both deliberate misconduct and inadvertent errors that compromise security protocols.

2.1. Nature and Scope of Insider Threats

In the healthcare sector, the implications of insider threats are considerably heightened due to the sensitive nature of patient data and the critical infrastructure underpinning healthcare delivery. The potential for harm extends beyond financial or reputational damage to encompass direct threats to patient safety and privacy, rendering the assessment of such threats a paramount concern (Roy Sarkar, 2010). These threats include a range of malicious activities, such as ransomware deployment, data exfiltration, and extortion, often exploiting intimate knowledge of organizational vulnerabilities to maximize impact. Furthermore, insider threats are a pervasive issue, with over 60% of organizations experiencing such incidents in the past year, and nearly a tenth encountering more than twenty attacks, underscoring the critical need for robust detection and mitigation strategies. The financial impact alone is substantial, with the average global cost of insider threats rising significantly, highlighting the urgent necessity for comprehensive security frameworks that extend beyond external threat models. This necessitates a nuanced understanding of insider motivations and behaviors, as well as the implementation of advanced analytical techniques to detect anomalous activities within privileged access domains (Ali et al., 2025). Such threats are particularly challenging to detect and mitigate compared to external attacks because insiders possess authorized access to an organization's sensitive assets, enabling them to bypass conventional security measures (Alsowail & Al-Shehari, 2022). This inherent trust relationship complicates early detection, as the actions of a malicious insider often blend seamlessly with legitimate operational activities until significant damage has occurred. The critical impact of insider threats underscores the urgent need for a more proactive and sophisticated approach to cybersecurity that transcends traditional perimeter defenses (Bertino & Ghinita, 2011). Moreover, insiders, whether malicious or negligent, often exploit their knowledge of internal systems and processes, posing a significant risk to organizational integrity and data confidentiality.

2.1.1. Characteristics of Insider Threats Specific to Healthcare

The operational environment of healthcare institutions is uniquely characterized by stringent regulatory compliance and the sensitive nature of patient data, which introduces distinct vulnerabilities that set insider threats apart from those in other sectors. This complexity is further compounded by the diverse array of personnel, including employees, consultants, and third-party vendors, each possessing varying levels of legitimate access to sensitive systems and protected health information, thereby rendering detection particularly challenging (Roy Sarkar, 2010). Moreover, the absence of a universally accepted definition of an "insider" across various organizational and governmental bodies exacerbates the difficulty in establishing coherent detection and prevention strategies within healthcare (Bishop & Gates, 2008). This necessitates the development of specialized detection systems, methods, and tools capable of accurately and rapidly identifying malicious insiders, as conventional security measures primarily target external adversaries and often prove insufficient against internal breaches (Ali et al., 2025). The increasing sophistication of insider threats, often involving the misuse of legitimate access, underscores the inadequacy of traditional security mechanisms and necessitates novel frameworks for real-time detection (Ali et al., 2025). Given that insiders possess intimate knowledge of an organization's systems, detecting their malicious activities through conventional rule-based approaches, typically designed by domain experts, is inherently challenging and often lacks flexibility and robustness (Kim et al., 2019).

The complex network of human interactions and digital access points within healthcare settings presents a conducive environment for malicious insiders to exploit system vulnerabilities through sophisticated methods that often resemble legitimate operations. This challenge is exacerbated by the necessity for extensive internal access to facilitate clinical and administrative functions, inadvertently creating opportunities for data exfiltration or system manipulation without triggering immediate alerts (Wasserman & Wasserman, 2022). Consequently, a significant portion of security incidents in healthcare organizations are attributed to internal sources, with many involving electronic data breaches (Omotosho et al., 2017). These incidents frequently arise from an insider's privileged understanding of internal security protocols, enabling them to bypass or disable detection mechanisms more effectively than external attackers (Colwill, 2009). This internal perspective allows malicious actors to exploit authorized access for illicit activities, often taking advantage of trust-based relationships and a deep familiarity with the system.

2.1.2. Types of Insiders

Employee: People who are employed by healthcare institutions, including doctors, nurses, administrative staff, IT specialists, or support personnel, and who have access to protected health information (PHI), electronic health records (EHRs), or operational systems.

Contractors: Individuals employed on a temporary basis or from outside the organization for specific tasks, such as locum tenens doctors, temporary nurses, IT consultants, or maintenance personnel, who have access to healthcare systems or facilities.

Partners: External entities, such as third-party vendors, business associates, or collaborators (e.g., billing companies, cloud service providers, or telehealth platforms), are granted authorized access to healthcare systems or data through agreements.

2.2. Types of Insider Threats

Insider threats in healthcare can manifest in various forms, each presenting unique challenges to organizational security. These threats can be categorized based on intent, ranging from unintentional actions due to negligence or lack of awareness to deliberate malicious activities aimed at personal gain or causing harm. Understanding the different types of insider threats is crucial for developing comprehensive security strategies that address the diverse risks posed by individuals with authorized access to sensitive healthcare information and systems.

2.2.1. Data theft and unauthorized access to electronic health records (EHR)

The vulnerabilities inherent in healthcare systems are critically exploited by insider threats for malicious purposes. The widespread adoption of electronic health records has transformed healthcare by streamlining data management; however, this digitization also presents significant cybersecurity challenges, rendering sensitive patient information vulnerable to breaches and unauthorized access (S & K R, 2025). This vulnerability is particularly concerning given that a substantial majority, 73% of information privacy and security incidents reported by health organizations over the years have involved electronic data, with millions of patient records being compromised or put at risk due to malicious actors (Omotosho et al., 2017). Such incidents underscore the urgent need for robust security measures, as the sensitive nature of patient data, including personal identification, medical history, and treatment plans, makes it a prime target for various illicit activities, ranging from financial fraud to identity theft (Odeh et al., 2024). The extensive aggregation of identified health data in electronic health records, while enhancing accessibility for clinical and research purposes, simultaneously amplifies its attractiveness to well-resourced adversaries, including nation-states and organized crime syndicates, for purposes ranging from espionage to illicit profiteering (Rutherford et al., 2018). Consequently, the imperative to safeguard this highly sensitive information is paramount, as its compromise can lead to severe repercussions for individuals, including identity theft, financial fraud, and even discrimination based on health status (Thapa & Camtepe, 2020). While paper records posed similar risks, the ease with which electronic health records can be transmitted globally exacerbates these concerns, making system breaches more prevalent despite existing security protocols (Sulmasy et al., 2017). The centralized nature of modern Electronic Health Record frameworks, while improving accessibility, also consolidates sensitive patient data, thereby increasing the potential impact of a single breach and making these systems attractive targets for malicious actors (Natarajan et al., 2025). This shift to digital platforms, though crucial for modern healthcare efficiency, inadvertently creates a larger attack surface, especially when medical information is accessed remotely, opening avenues for sophisticated cyberattacks (Rengamani et al., 2010).

2.2.2. Sabotage of medical devices and systems

The deliberate disruption or manipulation of these essential assets presents a significant threat to patient safety and the operational integrity of healthcare institutions. Furthermore, these acts of sabotage can trigger cascading failures within interconnected healthcare infrastructure, resulting in widespread service outages and compromising the delivery of essential medical care (Linnartz et al., 2022). The complex nature of these systems, often comprising proprietary hardware, software, and communication protocols, complicates their defense against sophisticated cyber-attacks, rendering them particularly vulnerable to targeted disruptions (Lekidis, 2023). The impact of such cyber-physical attacks on healthcare organizations remains under-investigated, despite the sector's high vulnerability to breaches that can compromise sensitive patient data and operational continuity (Abbou et al., 2024). Given the increasing reliance on networked medical devices and the pervasive integration of IT within clinical environments, insider threats represent a particularly insidious vector for sabotage, capable of exploiting vulnerabilities from within an organization's trusted perimeter (Wasserman & Wasserman, 2022). These insider-initiated incidents, whether driven by malice or negligence, can leverage privileged access to subvert security controls, manipulate critical system parameters, or exfiltrate sensitive information, thereby directly jeopardizing patient care and institutional stability.

The digital transformation of healthcare, while enhancing accessibility and treatment, has inadvertently expanded the attack surface for both external and internal threats, making data breaches a pervasive concern for all stakeholders (Seh et al., 2020). Furthermore, the inherent complexity of healthcare IT infrastructure, often integrating legacy systems with advanced technologies, creates an expansive attack surface susceptible to exploitation by insiders (Wasserman & Wasserman, 2022). This situation necessitates a multi-faceted approach to security that combines technological countermeasures with robust policy frameworks and continuous employee training to strengthen defenses against both malicious and negligent insider actions (Alsowail & Al-Shehari, 2022).

2.2.3. Misuse of Privileged Access for Personal Gain

This section investigates the misuse of legitimate system access by individuals within healthcare organizations for illicit personal gain, analyzing the various manifestations of such transgressions. This exploitation often capitalizes on the inherent trust placed in medical professionals and the extensive system privileges they are granted, frequently involving the manipulation or theft of sensitive patient data for financial enrichment or other self-serving objectives (Phyo et al., 2004). The sensitive nature of healthcare data, encompassing demographic details, Social Security numbers, and clinical diagnoses, necessitates stringent security measures, yet its centralized storage in both paper and electronic formats makes it a prime target for breaches (Rutherford et al., 2018). Consequently, the unauthorized disclosure of such protected health information can lead to severe personal repercussions for patients, including identity theft, financial fraud, and discrimination in employment or insurance, thereby underscoring the critical need for robust data protection frameworks (Thapa & Camtepe, 2020). This necessitates a comprehensive understanding of the mechanisms by which privileged access is misused, alongside the implementation of advanced security protocols to detect and deter such activities (Natarajan et al., 2025). Understanding these attack vectors is crucial for developing effective countermeasures, which must encompass not only technological safeguards but also comprehensive training programs and rigorous oversight to mitigate the risks associated with privileged access.

2.3. Impact on Healthcare

Financial Losses Due to Data Breaches and System Downtime

The financial ramifications of insider threats within the healthcare sector extend beyond immediate remediation expenses, encompassing long-term reputational damage and potential regulatory fines. In 2024, the average global cost per data breach reached $4.88 million, with the healthcare sector experiencing even greater losses, highlighting the severe financial consequences for affected entities (Cui & Song, 2025). Beyond these direct costs, organizations frequently incur substantial legal fees and may face significant penalties under stringent data privacy regulations such as the GDPR, further exacerbating the financial burden (Cui & Song, 2025). Furthermore, the pervasive nature of electronic data in healthcare amplifies these risks, as evidenced by reports indicating that 73% of information privacy and security incidents involve digital records, resulting in millions of compromised patient records (Omotosho et al., 2017). The sensitive nature of healthcare data, which includes personally identifiable information and protected health information, exacerbates the impact of breaches, as demonstrated by the average cost of a data breach in 2023 reaching $4.24 million, the highest in 17 years (Vitorino et al., 2023). This substantial financial impact is further compounded by the costs associated with identity theft, which can result in out-of-pocket losses and emotional distress for victims, alongside damage to organizational reputation and potential loss of business (Cao et al., 2024). Moreover, the vulnerability of healthcare data, which includes demographic data, Social Security numbers, and clinical information, renders it particularly attractive to cybercriminals, leading to further financial exploitation through activities such as loan applications or illicit sales on the Dark Web (Rutherford et al., 2018).

Patient Safety Risks from Compromised Medical Devices or Altered Records

The integrity of patient data, especially within Electronic Health Records, is crucial, as evidenced by cases where data entry errors have resulted in severe medical complications, including patient deaths due to incorrect treatments or medication overdoses. Such inaccuracies in medical records, whether accidental or intentional, can significantly compromise the quality of care and pose substantial patient safety risks (Bowman, 2013). These errors may arise from various sources, such as adjacency errors where clinicians select an item next to the intended one in a drop-down menu, or inconsistencies between structured data fields and free-text entries.

Conversely, the operational integrity of medical devices is of paramount importance, as vulnerabilities exploited by insider threats could result in device malfunction or the administration of inappropriate therapies, thereby directly endangering patient safety. These vulnerabilities extend beyond mere data breaches to include the potential for malicious insiders to manipulate device settings, which could lead to incorrect dosages, delayed critical alerts, or even complete device failure, thus transforming a device intended for healing into a source of harm (W Koczkodaj et al., 2019). The pervasive digitization of healthcare records and the increasing reliance on interconnected medical devices amplify the potential for widespread adverse events, necessitating robust cybersecurity measures that address both data integrity and device functionality (Odeh et al., 2024).

Reputational Damage and Loss of Trust in Healthcare Institutions

The impact of insider threats goes well beyond immediate financial setbacks, significantly affecting public trust and damaging an institution's reputation in both community and professional settings. This decline in trust is particularly severe in the healthcare sector, where the perception that sensitive patient information and well-being have been jeopardized directly undermines the organization's credibility (Syed, 2018). A breach in data security can severely damage an organization's reputation, leading to a notable loss of confidence among patients and the general public, often accompanied by adverse media coverage (Cole et al., 2017). Such events are especially harmful in healthcare, where maintaining the confidentiality and integrity of patient data is crucial, resulting in significant economic and social consequences (Cao et al., 2024). Research shows that organizations suffering data breaches, particularly those involving sensitive customer data, endure substantial financial impacts that often parallel the direct costs of the breach (Tanimura & Wehrly, 2015). This encompasses not only legal expenses and regulatory penalties but also less tangible losses such as reduced market share and increased customer attrition, which can amplify the overall economic effect (Cui & Song, 2025). The emotional distress and potential harm to individuals whose health information is exposed further exacerbate reputational damage, as such breaches undermine the essential trust patients have in healthcare providers to protect their most personal data (Omotosho et al., 2017). This erosion of trust can also lead to higher insurance premiums for those affected and even job loss if medical histories become public (Thapa & Camtepe, 2020).

3.0. SOCIAL ENGINEERING IN HEALTHCARE

This widespread threat capitalizes on human psychology rather than exploiting technical weaknesses, making it a particularly dangerous avenue for data breaches and service interruptions in the healthcare sector. The sector's heavy dependence on human interaction and trust, along with the sensitive nature of patient information, renders it especially susceptible to such deceptive strategies (Salahdine & Kaabouch, 2019). Social engineering, which is generally understood as the manipulation of people to take actions that result in harm or increase the likelihood of future harm, takes advantage of inherent human traits to exploit vulnerability to deceit (Stewart & Dawson, 2018). This type of cyberattack bypasses conventional technological defenses by focusing on the human factor, often considered the weakest link in any security system (Alzahrani, 2020). Unlike traditional cyberattacks that aim at system flaws, social engineering uses psychological manipulation to convince individuals to reveal confidential information or ignore security measures (Alzahrani, 2020). This creates an opportune environment for cybercriminals, as social engineering attacks achieve high success rates by exploiting natural human tendencies (Venkatesha et al., 2021).

These attacks frequently exploit elements of trust, authority, and urgency, which are heightened within the healthcare environment due to the critical nature of patient care and the fast-paced nature of operations (Chapagain et al., 2024). The effectiveness of these attacks relies on psychological manipulation, a strategy that takes advantage of human biases and cognitive shortcuts to bypass security protocols (R. Syed, 2018). This form of manipulation is particularly potent as it exploits inherent human characteristics, rendering individuals unwittingly complicit in the breach of sensitive information (Venkatesha et al., 2021). Typically orchestrated by external actors, these insidious attacks employ a range of psychological tactics to coerce individuals into revealing critical information necessary for accessing computer systems or networks (Peltier, 2006).

3.1. Overview of Social Engineering Techniques

Social engineering techniques exploit human psychology to manipulate individuals into revealing sensitive information or taking actions that compromise security, especially in healthcare, where protected health information (PHI) holds significant value. These attacks frequently target employees, contractors, and partners, heightening insider threats by exploiting trust within connected health ecosystems. Common methods, such as phishing, pretexting, and baiting, have surged in healthcare due to the sector's digital interconnectedness and the high stakes associated with its data.

Phishing

Phishing constitutes a form of fraudulent communication aimed at deceiving recipients into divulging credentials or installing malware, frequently by impersonating trusted entities. Within the healthcare sector, email phishing involves the use of deceptive messages containing malicious links or attachments, such as those imitating patient portals or vendor updates, which can result in breaches of electronic health records (EHRs). Voice phishing, or vishing, utilizes phone calls with spoofed caller IDs to extract protected health information (PHI), while SMS-based phishing, or smishing, dispatches text messages with urgent links, such as counterfeit appointment reminders or vaccine access offers during public health crises like COVID-19. The consequences of these activities include the deployment of ransomware, data theft affecting millions of individuals, and violations of regulations.

Pretexting

Pretexting involves the creation of plausible scenarios or personas to establish trust and obtain confidential information, typically without the use of technical tools. In the healthcare sector, perpetrators may impersonate patients, vendors, or auditors to solicit Protected Health Information (PHI). This may include posing as a government official requesting medical records or as a colleague requiring immediate access to Electronic Health Records (EHRs). Instances of pretexting also encompass romance scams or fraudulent IT support calls directed at staff. The consequences of such activities include unauthorized access, which can lead to identity theft, financial fraud, or more extensive network breaches.

Baiting

Baiting involves enticing individuals with attractive offers, such as complimentary downloads or physical media, to install malware or disclose sensitive information. In the healthcare sector, this tactic may involve leaving infected USB drives in hospital areas or sending emails purporting to offer "free software updates" that compromise systems upon download. The consequences of such attacks include system lockdowns, exposure of Protected Health Information (PHI), and operational disruptions, with the potential for extensive breaches in interconnected ecosystems, resulting in substantial recovery costs.

3.2. Vulnerabilities in Healthcare Environments

Healthcare organizations, with their complex operational structures and the sensitive data they handle, are particularly vulnerable to social engineering attacks. This vulnerability arises from several factors, including the extensive reliance on interconnected digital systems, the high value of protected health information, and the often-neglected human aspect of cybersecurity defenses (Omotosho et al., 2017). The inherent need for interoperability and constant accessibility in healthcare systems further heightens cyber risks, providing numerous entry points for malicious actors (Wasserman & Wasserman, 2022). Consequently, healthcare is one of the industries most at risk of cyber infiltration, experiencing a significant increase in security incidents in recent years (Wasserman & Wasserman, 2022).

High Pressure Work Environments and Time Constraints

The demanding nature of healthcare operations, marked by critical decision-making under pressure, creates an environment with exceptionally high cognitive load. This heightened cognitive burden, often intensified by severe time constraints and the inherent uncertainties of medical scenarios, significantly affects the decision-making processes of healthcare professionals (Reale et al., 2023). The constant pressure can lead to suboptimal decision-making efficiency, as clinicians may struggle to process complex information and thoroughly evaluate alternatives, especially when overwhelmed with numerous tasks (Shamszare & Choudhury, 2023). This phenomenon is further exacerbated by the need for rapid responses in emergency situations, where the margin for error is minimal and the consequences of delayed or erroneous decisions can be severe (Young et al., 2012). Such intense operational environments can lead to cognitive overload, a major contributor to medical errors and device-related incidents (Collins, 2019). The pervasive time pressure in these settings forces individuals to make swift choices, often limiting opportunities for comprehensive analysis and deliberation (Wu et al., 2022). This reliance on expedited decision-making frequently results in the adoption of heuristics, or cognitive shortcuts, which, while efficient in certain contexts, can introduce biases that compromise the accuracy and reliability of clinical judgments (Cook & Woods, 2018). Although these heuristics can be adaptive under time and resource constraints, particularly in emergency settings, their uncritical application can lead to significant cognitive errors (Croskerry, 2002).

Conversely, these pressures may compel decision-makers to prioritize immediate outcomes, potentially at the expense of long-term considerations or more comprehensive exploratory processes (Wu et al., 2022). This phenomenon is particularly evident in time-sensitive decision-making scenarios where the urgency of patient needs necessitates a rapid response, often precluding extensive consultation or reflection (Cohen, 2008). The inherent complexities of clinical reasoning, especially in the context of infectious diseases, frequently necessitate such shortcuts to manage overwhelming information, yet this can paradoxically increase the potential for diagnostic inaccuracies and suboptimal patient outcomes (Islam et al., 2015). This reliance on heuristics, while a necessary adaptation in high-stakes environments, introduces vulnerabilities in diagnostic reasoning, potentially leading to misdiagnoses (Vickrey et al., 2010). For instance, in emergency departments, diagnostic errors are notably frequent due to the chaotic and high-pressure environment, compelling clinicians to make rapid decisions with incomplete information under significant cognitive strain (Taylor et al., 2024). These cognitive biases are particularly insidious because even experienced clinicians may not be fully aware of how their decisions are influenced by such shortcuts.

Diverse Workforce with Varying Levels of Security Awareness

The inherent heterogeneity in cybersecurity literacy often results in a broad spectrum of understanding, ranging from advanced comprehension among IT professionals to basic knowledge among clinical or administrative staff. This variation creates uneven defensive postures against evolving threats. Consequently, there is a need for tailored security awareness training programs that consider varying levels of technical proficiency and cognitive processing. Such programs ensure that critical security information is accessible and actionable for all personnel, regardless of their departmental affiliation or digital acumen (Carreira et al., 2025). These customized educational initiatives are essential for mitigating human error, a significant factor in a substantial proportion of security breaches within healthcare environments (Khadka & Ullah, 2025). Moreover, the effectiveness of these training programs is often challenged by the dynamic nature of social engineering tactics and the high-pressure operational environments characteristic of healthcare, necessitating continuous reinforcement and adaptive learning modules (Branley-Bell et al., 2021).

Furthermore, the varied requirements of healthcare personnel, which range from basic users needing essential knowledge of the threat landscape to security experts requiring incident response training, demand dynamically adaptive programs that continuously adjust to individual performance and evolving threats (Hatzivasilis et al., 2020). This ongoing adaptation is instrumental in fostering self-efficacy among employees, a critical component for establishing a proactive cybersecurity posture throughout the organization (Stavrou & Piki, 2024). However, this proactive strategy encounters significant challenges, including a pronounced shortage of qualified cybersecurity professionals and inherent human biases that frequently compromise security protocols (Tahmasebi, 2024). Effectively overcoming these obstacles requires a paradigm shift from traditional compliance-focused training to an approach that nurtures intrinsically motivated security behaviors and recognizes the psychological factors that contribute to human susceptibility to social engineering (Haney et al., 2021).

Reliance on Email and Digital Communication for Patient Care

The widespread incorporation of email and digital communication into healthcare workflows, while enhancing efficiency and collaboration, simultaneously increases the vulnerability to sophisticated social engineering attacks. This increased dependence on digital channels, including electronic health records, telemedicine platforms, and mobile health applications, necessitates robust cybersecurity measures to address the inherent vulnerabilities associated with the increased volume of sensitive patient data being transmitted and stored digitally (Odeh et al., 2024). The digitization of healthcare systems has fundamentally transformed the management and sharing of Electronic Health Records, which, despite their critical role in modern healthcare, are particularly susceptible to security breaches due to their sensitive nature (S & K R, 2025). This expanding digital footprint in healthcare presents an attractive target for cybercriminals seeking to exploit system weaknesses and human factors (Omotosho et al., 2017).

The intrinsic value and sensitivity of health data make the healthcare sector a prime target for malicious actors, with the potential consequences of successful attacks extending far beyond financial losses to include direct threats to patient care and public trust (Lorenzini et al., 2022). This vulnerability is exacerbated by the complex interoperability requirements and constant accessibility demands within healthcare environments, which often inadvertently introduce additional cyber risks (Wasserman & Wasserman, 2022). The healthcare sector, already managing a vast and intricate array of digital systems, has seen a significant rise in security incidents, placing it among the industries most susceptible to cyber infiltration (Wasserman & Wasserman, 2022). Indeed, the industry's growing reliance on computerized systems for operations and data management exposes it to substantial cyber threats, resulting in a higher incidence of hacks and malware attacks compared to other sectors (Abbou et al., 2024).

3.3. Case Studies of Social Engineering Attacks

These cyber threats manifest in various forms, with social engineering attacks emerging as a particularly insidious method employed by malicious actors. Social engineering exploits human psychology and behavior rather than technical vulnerabilities, making it a challenging threat to defend against in healthcare settings. By examining specific case studies of social engineering attacks in the healthcare sector, we can gain valuable insights into the tactics used by attackers and the potential consequences of successful breaches.

3.3.1. Analysis of Notable Social Engineering Incidents in Healthcare

Social engineering incidents in healthcare underscore the sector's susceptibility to psychological manipulation, often exploiting trust in high-stakes environments to gain unauthorized access to protected health information (PHI). An analysis of these cases reveals patterns such as phishing and pretexting as primary vectors, exacerbated by the interconnected nature of electronic health records (EHRs) and third-party dependencies. In 2025, social engineering continued to be a leading initial access method in 36% of incident response cases, contributing to breaches costing up to $11 million on average. Below, we examine three notable incidents, focusing on the tactics employed, insider involvement, impacts, and lessons for mitigation.

1. Change Healthcare Ransomware Attack (2024, with Ongoing Impacts into 2025)

The ransomware attack on Change Healthcare, a subsidiary of UnitedHealth Group, in February 2024 serves as a pertinent example of how social engineering can lead to extensive disruptions. Executed by the ALPHV/BlackCat group, the breach was initiated through phishing or pretexting strategies that deceived an insider, likely an employee or contractor, into providing remote access via compromised credentials. This breach facilitated the exfiltration of personal health information (PHI) of up to 100 million individuals, encompassing medical records and payment details, and resulted in system outages that delayed prescription and claims processing across hospitals in the United States. The financial impact exceeded $2.4 billion, with broader implications including heightened patient mortality risks due to delays in care.

Analysis indicates the significant role of negligent insiders, exemplified by individuals who fall victim to phishing emails that imitate vendor communications, exacerbated by insufficient multi-factor authentication (MFA) measures. This incident highlights vulnerabilities within the supply chain, as third-party partners contributed to the expansion of the breach's impact. The findings suggest the necessity of implementing mandatory security awareness training and adopting zero-trust architectures to authenticate all access requests, thereby mitigating the 279% increase in business email compromise (BEC) incidents observed in the healthcare sector.

2. Highmark Health Phishing Breach (2023)

In December 2022, Highmark Health, a prominent integrated healthcare system in the U.S., experienced a phishing attack that impacted 300,000 individuals. An employee, either disgruntled or negligent, clicked on a malicious link in a spoofed email, allowing unauthorized access to their account for two days. This breach exposed PHI, including personal and medical information, underscoring how easily email-based social engineering can circumvent defenses in busy clinical environments.

The analysis highlights human factors, noting that healthcare staff, often working under pressure, are susceptible to exploiting trust and urgency in communications. Insider threats were apparent, as the breach involved the misuse of credentials without immediate detection. The consequences included regulatory fines under HIPAA and damage to reputation. Key lessons underscore the importance of simulated phishing exercises and real-time monitoring, given that phishing accounted for 45% of healthcare incidents in similar surveys.

3. Magellan Health Pretexting Incident (2020)

In December 2020, Magellan Health, a provider of behavioral health services, fell victim to a pretexting attack. Attackers, posing as a trusted client, tricked an employee into divulging credentials, which led to a ransomware attack and the exposure of over two million records, including PHI and PII. This breach, attributed to the REvil group, highlighted how fabricated scenarios can exploit the collaborative nature of the healthcare sector.

Analysis indicates that pretexting is particularly effective in targeting partners and contractors, with 94% of organizations granting high-privilege access to third parties. The consequences include heightened risks of identity theft and operational disruptions, leading to recovery costs that can reach millions. Key lessons involve implementing identity verification protocols and conducting awareness training, as similar tactics were evident in 2025 incidents like the IMSS Mexico breach, where 350,000 records were stolen for social engineering exploitation.

These incidents highlight recurring themes: a heavy reliance on human error, with 61% of breaches attributed to negligence, escalation through insider threats, and heightened risks within interconnected ecosystems. To address these issues, healthcare organizations must implement comprehensive training, multi-factor authentication (MFA), and incident response plans, as underscored in HHS advisories regarding IT help desk scams.

3.3.2. Lessons Learned and Implications for Future Prevention

The examination of historical social engineering incidents within the healthcare sector yields essential insights into the vulnerabilities exploited and their subsequent impact on patient safety and data integrity. Despite the implementation of advanced health information technology systems, security breaches continue to affect numerous hospitals and compromise the data of thousands of patients, suggesting that other hospital factors, such as area characteristics, region, bed size, health system membership, hospital type, hospital governance, and market concentration, may significantly influence breach risk (Rutherford et al., 2018). Moreover, while network servers were among the least frequent locations for data breaches, incidents originating from them invariably affected the largest number of patients (Rutherford et al., 2018). The widespread use of electronic health records and interconnected systems introduces numerous attack vectors, highlighting the necessity for robust cybersecurity frameworks that extend beyond mere technical controls to include human elements (Wasserman & Wasserman, 2022). The increasing threat of cyberattacks further underscores the urgent need for comprehensive cybersecurity strategies within healthcare, as the industry remains a prime target for malicious actors (Wasserman & Wasserman, 2022). The sensitive nature and high value of health data render healthcare an attractive target for cybercriminals, with potential consequences ranging from substantial financial losses to severe disruptions in patient care (Lorenzini et al., 2022). These breaches often result in significant monetary and privacy losses, impacting not only the directly involved populations but also the broader healthcare environment (Raghupathi et al., 2023). Consequently, identifying recurring vulnerabilities, particularly those arising from social engineering tactics, is crucial for strengthening defenses and ensuring the continuous delivery of secure and reliable healthcare services. Thus, understanding the modalities through which these attacks manifest, especially those exploiting human susceptibility rather than technical vulnerabilities, becomes a foundational step in crafting effective preventative measures.

3.4. Psychological and Behavioral Aspects

Social engineering exploits fundamental psychological vulnerabilities in humans to manipulate individuals into performing actions or disclosing confidential information, often leveraging cognitive biases such as the principle of reciprocity or the halo effect. These attacks primarily aim to alter normal and rational decision-making processes, as described in behavioral decision theory, by exploiting the inherent human trust in other individuals over technological safeguards (Salahdine & Kaabouch, 2019). This reliance on human interaction distinguishes social engineering from purely technical cyberattacks, rendering conventional cybersecurity defenses less effective (Alzahrani, 2020). Indeed, while technical solutions remain crucial, they are inherently limited in preventing manipulations that exploit human susceptibility (Alzahrani, 2020).

Exploitation of Trust, Authority, and Urgency in Healthcare Settings

In this context, social engineering exploits the intrinsic trust that patients place in healthcare professionals and institutions, alongside the often-urgent nature of medical situations, to manipulate individuals into disclosing sensitive information or engaging in actions that compromise security (Touchie et al., 2021). This manipulation takes advantage of human vulnerabilities, as individuals are inherently more trusting of other humans than of technological safeguards, making them the most susceptible link in any security chain (Salahdine & Kaabouch, 2019). The effectiveness of social engineering attacks often depends on the attacker's ability to adeptly apply psychological manipulation, customizing techniques to specific victims and exploiting traits such as susceptibility to deception (Alzahrani, 2020). These attacks are broadly categorized into physical, technical, social, and socio-technical approaches, employing both human-based and computer-based methodologies to illicitly obtain information or access (Alzahrani, 2020). Notably, these insidious tactics frequently involve outsiders who exploit psychological tricks to gain unauthorized access to computer systems or networks . This contrasts with traditional hacking, which directly targets technological vulnerabilities, as social engineering instead exploits human elements that often circumvent robust technical defenses (Venkatesha et al., 2021).

Social engineering poses a particularly significant threat within the healthcare sector, where the necessity for prompt decision-making and a culture of immediate response can supersede security protocols, rendering the environment susceptible to exploitation (Venkatesha et al., 2021). This threat often involves psychological manipulation, wherein attackers exploit emotional states and cognitive biases to circumvent otherwise robust security measures. Addressing these threats effectively requires a nuanced understanding of human behavior, as traditional cybersecurity solutions frequently fail to account for the human element of security (Alzahrani, 2020). The core principle of social engineering is its capacity to bypass technological safeguards, such as firewalls, by exploiting the inherent human element through deception and persuasion (Hijji & Alam, 2021). The success of such attacks often hinges on the attacker's skill in leveraging cognitive biases and emotional responses, thereby leading victims to inadvertently compromise data confidentiality, integrity, or availability (Chapagain et al., 2024).

Cognitive Biases That Make Healthcare Workers Susceptible to Social Engineering

Cognitive biases are systematic patterns of deviation from rational judgment, often resulting in mistakes in processing information and making decisions. These biases are particularly vulnerable to exploitation in social engineering attacks within healthcare environments (O'Sullivan & Schofield, 2018). Human tendencies like heuristics, or mental shortcuts, are generally adaptive, especially when quick decisions are necessary under pressure. However, they can also lead to significant diagnostic and clinical errors if misapplied or if they result in incorrect interpretations of complex situations (Croskerry, 2002). While these heuristics facilitate efficient decision-making and streamline clinical workflows, they also make healthcare professionals susceptible to cognitive biases. These biases are not linked to intelligence or cognitive ability but are common phenomena (Vickrey et al., 2010). A notable lack of awareness of one's own biases is widespread among healthcare practitioners, even among those who consider themselves adept decision-makers, thereby increasing their vulnerability to manipulation (O'Sullivan & Schofield, 2018).

4.0. THREAT INTELLIGENCE FOR MITIGATING INSIDER THREATS AND SOCIAL ENGINEERING

Organizations encounter significant challenges in managing insider threats due to the diverse composition of employees, consultants, and complex infrastructure, which can lead to substantial damage, including financial losses, reputational harm, or compromise of intellectual property. This multifaceted risk necessitates a robust threat intelligence framework to identify, analyze, and mitigate the subtle yet pervasive indicators of malicious insider activity (Tsiostas et al., 2020). The increasing prevalence and cost of cyberattacks originating from insider threats underscore the inadequacy of current detection methods, highlighting the urgent need for advanced systems capable of accurate and rapid identification (Sergiu, 2020).

4.1. Role of Threat Intelligence

Threat intelligence is crucial in addressing insider threats and social engineering attacks within the healthcare sector by offering actionable insights into potential risks, attacker strategies, and vulnerabilities associated with the sector's sensitive data and interconnected systems. In a context where 36% of healthcare incidents in 2025 originated from social engineering, the utilization of threat intelligence is essential for anticipating and responding to threats targeting protected health information (PHI).

4.1.1. Definition and components of threat intelligence frameworks

Threat intelligence involves the systematic collection, analysis, and dissemination of information regarding current and emerging threats, with the aim of identifying, preventing, and mitigating cyberattacks. Within the healthcare sector, frameworks are composed of three fundamental components:

Strategic Intelligence: High-level insights into threat actors, their motives, and emerging trends reveal that state-sponsored groups often target PHI for espionage or financial gain. Notably, 80% of malicious insider incidents are driven by financial motives.

Tactical Intelligence: Details on specific attack methods, such as phishing or pretexting techniques, facilitate the development of targeted defenses against social engineering.

Operational Intelligence: Real-time data on indicators of compromise (IoCs), such as malicious IP addresses or phishing email signatures, is crucial for detecting and responding to active threats. These components create a structured approach to anticipating insider threats, with frameworks like MITRE ATT&CK mapping tactics to healthcare-specific vulnerabilities, such as weak access controls in EHR systems.

4.1.2. Sources of threat intelligence in healthcare

Healthcare organizations rely on diverse sources to build robust threat intelligence:

Internal Logs: System logs, EHR access records, and employee activity monitoring offer valuable insights into insider behavior. For instance, anomaly detection in access logs can identify unauthorized PHI access by employees or contractors. Additionally, network traffic analysis and endpoint monitoring uncover patterns such as unusual data downloads.

External Feeds: Industry-specific feeds from the Health Information Sharing and Analysis Center (H-ISAC), along with government alerts such as those from

HHS or FBI advisories, and commercial platforms like Recorded Future, deliver real-time data on phishing campaigns or ransomware groups like ALPHV/BlackCat. Open-source intelligence (OSINT), which includes dark web monitoring, keeps track of stolen PHI sales, while posts on online platforms offer early warnings of emerging threats.

4.1.3. Integration of threat intelligence into security operations

Incorporating threat intelligence into healthcare security operations enhances defenses against insider threats and social engineering attacks. Essential practices include:

Real-Time Monitoring and Response

Threat intelligence feeds are integrated into Security Information and Event Management (SIEM) systems to correlate Indicators of Compromise (IoCs) with internal logs, thereby facilitating the prompt detection of phishing or unauthorized access attempts.

Automated Defenses

Intelligence-driven tools, such as firewalls and intrusion detection systems, utilize Indicators of Compromise (IoCs) to block malicious IP addresses or email domains. This approach effectively reduces the success rate of phishing attacks.

Training and Awareness

Tactical intelligence plays a crucial role in simulated phishing exercises and employee training, specifically targeting the 27% of personnel who infrequently review security policies.

Incident Response Planning

Operational intelligence plays a crucial role in guiding incident response by prioritizing threats according to their severity. Integration challenges, such as data overload and interoperability with legacy systems, persist; however, frameworks like the NIST Cybersecurity Framework facilitate streamlined adoption, thereby enhancing resilience within connected health ecosystems.

4.2. Behavioral Analytics and Anomaly Detection

Behavioral analytics and anomaly detection systems are crucial for identifying deviations from established baselines of user activity, thereby signaling potential insider threats. This approach utilizes the analysis of digital footprints to detect anomalous patterns that may indicate malicious intent or inadvertent security breaches. Anomaly detection, fundamentally, identifies rare events or observations that significantly deviate from normal behavior within a dataset, often raising suspicion regarding their origin or consistency. These anomalies can manifest in various forms, such as unusual login times, access to sensitive data outside typical work parameters, or uncharacteristic data transfers. This method surpasses traditional signature-based intrusion detection systems by concentrating on behavioral indicators rather than predefined attack patterns, which often prove ineffective against novel or sophisticated insider threats (Sowmya & Mary Anita, 2023). This enables the identification of previously unknown threats by establishing a baseline of normal user behavior and flagging deviations from this norm as potential security incidents (Alhayan et al., 2025). The integration of machine learning and artificial intelligence into anomaly detection further refines this process, allowing systems to autonomously learn and adapt to evolving behavioral patterns, thereby enhancing accuracy and reducing false positives.

This refinement is particularly crucial because traditional anomaly detection methods, such as statistical approaches or distance-based techniques, often struggle with high-dimensional and complex data, resulting in elevated false positive rates that can overwhelm security teams (Olateju et al., 2024). However, advancements in unsupervised algorithms offer a promising solution by adapting to dynamic system contexts and effectively identifying unknown attacks, although their efficacy depends on accurately characterizing expected behavior (Zoppi et al., 2021). In the context of insider threats within healthcare, this involves meticulously modeling typical user interactions with electronic health records and other sensitive systems to detect any deviations that could signal data exfiltration or unauthorized access (Ali et al., 2025).

Machine Learning Algorithms for Detecting Unusual User Behavior

Machine learning algorithms are increasingly utilized to identify anomalous patterns in user behavior that deviate from established baselines, thereby enhancing the proactive detection of potential insider threats. This analytical capability is particularly critical given the dynamic and sophisticated nature of insider attacks, which often exploit legitimate access permissions, rendering them difficult to detect through traditional security measures (Alatawi & Albalawi, 2025). Moreover, machine learning excels at identifying subtle deviations in large and complex datasets, a task where traditional statistical models often fall short, especially as data volumes grow (Davis et al., 2020). The inherent adaptability of machine learning models allows them to continuously learn from new data, refining their accuracy in distinguishing between benign fluctuations and genuine indicators of malicious intent over time. This facilitates the dynamic identification of novel attack vectors that static, signature-based detection systems would inevitably miss (Mane & Rao, 2021). Furthermore, these models can discern varying network attacks as anomalies by establishing a baseline of normal network traffic (Campazas-Vega et al., 2023).

Establishing Baselines for Normal Activity in Healthcare Systems

Creating detailed baselines is essential for differentiating normal operational activities from unusual behaviors that may indicate insider threats or social engineering attacks within the intricate healthcare IT environment. This initial step requires a thorough documentation of standard system performance, user access habits, and data movement to establish a solid benchmark for detecting deviations. These baselines cover a broad range of metrics, such as network traffic levels, typical access times for various user roles, commonly accessed databases, and regular data modification records (Abouelmehdi et al., 2018). By setting these baselines, it becomes possible to proactively identify anomalies, like unexpected data access requests outside normal working hours or attempts by staff to access highly sensitive patient information without a clear clinical justification, which could indicate a compromised account or malicious intent (Wasserman & Wasserman, 2022). Additionally, these baselines must consider the dynamic nature of healthcare operations, incorporating elements such as emergency protocols, shift changes, and surge events to avoid false positives while remaining alert to real threats.

Real-time Monitoring and Alerting for Potential Insider Threats

This strategy entails the ongoing gathering and examination of various data streams, such as network traffic, system logs, and user behavior analytics, to detect unusual patterns that may suggest malicious insider actions. This requires the implementation of advanced monitoring tools that can ingest and process data in real-time, often utilizing artificial intelligence and machine learning algorithms to identify subtle deviations from established norms (Ali et al., 2025). These systems frequently combine security event log data with access control lists and other network information to create a comprehensive threat landscape, thereby improving the accuracy of anomaly detection (Tall et al., 2016). By adopting this proactive approach, organizations can detect potential insider threats early, allowing for timely intervention and mitigation before significant harm occurs (Al-Mhiqani et al., 2020). Additionally, the effectiveness of real-time monitoring is greatly enhanced by incorporating user and entity behavior analytics, which establish baselines for normal activity and highlight deviations that might indicate an insider threat, thus providing a more nuanced understanding of behavioral anomalies within the organizational environment (Al-Muntaser et al., 2023). The challenge lies in sifting through large volumes of data to pinpoint genuine threats amidst numerous false positives, necessitating intelligent filtering and correlation mechanisms (Yuan & Wu, 2020). The inherent authorized access of insiders makes it difficult to distinguish their malicious activities from legitimate operations, posing a significant challenge to automated threat detection systems in reducing false alarms without impeding employee productivity (Singh & Sharma, 2022).

4.3. Integration with Cloud-Based Systems

The growing adoption of cloud computing demands robust integration strategies for threat intelligence platforms to effectively monitor and safeguard sensitive healthcare data stored off-premise. This integration is essential for harnessing the extensive computational power and data storage capabilities offered by cloud environments, which are increasingly used for real-time patient monitoring and health information exchange (Kang et al., 2018). For instance, integrating cloud-based Internet of Things systems enhances telemedicine services by enabling real-time data analysis and patient management on an unprecedented scale, thereby requiring sophisticated threat intelligence to secure these interconnected ecosystems (Dike & Jackson, 2024).

Advantages of Cloud-based Threat Intelligence Platforms

These platforms provide enhanced scalability and accessibility, enabling organizations to swiftly adapt to evolving threat landscapes and access critical intelligence from any location. Moreover, cloud-based solutions facilitate the integration of advanced security services, such as machine learning algorithms for threat detection and automated orchestration tools, which would be financially prohibitive or technically challenging to implement in traditional on-premise infrastructures (Hassan et al., 2024). This shift allows for a proactive rather than reactive cybersecurity posture, transforming how organizations predict and neutralize threats before they can inflict significant damage (Ovabor et al., 2024). The transition to cloud platforms also offers substantial economic benefits alongside technological advantages, enabling businesses to leverage robust analytics and AI services for real-time data processing and predictive decision-making (Amajuoyi et al., 2024).

Challenges in Implementing Cloud Solutions in Healthcare

The integration of cloud technologies within the healthcare sector presents a multifaceted array of challenges, primarily arising from stringent regulatory compliance, data privacy concerns, and the prevalent legacy infrastructure in many medical institutions. A significant challenge is ensuring the confidentiality and privacy of sensitive patient data, which is of paramount importance in healthcare and often compromised in cloud environments (Gitonga et al., 2020). This issue is further complicated by the necessity for compliance with regulations such as HIPAA and GDPR, which impose strict requirements on the storage, processing, and sharing of health data, rendering cloud adoption risky and potentially costly due to the possibility of data loss and subsequent fines (Georgiou & Lambrinoudakis, 2021). The centralized data storage models commonly employed by cloud services also introduce vulnerabilities, including data breaches, a lack of transparency, and elevated operational costs, alongside diminishing patient-centric control over their health information (Hiwale et al., 2023). Furthermore, the transition of protected health information to cloud platforms introduces significant security concerns, necessitating robust frameworks to ensure data protection, privacy, and adherence to regulatory mandates (Seth et al., 2024). Specifically, the outsourcing of Protected Health Records to cloud environments necessitates advanced encryption prior to storage, as direct control over such data is relinquished by the patient upon upload (Ramesh et al., 2020). This shift necessitates a re-evaluation of established privacy concepts and legal frameworks to harmonize them with the technological advancements offered by cloud computing in the health domain (Zandesh, 2024).

5.0. CLOUD TRUST MODELS FOR HEALTHCARE SECURITY

The growing dependence on cloud infrastructure within the healthcare sector necessitates the establishment of robust trust models to protect sensitive patient data and ensure operational continuity. These models must address the specific security and privacy requirements of healthcare data, including confidentiality, integrity, and availability, while also adhering to stringent regulatory compliance such as HIPAA (Ermakova et al., 2020). The inherent sensitivity of personal health information, combined with the potential for significant financial penalties and reputational damage resulting from breaches, highlights the critical need for advanced security paradigms in cloud-based healthcare systems (Georgiou & Lambrinoudakis, 2021). This necessity drives the development of specialized cloud security frameworks that incorporate multifactor authentication and attribute-based encryption to control access to electronic health records, thereby mitigating the risks of unauthorized access (Gitonga et al., 2020). Moreover, the development of comprehensive security maturity models for cloud-based healthcare systems is essential to provide a structured approach for the continuous assessment and improvement of an organization's security posture (Akinsanya et al., 2020).

5.1. Overview of Cloud Trust Models

This section offers an in-depth analysis of various cloud trust models, exploring their architectural foundations, security mechanisms, and relevance within complex distributed systems. These models are essential for maintaining data integrity and confidentiality in cloud environments, particularly given the inherently distributed and multi-tenant nature of cloud computing. The creation of robust trust models is further complicated by the necessity to manage identities and access controls across different trust domains, a critical challenge in an environment where users and service providers often operate under distinct security policies. Moreover, effective trust models must continuously assess risk and trustworthiness, adapting to emerging threats and vulnerabilities across diverse architectural stacks within the cloud ecosystem.

Zero Trust Model

The Zero Trust model represents a fundamental shift in cybersecurity paradigms, transitioning from a perimeter-based defense to a continuous verification approach. This model posits that no user or device, whether internal or external to the network, should be inherently trusted. It operates on the core principle of "never trust, always verify," necessitating rigorous authentication and authorization for every access request, regardless of its origin (Daah et al., 2024). This stands in stark contrast to traditional security models, which assume inherent trust for entities within the corporate network (Dhiman et al., 2024). Instead, Zero Trust underscores the importance of verifying and authenticating every user and device, restricting access to resources based on the principle of least privilege (Azad et al., 2024). This strategic approach permeates the entire digital estate, encompassing user accounts, devices, applications, and data, irrespective of their location (Garbis & Chapman, 2021). It aims to eliminate implicit trust and continuously validate every stage of digital interaction, acknowledging that most business applications and resources now exist beyond traditional network perimeters (Paul & Rao, 2022). This necessitates a comprehensive policy framework that dynamically governs the authentication and authorization of all entities, including users, services, and requested resources, through continuous status assessments (Chandramouli, 2023). This architectural shift is crucial for securing cloud environments and remote workforces, as it addresses the increasing complexity of cybersecurity threats and the sophistication of attack vectors by reducing the attack surface through micro-segmentation (Reddy, 2025). Furthermore, Zero Trust seeks to prevent data breaches and restrict internal lateral movement by meticulously identifying and classifying data, enumerating traffic flows, and constructing access policies based on these insights. The comprehensive policy framework underpinning Zero Trust Architecture dynamically governs the authentication and authorization of all entities, leveraging continuous status assessments for users, services, and requested resources (Chandramouli, 2023).

Federated Trust Model

A federated trust model constitutes a decentralized security framework wherein multiple, independently managed trust domains collaborate to establish and maintain trust relationships without reliance on a singular, centralized authority. This paradigm facilitates secure and seamless interactions across disparate systems by enabling identity providers to authenticate users and service providers to authorize access based on established trust agreements (Ribeiro De Mello et al., 2020). This distributed approach minimizes the attack surface associated with a single point of failure, thereby enhancing overall system resilience and confidentiality (Hussain et al., 2021). Furthermore, within a federated identity management context, entities across different organizational boundaries can securely share resources and services, which is particularly pertinent in healthcare for interoperability (Pöhn & Hillmann, 2021). This framework is critical for enabling secure data exchange and collaborative care, allowing healthcare providers to access patient information across various institutions while upholding stringent privacy regulations (Hardjono, 2019). The complexities of integrating diverse identity models within a federated healthcare environment necessitate robust mechanisms for attribute alignment and dynamic levels of assurance to mitigate potential risks (Shemshi & Jakimovski, 2025).

Shared Responsibility Model

This model is essential for comprehending cloud security, as it distinctly separates the responsibilities of the cloud service provider, referred to as "security of the cloud," from those of the customer, known as "security in the cloud." This distinction is vital because it assigns the cloud provider the duty of ensuring the physical security and network controls of the underlying infrastructure, while the user is responsible for application-level security, data encryption, and access management within their deployed services (Jaatun et al., 2018). For example, in the Software as a Service model, the consumer has limited insight into the underlying infrastructure and maintenance processes, thereby placing a greater security burden on the cloud provider (Farnga, 2018). Conversely, in the Infrastructure as a Service model, the user maintains significant control over operating systems, applications, and network configurations, which necessitates strong internal security protocols. The complexity of cryptographic key management further complicates this shared responsibility in cloud environments, differing markedly from traditional enterprise IT due to the varied ownership and control over infrastructure components (Chandramouli et al., 2013).

5.2. Compliance with Regulatory Standards

Compliance with stringent regulatory frameworks, such as HIPAA in the United States and GDPR in Europe, is essential for healthcare organizations transitioning sensitive patient data to cloud environments. These regulations impose rigorous requirements for data protection, privacy, and the secure processing of health information, rendering compliance a significant challenge for entities operating within highly regulated sectors like healthcare. The complexity of navigating these legal landscapes necessitates a robust framework that facilitates not only data protection and privacy but also the capacity for comprehensive incident investigation and reporting (Seth et al., 2024). Furthermore, any cloud-based solution must effectively address data privacy and security concerns, particularly given the increased risk of data breaches, lack of transparency, and high costs associated with centralized data storage (Hiwale et al., 2023).

General Data Protection Regulation (GDPR)

This regulation significantly impacts healthcare organizations by imposing strict requirements on the processing and safeguarding of personal health information. Adopted on April 27, 2016, the GDPR became enforceable on May 25, 2018, requiring healthcare institutions to analyze their obligations and implement measures to ensure compliance with its provisions (Gonçalves-Ferreira et al., 2018). This includes adherence to principles such as explicit consent for data processing, the right to data portability, and enhanced accountability for data controllers and processors (Neisse et al., 2018). The regulation, notably Article 15, bolsters individual privacy rights by granting data subjects the right to access their personal data in an understandable format, compelling organizations to optimize their data handling processes (Pöhn et al., 2023). This comprehensive framework standardizes data protection across the European Union, influencing global data management practices, especially concerning sensitive data like health records. The GDPR's core principles mandate obtaining explicit consent from individuals for data collection, storage, and processing, while also emphasizing data anonymization to protect identity and privacy (Al-Fayad, 2020). Furthermore, it establishes severe penalties for non-compliance, thereby incentivizing robust data governance frameworks within healthcare IT infrastructures (Birnstill et al., 2018). The hefty fines, potentially reaching €20 million or 4% of annual global turnover, underscore the critical need for meticulous adherence to GDPR stipulations within healthcare systems, particularly those managing sensitive patient data (Kammüller et al., 2019). In light of these stringent requirements, healthcare entities must implement robust data minimization strategies, ensuring that only the essential personal data is collected and shared for its intended purpose (Milani et al., 2020).

Health Insurance Portability and Accountability Act (HIPAA)

The Health Insurance Portability and Accountability Act (HIPAA), enacted in 1996, mandates stringent safeguards for the privacy and security of protected health information, significantly impacting the design and operation of cloud-based healthcare systems. This foundational legislation established regulations to protect patient privacy, which were further enhanced by the Federal Information Security Management Act of 2002 (Ahmed, 2019). HIPAA's primary aim was to regulate health plans, healthcare clearinghouses, and healthcare providers involved in electronic financial and administrative transactions, thereby simplifying administrative processes while ensuring robust data protection (Rocchiccioli, 2003). The Health Information Technology for Economic and Clinical Health Act of 2009 subsequently expanded HIPAA's scope, introducing more stringent regulations and increased penalties for non-compliance, with a particular focus on the adoption of electronic health records (Peterson & Watzlaf, 2015). This legislative framework requires healthcare organizations to implement comprehensive technical, administrative, and physical safeguards to ensure the confidentiality, integrity, and availability of electronic protected health information (ePHI) (Elkourdi et al., 2024). Ensuring information integrity, which involves maintaining the accuracy and consistency of data throughout its lifecycle, is crucial for effective patient care and compliance (Fedorowicz & Ray, 2004). Given HIPAA's extensive scope, encompassing most health plans and practitioners, it regulates privacy and security across electronic, paper, and oral communications (Feld, 2005). Consequently, healthcare entities must develop and maintain robust compliance programs to consistently execute HIPAA's intricate requirements, adapting their internal processes to meet evolving regulatory demands (Brown, 2005). This regulatory landscape has compelled healthcare organizations to prioritize data security, particularly when considering the outsourcing of information technology services to cloud environments (Haufe et al., 2014). The complexities of HIPAA compliance necessitate a thorough evaluation of cloud trust models, especially given the sensitive nature of protected health information and the heightened risk of data breaches (Jiang & Bai, 2019). Despite these comprehensive legal frameworks, including the Omnibus Rule, the frequency and impact of data breaches within the US healthcare system have demonstrably increased, indicating that regulatory measures alone are insufficient to curb security incidents.

6.0. FUTURE DIRECTIONS AND EMERGING CHALLENGES

The cybersecurity landscape in the healthcare sector is swiftly changing, propelled by technological advancements, increasingly sophisticated threats, and evolving regulatory demands. As insider threats and social engineering attacks continue to jeopardize patient data integrity and operational continuity, future strategies must emphasize proactive, adaptive measures. This section delves into emerging technologies for threat detection, the evolution of attack tactics, and the ethical and regulatory implications, building on current vulnerabilities such as those found in electronic health records (EHRs) and interconnected medical devices (Odeh et al., 2024).

6.1. Advancements in Threat Detection Technologies

Integrating cutting-edge technologies holds the promise of enhancing predictive capabilities while safeguarding sensitive healthcare data from insider threats and social engineering exploits.

AI and Machine Learning for Predictive Threat Analysis

Artificial intelligence (AI) and machine learning (ML) algorithms are set to transform insider threat detection by analyzing behavioral patterns and predicting anomalies before they escalate into breaches. These tools can establish baselines for normal user activity in healthcare systems, identifying deviations such as unusual access to electronic health records (EHRs) or attempts at data exfiltration (Ali et al., 2025). For example, ML models are adept at processing large datasets to detect subtle indicators of malicious intent, thereby reducing false positives and enabling real-time alerting (Alhayan et al., 2025). As healthcare organizations contend with increasing costs from data breaches, averaging $4.88 million globally, predictive analytics could mitigate financial and patient safety risks by anticipating threats such as ransomware deployment (Cui & Song, 2025).

Blockchain for Secure Identity Management in Healthcare

Blockchain technology provides decentralized and tamper-resistant solutions for identity management and secure data sharing within healthcare ecosystems. By facilitating federated learning and attribute-based encryption, blockchain can prevent unauthorized access to protected health information (PHI) while promoting interoperability across cloud-based systems (Natarajan et al., 2025). This capability is particularly pertinent for mitigating insider threats, as it supports multi-factor authentication and dynamic trust models, thereby reducing vulnerabilities in federated environments where contractors and partners have access (Suleski et al., 2023). Future implementations could address existing gaps in electronic health record (EHR) security, where 73% of breaches involve electronic data (Omotosho et al., 2017).

Quantum Computing Implications for Healthcare Cybersecurity

Quantum computing presents both opportunities and challenges, as it could make current encryption techniques obsolete while facilitating the development of advanced secure systems. Quantum-secure protocols, like those used for patient login credentials, can bolster data protection in EHR frameworks against sophisticated attacks (Natarajan et al., 2025). Nonetheless, this advancement also poses increased risks to legacy systems in healthcare, necessitating the implementation of quantum-resistant algorithms to defend against future threats such as insider data exfiltration (Thapa & Camtepe, 2020). As quantum technologies evolve, the healthcare sector must incorporate them into threat intelligence frameworks to ensure confidentiality and integrity in high-stakes environments (Lekidis, 2023).

6.2. Evolving Social Engineering Tactics

In healthcare environments, social engineering attacks are becoming increasingly sophisticated, leveraging new technologies to exploit human weaknesses.

Deepfake Technology in Social Engineering Attacks

Deepfakes, which are AI-generated synthetic media, have the potential to enhance pretexting and vishing strategies by impersonating trusted individuals such as physicians or administrators to illicitly obtain Protected Health Information (PHI). This development builds upon existing social engineering techniques that exploit trust and urgency within high-pressure healthcare settings (Chapagain et al., 2024). As demonstrated by incidents such as the Magellan Health breach, where impersonation facilitated the deployment of ransomware, deepfakes may intensify attacks facilitated by insiders, thereby necessitating the implementation of AI-driven detection tools to verify authenticity (Alzahrani, 2020).

AI-Generated Phishing Content and Its Detection

AI technologies are capable of generating highly personalized phishing emails or smishing messages that closely resemble legitimate communications, such as patient portal updates, thereby increasing their success rates in the healthcare sector, where 36% of incidents are attributed to social engineering (Venkatesha et al., 2021). To effectively counter these threats, detection strategies must advance to incorporate machine learning-based anomaly analysis of content patterns, in conjunction with threat intelligence feeds (Alatawi & Albalawi, 2025). Insights from breaches, such as the Change Healthcare ransomware attack, underscore the necessity for real-time monitoring systems to detect AI-generated deceptions before they compromise electronic health records (Abbou et al., 2024).

Emerging Attack Vectors in IoT Medical Devices

The widespread adoption of Internet of Things (IoT) devices in healthcare, including connected monitors and wearable technology, introduces novel vulnerabilities for social engineering and sabotage. Insiders may exploit these vulnerabilities for data theft or manipulation, as IoT increases the attack surface within interconnected systems (Kang et al., 2018). Future challenges involve securing against tactics such as baiting through infected devices, necessitating the implementation of integrated threat intelligence and zero-trust models to avert cascading failures that could compromise patient safety (Azad et al., 2024).

6.3. Ethical and Regulatory Considerations

As cybersecurity measures progress, they must carefully navigate ethical dilemmas and evolving regulations to strike a balance between protection and rights.

Balancing Security Monitoring with Employee Privacy Rights

Enhanced monitoring for insider threats, such as behavioral analytics, poses a risk of infringing on employee privacy, especially within diverse healthcare workforces that exhibit varying levels of security awareness (Khadka & Ullah, 2025). Ethical frameworks must ensure transparency and consent, drawing from GDPR principles that emphasize data minimization and individuals' rights to access their personal data (Pöhn et al., 2023). Striking this balance is crucial to prevent the erosion of trust while addressing threats that could cause reputational damage (R. Syed, 2018).

Evolving Legal Landscape for Healthcare Data Protection

Regulations such as GDPR and HIPAA are evolving to accommodate cloud and AI integrations, enforcing stricter compliance measures for data breaches and necessitating robust incident response (Elkourdi et al., 2024). Future initiatives aim to harmonize global standards for healthcare cloud security, as breaches continue to escalate despite existing frameworks (Zandesh, 2024). This progression requires proactive assessments to mitigate fines and ensure patient data privacy within federated systems (Al-Fayad, 2020).

Ethical Implications of AI-Driven Security Measures

AI's role in threat detection brings up concerns about bias, accountability, and over-reliance, which could result in discriminatory monitoring within healthcare (O'Sullivan & Schofield, 2018). Ethical considerations involve ensuring fairness in ML models and addressing cognitive biases that make workers vulnerable to attacks (Vickrey et al., 2010). As AI becomes more integral, guidelines must encourage responsible use to safeguard patient outcomes without compromising ethical standards (Lorenzini et al., 2022).

7.0. CONCLUSION

The increasing complexity of cybersecurity challenges within the healthcare sector highlights the necessity for integrated strategies that address both insider threats and vulnerabilities related to social engineering. By synthesizing insights from the diverse risks associated with electronic health records (EHRs), medical devices, and the integrity of patient data, this conclusion summarizes key findings, outlines proposed solutions, and underscores the importance of a comprehensive approach. Looking forward, the evolution of threats demands continuous innovation, with emerging technologies offering promising defenses amidst persistent calls for collaborative research to protect healthcare ecosystems (Alsowail & Al-Shehari, 2022).

7.1. Summary of Key Points

Recap of Major Insider Threats and Social Engineering Risks in Healthcare

Insider threats within the healthcare sector, which include malicious data theft, unauthorized access to electronic health records (EHR), and the sabotage of medical devices, exploit the privileged positions of employees, contractors, and partners. These actions result in significant breaches, with 73% involving electronic data and compromising millions of records (Omotosho et al., 2017). The unique environment of the healthcare sector, characterized by regulatory compliance requirements and extensive access needs, exacerbates these threats, making detection difficult as insiders circumvent traditional defenses (Ali et al., 2025). Simultaneously, social engineering tactics such as phishing, pretexting, and baiting exploit human psychology by targeting trust and urgency in high-stakes settings to extract protected health information (PHI). This is exemplified by incidents like the Anthem breach, which exposed 79 million records, and the Magellan Health attack (Salahdine & Kaabouch, 2019). These risks result in financial losses averaging $4.88 million per breach, pose patient safety hazards due to altered records or device malfunctions, and lead to reputational damage that undermines public trust (Cui & Song, 2025).

Overview of Threat Intelligence and Cloud Trust Model Solutions

In the healthcare sector, threat intelligence frameworks incorporate sources such as behavioral analytics and real-time monitoring to establish baselines for normal activity, thereby facilitating the proactive detection of anomalies, including insider misuse or breaches induced by social engineering (Ovabor et al., 2024). These frameworks comprise components such as the definition of intelligence cycles, aggregation from internal logs and external feeds, and operational integration for alerting, which address deficiencies in traditional perimeter security (Tahmasebi, 2024). Cloud trust models, including zero-trust architectures and multi-factor authentication (MFA), enhance security in interconnected environments by continuously verifying access and utilizing blockchain for identity management, thereby mitigating risks associated with IoT devices and remote access (Daah et al., 2024). These solutions also extend to privacy-preserving techniques such as federated learning, ensuring compliance with regulations like HIPAA and GDPR while reducing the attack surface in cloud-based EHR systems (Elkourdi et al., 2024).

Importance of a Holistic Approach to Healthcare Cybersecurity

A comprehensive strategy is imperative, integrating technological safeguards, employee training, and policy frameworks to address the complex interplay of insider threats and social engineering, wherein human factors constitute the most vulnerable element (Khadka & Ullah, 2025). This approach surpasses isolated measures by incorporating ethical considerations, continuous adaptation, and multi-stakeholder collaboration to safeguard patient safety, data integrity, and operational continuity in the face of escalating cyber incidents (Lorenzini et al., 2022). By addressing both intentional misconduct and negligent actions, healthcare institutions can mitigate cascading impacts, ranging from financial penalties to reputational harm, thereby fostering resilience in an increasingly digitized sector (Cao et al., 2024).

7.2. Future Outlook

Predictions for the Evolution of Insider Threats and Social Engineering

Insider threats are expected to become increasingly sophisticated, utilizing artificial intelligence for behavioral mimicry and exploiting the expanded Internet of Things ecosystems within healthcare. This development may lead to heightened breach costs and increased risks to patients as remote access becomes more prevalent (Chapagain et al., 2024). Social engineering tactics are anticipated to evolve through the use of deepfakes and AI-generated content, thereby enhancing the effectiveness of phishing attacks during crises and targeting a diverse range of personnel. This evolution could result in higher success rates unless countered by adaptive defense mechanisms (Venkatesha et al., 2021). As the digitization of healthcare accelerates, hybrid threats that combine internal access with external manipulation are likely to increase, necessitating the development of predictive models to anticipate motivations such as financial gain or negligence (Ali et al., 2025).

Emerging Technologies and Their Potential Impact on Healthcare Security

Technological advancements, including AI-driven anomaly detection, blockchain-enabled identity management, and quantum-secure protocols, hold the potential to revolutionize threat mitigation. These innovations offer real-time predictive analysis and tamper-proof data sharing to address vulnerabilities in electronic health records (EHR) and prevent device sabotage (Alhayan et al., 2025). Nevertheless, these technologies also present challenges, such as algorithmic bias and quantum risks to encryption, necessitating their integration with zero-trust frameworks to bolster cloud security while preserving privacy (Thapa & Camtepe, 2020). While their adoption could substantially mitigate the impacts of breaches, it requires ethical implementation to prevent over-reliance or violations of privacy (Shamszare & Choudhury, 2023).

Call to Action for Continued Research and Collaboration in the Field

It is imperative for stakeholders to prioritize interdisciplinary research concerning human factors, regulatory developments, and technological integration. This approach should foster collaborations among academia, industry, and policymakers to establish standardized frameworks, such as maturity models for cloud security (Stavrou & Piki, 2024). Furthermore, the enhancement of training programs and the promotion of ethical hacking initiatives are essential for cultivating a robust cybersecurity culture. Global collaboration in threat intelligence sharing is also crucial to address emerging threats in telehealth and the Internet of Things (Dike & Jackson, 2024). Immediate investment in these domains is necessary to ensure proactive resilience, thereby safeguarding vulnerable healthcare systems from evolving threats (Ovabor et al., 2024).

REFERENCES

Abbou, B., Klein, A., Dudkiewicz, M., Goldschmid, N., Dahan Shriki, D., Gabbay-Benziv, R., Ophir, A., Kessel, B., Ben Natan, M., & Roguin, A. (2024). When all computers shut down: The clinical impact of a major cyber-attack on a general hospital. *Frontiers in Digital Health, 6*, 1321485. Advance online publication. DOI: 10.3389/fdgth.2024.1321485 PMID: 38433989

Abouelmehdi, K., Khaloufi, H., & Beni-Hessane, A. (2018). Big healthcare data: Preserving security and privacy. *Journal of Big Data, 5*(1), 1. Advance online publication. DOI: 10.1186/s40537-017-0110-7

Ahmed, S. (2019). *BYOD, Personal Area Networks (PANs) and IOT: Threats to Patients Privacy*. Cornell University. https://doi.org//arxiv.1902.06462DOI: 10.48550

Akinsanya, O. O., Papadaki, M., & Sun, L. (2020). Towards a maturity model for health-care cloud security (M2HCS). *Information &amp. Information and Computer Security, 28*(3), 321–345. DOI: 10.1108/ICS-05-2019-0060

Al-Fayad, F. S. (2020). The European Union's GDPR and Its Effect on Data-Driven Marketing Strategies. *International Journal of Marketing Studies, 12*(1), 39. DOI: 10.5539/ijms.v12n1p39

Al-Mhiqani, M. N., Zainal Abidin, Z., Ali, N. S., Hassan, A., Ahmad, R., Yunos, Z., Abdulkareem, K. H., & Yassin, W. (2020). A Review of Insider Threat Detection: Classification, Machine Learning Techniques, Datasets, Open Challenges, and Recommendations. *Applied Sciences (Basel, Switzerland), 10*(15), 5208. DOI: 10.3390/app10155208

Al-Muntaser, B., Mohamed, M. A., & Tuama, A. Y. (2023). Real-Time Intrusion Detection of Insider Threats in Industrial Control System Workstations Through File Integrity Monitoring. *International Journal of Advanced Computer Science and Applications, 14*(6). Advancc online publication. DOI: 10.14569/IJACSA.2023.0140636

Alatawi, E., & Albalawi, U. (2025). Harnessing AI for Cyber Defense: Honeypot-Driven Intrusion Detection Systems. *Symmetry, 17*(5), 628. DOI: 10.3390/sym17050628

Alhayan, F., Alshuhail, A., Ismail, A. O. A., Alrusaini, O., Alahmari, S., Yahya, A. E., Albouq, S. S., & Al Sadig, M. (2025). Enhanced anomaly network intrusion detection using an improved snow ablation optimizer with dimensionality reduction and hybrid deep learning model. *Scientific Reports, 15*(1), 13270. Advance online publication. DOI: 10.1038/s41598-025-97398-1 PMID: 40247081

Ali, A., Husain, M., & Hans, P. (2025). *Real-Time Detection of Insider Threats Using Behavioral Analytics and Deep Evidential Clustering*. https://doi.org//arxiv.2505.15383DOI: 10.48550

Alsowail, R. A., & Al-Shehari, T. (2022). Techniques and countermeasures for preventing insider threats. *PeerJ. Computer Science*, *8*(12), e938. DOI: 10.7717/peerj-cs.938 PMID: 35494800

Alzahrani, A. (2020). Coronavirus Social Engineering Attacks: Issues and Recommendations. *International Journal of Advanced Computer Science and Applications*, *11*(5). Advance online publication. DOI: 10.14569/IJACSA.2020.0110523

Amajuoyi, C., Nwobodo, L., & Adegbola, M.Chinazor Prisca AmajuoyiLuther Kington NwobodoMayokun Daniel Adegbola. (2024). Transforming business scalability and operational flexibility with advanced cloud computing technologies. *Computer Science &amp. IT Research Journal*, *5*(6), 1469–1487. DOI: 10.51594/csitrj.v5i6.1248

Azad, M. A., Abdullah, S., Arshad, J., Lallie, H., & Ahmed, Y. H. (2024). Verify and trust: A multidimensional survey of zero-trust security in the age of IoT. *Internet of Things : Engineering Cyber Physical Human Systems*, *27*, 101227. DOI: 10.1016/j.iot.2024.101227

Bertino, E., & Ghinita, G. (2011). *Towards mechanisms for detection and prevention of data exfiltration by insiders*. 10–19. DOI: 10.1145/1966913.1966916

Birnstill, P., Wagner, P. G., Krempel, E., & Beyerer, J. (2018). Identity Management and Protection Motivated by the General Data Protection Regulation of the European Union—A Conceptual Framework Based on State-of-the-Art Software Technologies. *Technologies*, *6*(4), 115. DOI: 10.3390/technologies6040115

Bishop, M., & Gates, C. (2008). *Defining the insider threat*. 1–3. DOI: 10.1145/1413140.1413158

Bowman, S. (2013). Impact of electronic health record systems on information integrity: Quality and safety implications. *Perspectives in Health Information Management*, •••, 10. PMID: 24159271

Branley-Bell, D., Sillence, E., & Coventry, L. (2021). *Promoting Cybersecurity Culture Change in Healthcare*. 544–549. DOI: 10.1145/3453892.3461622

Brown, C. (2005). HIPAA Programs: Design and Implementation. *Information Systems Security : ... International Conference, ICISS ... : Proceedings*, *14*(1), 10–20. DOI: 10.1201/1086/45098.14.1.20050301/87267.3

Campazas-Vega, A., Crespo-Martínez, I. S., Guerrero-Higueras, Á. M., Álvarez-Aparicio, C., Matellán, V., & Fernández-Llamas, C. (2023). Malicious traffic detection on sampled network flow data with novelty-detection-based models. *Scientific Reports, 13*(1), 15446. Advance online publication. DOI: 10.1038/s41598-023-42618-9 PMID: 37723267

Cao, H., Phan, H. V., & Silveri, S. (2024). Data breach disclosures and stock price crash risk: Evidence from data breach notification laws. *International Review of Financial Analysis, 93*, 103164. DOI: 10.1016/j.irfa.2024.103164

Carreira, C., Mendes, A., Ferreira, J., & Christin, N. (2025). *A Systematic Review of Security Communication Strategies: Guidelines and Open Challenges*. https://doi.org//arxiv.2504.02109DOI: 10.48550

Chandramouli, R. (2023). *A Zero Trust Architecture Model for Access Control in Cloud Native Applications in Multi-Cloud Environments*. National Institute Of Standards Technology., DOI: 10.6028/NIST.SP.800-207A.ipd

Chandramouli, R., Iorga, M., & Chokhani, S. (2013). *Cryptographic Key Management Issues and Challenges in Cloud Services*. National Institute Of Standards Technology., DOI: 10.6028/NIST.IR.7956

Chapagain, D., Kshetri, N., Aryal, B., & Dhakal, B. (2024). *SEAtech: Deception Techniques in Social Engineering Attacks: An Analysis of Emerging Trends and Countermeasures*. https://doi.org//arxiv.2408.02092DOI: 10.48550

Cohen, I. (2008). Improving Time-Critical Decision Making in Life-Threatening Situations: Observations and Insights. *Decision Analysis, 5*(2), 100–110. DOI: 10.1287/deca.1080.0111

Cole, I., Sibamba, L., Hilowle, A., & Jallow, J. (2017). *IT Risk Assessment for Group6 Healthcare Clinic Report*. https://doi.org//arxiv.1712.04560DOI: 10.48550

Collins, R. (2019). Clinician Cognitive Overload and Its Implications for Nurse Leaders. *Nurse Leader, 18*(1), 44–47. DOI: 10.1016/j.mnl.2019.11.007

Colwill, C. (2009). Human factors in information security: The insider threat – Who can you trust these days? *Information Security Technical Report, 14*(4), 186–196. DOI: 10.1016/j.istr.2010.04.004

Cook, R. I., & Woods, D. D. (2018). *Operating at the Sharp End: The Complexity of Human Error* (pp. 255–310). Crc. DOI: 10.1201/9780203751725-13

Croskerry, P. (2002). Achieving Quality in Clinical Decision Making: Cognitive Strategies and Detection of Bias. *Academic Emergency Medicine*, *9*(11), 1184–1204. DOI: 10.1197/aemj.9.11.1184 PMID: 12414468

Cui, Z., & Song, Z. (2025). *Enterprise Security Incident Analysis and Countermeasures Based on the T-Mobile Data Breach*. https://doi.org//arxiv.2507.12937DOI: 10.48550

Daah, C., Awan, I., Konur, S., & Qureshi, A. (2024). Enhancing Zero Trust Models in the Financial Industry through Blockchain Integration: A Proposed Framework. *Electronics (Basel)*, *13*(5), 865. DOI: 10.3390/electronics13050865

Davis, N., Raina, G., & Jagannathan, K. (2020). A framework for end-to-end deep learning-based anomaly detection in transportation networks. *Transportation Research Interdisciplinary Perspectives*, *5*, 100112. DOI: 10.1016/j.trip.2020.100112

Dhiman, P., Hamid, Y., Kaur, A., Saini, N., Nisa, K. U., Gulzar, Y., & Turaev, S. (2024). A Review and Comparative Analysis of Relevant Approaches of Zero Trust Network Model. *Sensors (Basel)*, *24*(4), 1328. DOI: 10.3390/s24041328 PMID: 38400486

Dike, U., & Jackson, V.Uzondu C. DikeVictor M. Jackson. (2024). Telemedicine integration with cloud-based IoT: A literature review approach. *World Journal of Advanced Research and Reviews*, *24*(2), 723–131. DOI: 10.30574/wjarr.2024.24.2.3355

Elkourdi, F., Xiao, L., Yu, Z., Wei, C., & Asan, O. (2024). Exploring Current Practices and Challenges of HIPAA Compliance in Software Engineering: Scoping Review. *IEEE Open Journal of Systems Engineering*, *2*, 94–104. DOI: 10.1109/OJSE.2024.3392691

Ermakova, T., Sunyaev, A., Fabian, B., Thiebes, S., & Kornacka, M. (2020). Security and Privacy Requirements for Cloud Computing in Healthcare. *ACM Transactions on Management Information Systems*, *11*(2), 1–29. DOI: 10.1145/3386160

Farnga, M. (2018). *Cloud Security Architecture and Implementation - A practical approach*. Cornell University. https://doi.org//arxiv.1808.03892DOI: 10.48550

Fedorowicz, J., & Ray, A. W. (2004). Impact of HIPAA on the integrity of healthcare information. *International Journal of Healthcare Technology and Management*, *6*(2), 142. DOI: 10.1504/IJHTM.2004.004954

Feld, A. D. (2005). The Health Insurance Portability and Accountability Act (HIPAA): Its Broad Effect on Practice. *The American Journal of Gastroenterology*, *100*(7), 1440–1443. DOI: 10.1111/j.1572-0241.2005.50621.x PMID: 15984962

Garbis, J., & Chapman, J. W. (2021). *What Is Zero Trust?* Apress., DOI: 10.1007/978-1-4842-6702-8_2

Georgiou, D., & Lambrinoudakis, C. (2021). Data Protection Impact Assessment (DPIA) for Cloud-Based Health Organizations. *Future Internet, 13*(3), 66. DOI: 10.3390/fi13030066

Gitonga, N. K., Muketha, G. M., & Kamau, G. (2020). Cloud Data Privacy Preserving Model for Health Information Systems Based on Multi Factor Authentication. [IJRTE]. *International Journal of Recent Technology and Engineering*, *9*(3), 360–367. DOI: 10.35940/ijrte.C4458.099320

Gonçalves-Ferreira, D., Bacelar-Silva, G. M., Sousa, M., Cruz-Correia, R., Beale, T., Frade, S., & Antunes, L. F. (2018). *OpenEHR and General Data Protection Regulation: Evaluation of Principles and Requirements (Preprint)*. Jmir. DOI: 10.2196/preprints.9845

Haney, J., Jacobs, J., & Lutters, W. (2021). Cybersecurity Advocates: Force Multipliers in Security Behavior Change. *IEEE Security and Privacy, 19*(4), 54–59. DOI: 10.1109/MSEC.2021.3077405 PMID: 37051374

Hardjono, T. (2019). *A Federated Authorization Framework for Distributed Personal Data and Digital Identity*. Cornell University. https://doi.org//arxiv.1906.03552DOI: 10.48550

Hassan, O. F., Fatai, F. O., Sanusi, M. A., Akinde, A. O., Aderibigbe, O., Onasanya, T., & Odukoya, O. (2024). Enhancing Cybersecurity through Cloud Computing Solutions in the United States. *Intelligent Information Management, 16*(04), 176–193. DOI: 10.4236/iim.2024.164011

Hatzivasilis, G., Goeke, L., Hildebrandt, T., Ioannidis, S., Spanoudakis, G., Leftheriotis, G., Koshutanski, H., Oikonomou, F., Frati, F., Tsakirakis, G., & Smyrlis, M. (2020). Modern Aspects of Cyber-Security Training and Continuous Adaptation of Programmes to Trainees. *Applied Sciences (Basel, Switzerland), 10*(16), 5702. DOI: 10.3390/app10165702

Haufe, K., Dzombeta, S., & Brandis, K. (2014). Proposal for a Security Management in Cloud Computing for Health Care. *TheScientificWorldJournal, 2014*(6), 1–7. DOI: 10.1155/2014/146970 PMID: 24701137

Hijji, M., & Alam, G. (2021). A Multivocal Literature Review on Growing Social Engineering Based Cyber-Attacks/Threats During the COVID-19 Pandemic: Challenges and Prospective Solutions. *IEEE Access : Practical Innovations, Open Solutions, 9*(3), 7152–7169. DOI: 10.1109/ACCESS.2020.3048839 PMID: 34786300

Hiwale, M., Walambe, R., Potdar, V., & Kotecha, K. (2023). A systematic review of privacy-preserving methods deployed with blockchain and federated learning for the telemedicine. *Healthcare Analytics (New York, N.y.), 3*, 100192. DOI: 10.1016/j.health.2023.100192

Hussain, M. I., Razque, F., He, J., Zardari, Z. A., Sabah, F., Zhu, N., & Hussain, S. (2021). AAAA: SSO and MFA Implementation in Multi-Cloud to Mitigate Rising Threats and Concerns Related to User Metadata. *Applied Sciences (Basel, Switzerland), 11*(7), 3012. DOI: 10.3390/app11073012

Islam, R., Weir, C. R., Jones, M., Del Fiol, G., & Samore, M. H. (2015). Understanding complex clinical reasoning in infectious diseases for improving clinical decision support design. *BMC Medical Informatics and Decision Making, 15*(1), 101. Advance online publication. DOI: 10.1186/s12911-015-0221-z PMID: 26620881

Jaatun, M. G., Cruzes, D. S., Moe, N. B., Tøndel, I. A., Bernsmed, K., & Haugset, B. (2018). Accountability Requirements in the Cloud Provider Chain. *Symmetry, 10*(4), 124. DOI: 10.3390/sym10040124

Jiang, J., & Bai, G. (2019). Types of Information Compromised in Breaches of Protected Health Information. *Annals of Internal Medicine, 172*(2), 159–160. DOI: 10.7326/M19-1759 PMID: 31546251

Kammüller, F., Ogunyanwo, O., & Probst, C. (2019). *Designing Data Protection for GDPR Compliance into IoT Healthcare Systems*. Cornell University. https://doi.org//arxiv.1901.02426DOI: 10.48550

Kang, M., Park, E., Cho, B. H., & Lee, K.-S. (2018). Recent Patient Health Monitoring Platforms Incorporating Internet of Things-Enabled Smart Devices. *International Neurourology Journal, 22*(4), 313. DOI: 10.5213/inj.1820corr.001 PMID: 30599503

Khadka, K., & Ullah, A. B. (2025). Human factors in cybersecurity: An interdisciplinary review and framework proposal. *International Journal of Information Security, 24*(3), 119. Advance online publication. DOI: 10.1007/s10207-025-01032-0

Kim, J., Kim, H., Cho, S., Kang, P., & Park, M. (2019). Insider Threat Detection Based on User Behavior Modeling and Anomaly Detection Algorithms. *Applied Sciences (Basel, Switzerland), 9*(19), 4018. DOI: 10.3390/app9194018

Koczkodaj, , W., Masiak, J., F Zabrodskii, P., Strzałka, D., & Mazurek, M. (2019). Massive Health Record Breaches Evidenced by the Office for Civil Rights Data. *Iranian Journal of Public Health, 48*(2). Advance online publication. DOI: 10.18502/ijph.v48i2.826 PMID: 31205882

Lekidis, A. (2023). *Cyber-attack TTP analysis for EPES systems*. https://doi.org//arxiv.2302.09164DOI: 10.48550

Linnartz, P., Winkens, A., & Ulbig, A. (2022). *Assessing the impact of cyber attacks manipulating distributed energy resources on power system operation*. Cornell University. https://doi.org//arxiv.2207.07968DOI: 10.48550

Lorenzini, G., Shaw, D. M., & Elger, B. S. (2022). It takes a pirate to know one: Ethical hackers for healthcare cybersecurity. *BMC Medical Ethics*, *23*(1), 131. Advance online publication. DOI: 10.1186/s12910-022-00872-y PMID: 36494715

Mane, S., & Rao, D. (2021). *Explaining Network Intrusion Detection System Using Explainable AI Framework*. https://doi.org//arxiv.2103.07110DOI: 10.48550

Milani, M., Huang, Y., & Chiang, F. (2020). *Diversifying Anonymized Data with Diversity Constraints*. https://doi.org//arxiv.2007.09141DOI: 10.48550

Natarajan, M., Bharathi, A., Varun, C. S., & Selvarajan, S. (2025). Quantum secure patient login credential system using blockchain for electronic health record sharing framework. *Scientific Reports*, *15*(1), 4023. Advance online publication. DOI: 10.1038/s41598-025-86658-9 PMID: 39894869

Neisse, R., Fovino, I. N., & Steri, G. (2018). *Blockchain-based Identity Management and Data Usage Control (Extended Abstract)*. Springer., DOI: 10.1007/978-3-319-92925-5_15

O'Sullivan, E., & Schofield, S. (2018). Cognitive Bias in Clinical Medicine. *Journal of the Royal College of Physicians of Edinburgh*, *48*(3), 225–232. DOI: 10.4997/jrcpe.2018.306 PMID: 30191910

Odeh, A., Abdelfattah, E., & Salameh, W. (2024). Privacy-Preserving Data Sharing in Telehealth Services. *Applied Sciences (Basel, Switzerland)*, *14*(23), 10808. DOI: 10.3390/app142310808

Olateju, O. O., Olaniyi, O. O., Oladoyinbo, T. O., Okon, S. U., Salami, A. A., & Igwenagu, U. T. I. (2024). Combating the Challenges of False Positives in AI-Driven Anomaly Detection Systems and Enhancing Data Security in the Cloud. *Asian Journal of Research in Computer Science*, *17*(6), 264–292. DOI: 10.9734/ajrcos/2024/v17i6472

Omotosho, A., Emuoyibofarhe, J., & Meinel, C. (2017). Ensuring patients' privacy in a cryptographic-based-electronic health records using bio-cryptography. *International Journal of Electronic Healthcare*, *9*(4), 227. DOI: 10.1504/IJEH.2017.085800

Ovabor, K., Atkison, T., Benedict, J., Fabusoro, A., & Sule-Odu, I. (2024). AI-driven threat intelligence for real-time cybersecurity: Frameworks, tools, and future directions. *Open Access Research Journal of Science and Technology, 12*(2), 040–048. DOI: 10.53022/oarjst.2024.12.2.0135

Paul, B., & Rao, M. (2022). Zero-Trust Model for Smart Manufacturing Industry. *Applied Sciences (Basel, Switzerland), 13*(1), 221. DOI: 10.3390/app13010221

Peltier, T. R. (2006). Social Engineering: Concepts and Solutions. *Information Systems Security : ... International Conference, ICISS ... : Proceedings, 15*(5), 13–21. DOI: 10.1201/1086.1065898X/46353.15.4.20060901/95427.3

Peterson, C., & Watzlaf, V. (2015). Telerehabilitation Store and Forward Applications: A Review of Applications and Privacy Considerations in Physical and Occupational Therapy Practice. *International Journal of Telerehabilitation, 6*(2), 75–84. DOI: 10.5195/ijt.2014.6161 PMID: 25945231

Phyo, A. H., Furnell, S. M., & Portilla, F. (2004). *A Framework for Role-Based Monitoring of Insider Misuse.* Kluwer Academic., DOI: 10.1007/1-4020-8145-6_4

Pöhn, D., & Hillmann, P. (2021). *Reference Service Model for Federated Identity Management.* Springer., DOI: 10.1007/978-3-030-79186-5_13

Pöhn, D., Mörsdorf, N., & Hommel, W. (2023). *Needle in the Haystack: Analyzing the Right of Access According to GDPR Article 15 Five Years after the Implementation.* https://doi.org//arxiv.2308.15166DOI: 10.48550

Raghupathi, W., Saharia, A., & Raghupathi, V. (2023). Analyzing Health Data Breaches: A Visual Analytics Approach. *AppliedMath, 3*(1), 175–199. DOI: 10.3390/appliedmath3010011

Ramesh, D., Sharma, R. P., & Edla, D. R. (2020). HHDSSC: Harnessing healthcare data security in cloud using ciphertext policy attribute-based encryption. *International Journal of Information and Computer Security, 13*(3/4), 322. DOI: 10.1504/IJICS.2020.109480

Reale, C., Andreae, M. H., Sushereba, C., Banerjee, A., Militello, L. G., Slagle, J., Weinger, M. B., Anders, S., Mcivor, W. R., Gaba, D. M., Salwei, M. E., Torsher, L. C., & Burden, A. (2023). Decision-Making During High-Risk Events: A Systematic Literature Review. *Journal of Cognitive Engineering and Decision Making, 17*(2), 188–212. DOI: 10.1177/15553434221147415 PMID: 37823061

Reddy, R. P. (2025). Zero Trust Architectures in Modern Enterprises: Principles, Implementation Challenges, and Best Practices. *International Journal of Computer Trends and Technology, 73*(6), 48–57. DOI: 10.14445/22312803/IJCTT-V73I6P107

Rengamani, H., Upadhyaya, S., Kumaraguru, P., & Rao, H. R. (2010). *Protecting senior citizens from cyber security attacks in the e-health scenario*. 1–4. DOI: 10.1145/1852666.1852759

Ribeiro De Mello, E., Silva Wangham, M., Da Silva, C. E., Cavalcanti Da Silva, G., De Chaves, S. A., Bristot Loli, S., & Bristot Loli, B. (2020). Multi-factor authentication for shibboleth identity providers. *Journal of Internet Services and Applications, 11*(1), 8. Advance online publication. DOI: 10.1186/s13174-020-00128-1

Rocchiccioli, J. (2003). Health Insurance Portability and Accountability Act: Administrative Simplification to Understand the Revised Proposed Privacy Standards—A Policy Update. *The Journal of the Association of Nurses in AIDS Care: JANAC, 14*(2), 63–66. DOI: 10.1177/1055329002251000 PMID: 12698767

Roy Sarkar, K. (2010). Assessing insider threats to information security using technical, behavioural and organisational measures. *Information Security Technical Report, 15*(3), 112–133. DOI: 10.1016/j.istr.2010.11.002

Rutherford, A., Walden, A., Noblin, A., Gabriel, M. H., & Cortelyou-Ward, K. (2018). Data breach locations, types, and associated characteristics among US hospitals. *The American Journal of Managed Care, 24*(2), 78–84. PMID: 29461854

S, M., & K R, J. (2025). Blockchain-enabled federated learning with edge analytics for secure and efficient electronic health records management. *Scientific Reports, 15*(1). DOI: 10.1038/s41598-025-12225-x

Salahdine, F., & Kaabouch, N. (2019). Social Engineering Attacks: A Survey. *Future Internet, 11*(4), 89. DOI: 10.3390/fi11040089

Seh, A. H., Zarour, M., Alenezi, M., Sarkar, A. K., Agrawal, A., Kumar, R., & Ahmad Khan, R. (2020). Healthcare Data Breaches: Insights and Implications. *Health Care, 8*(2), 133. DOI: 10.3390/healthcare8020133 PMID: 32414183

Sergiu, E. (2020). Insider threats and thermal stress in the working environment. *Scientific Bulletin of Naval Academy, 23*(1), 271–276. DOI: 10.21279/1454-864X-20-I1-038

Seth, D., Najana, M., & Ranjan, P. (2024). Compliance and Regulatory Challenges in Cloud Computing: A Sector-Wise Analysis. *International Journal of Global Innovations and Solutions (IJGIS)*. DOI: 10.21428/e90189c8.68b5dea5

Shamszare, H., & Choudhury, A. (2023). Clinicians' Perceptions of Artificial Intelligence: Focus on Workload, Risk, Trust, Clinical Decision Making, and Clinical Integration. *Health Care, 11*(16), 2308. DOI: 10.3390/healthcare11162308 PMID: 37628506

Shemshi, V., & Jakimovski, B. (2025). Extended Model for Efficient Federated Identity Management with Dynamic Levels of Assurance Across eIDAS, REFEDS, and Kantara Frameworks for Educational Institutions. *Information (Basel), 16*(5), 385. DOI: 10.3390/info16050385

Singh, A., & Sharma, A. (2022). *A systematic literature review on insider threats*. Cornell University. https://doi.org//arxiv.2212.05347DOI: 10.48550

Sowmya, T., & Mary Anita, E. A. (2023). A comprehensive review of AI based intrusion detection system. *Measurement. Sensors, 28*, 100827. DOI: 10.1016/j.measen.2023.100827

Stavrou, E., & Piki, A. (2024). Cultivating self-efficacy to empower professionals' re-up skilling in cybersecurity. *Information &amp. Information and Computer Security, 32*(4), 523–541. DOI: 10.1108/ICS-02-2024-0038

Stewart, J., & Dawson, M. (2018). How the modification of personality traits leave one vulnerable to manipulation in social engineering. *International Journal of Information Privacy. Security and Integrity, 3*(3), 187. DOI: 10.1504/IJIPSI.2018.10013213

Suleski, T., Ahmed, M., Yang, W., & Wang, E. (2023). A review of multi-factor authentication in the Internet of HealthcareThings. *Digital Health, 9*, 205520762311771. DOI: 10.1177/20552076231177144 PMID: 37252257

Sulmasy, L. S., Horwitch, C. A., & López, A. M. (2017). Ethical Implications of the Electronic Health Record: In the Service of the Patient. *Journal of General Internal Medicine, 32*(8), 935–939. DOI: 10.1007/s11606-017-4030-1 PMID: 28321550

Syed, R. (2018). Enterprise reputation threats on social media: A case of data breach framing. *The Journal of Strategic Information Systems, 28*(3), 257–274. DOI: 10.1016/j.jsis.2018.12.001

Tahmasebi, M. (2024). Beyond Defense: Proactive Approaches to Disaster Recovery and Threat Intelligence in Modern Enterprises. *Journal of Information Security, 15*(02), 106–133. DOI: 10.4236/jis.2024.152008

Tall, A., Wang, J., & Han, D. (2016). *Survey of data intensive computing technologies application to to security log data management*. 268–273. DOI: 10.1145/3006299.3006336

Tanimura, J. K., & Wehrly, E. W. (2015). The Market Value and Reputational Effects from Lost Confidential Information. *International Journal of Financial Management, 5*(4). Advance online publication. DOI: 10.21863/ijfm/2015.5.4.020

Taylor, R. A., Sangal, R. B., Smith, M. E., Haimovich, A. D., Rodman, A., Iscoe, M. S., Pavuluri, S. K., Rose, C., Janke, A. T., Wright, D. S., Socrates, V., & Declan, A. (2024). Leveraging artificial intelligence to reduce diagnostic errors in emergency medicine: Challenges, opportunities, and future directions. *Academic Emergency Medicine*, *32*(3), 327–339. DOI: 10.1111/acem.15066 PMID: 39676165

Thapa, C., & Camtepe, S. (2020). *Precision Health Data: Requirements, Challenges and Existing Techniques for Data Security and Privacy*. https://doi.org//arxiv.2008.10733DOI: 10.48550

Touchie, C., Kinnear, B., Schumacher, D., Caretta-Weyer, H., Hamstra, S. J., Hart, D., Gruppen, L., Ross, S., Warm, E., & Ten Cate, O. (2021). On the validity of summative entrustment decisions. *Medical Teacher*, *43*(7), 780–787. DOI: 10.1080/0142159X.2021.1925642 PMID: 34020576

Tsiostas, D., Chouliaras, N., Douligeris, C., Kittes, G., Maglaras, L., Vlachos, V., & Kantzavelou, I. (2020). *The Insider Threat: Reasons, Effects and Mitigation Techniques*. 340–345. DOI: 10.1145/3437120.3437336

Venkatesha, S., Reddy, K. R., & Chandavarkar, B. R. (2021). Social Engineering Attacks During the COVID-19 Pandemic. *SN Computer Science*, *2*(2), 78. Advance online publication. DOI: 10.1007/s42979-020-00443-1 PMID: 33585823

Vickrey, B. G., Samuels, M. A., & Ropper, A. H. (2010). How neurologists think: A cognitive psychology perspective on missed diagnoses. *Annals of Neurology*, *67*(4), 425–433. DOI: 10.1002/ana.21907 PMID: 20437577

Vitorino, J., Praça, I., & Maia, E. (2023). SoK: Realistic adversarial attacks and defenses for intelligent network intrusion detection. *Computers &amp. Computers & Security*, *134*, 103433. DOI: 10.1016/j.cose.2023.103433

Wasserman, L., & Wasserman, Y. (2022). Hospital cybersecurity risks and gaps: Review (for the non-cyber professional). *Frontiers in Digital Health*, *4*(Suppl 6), 862221. Advance online publication. DOI: 10.3389/fdgth.2022.862221 PMID: 36033634

Wu, C. M., Schulz, E., Speekenbrink, M., & Pleskac, T. J. (2022). Time pressure changes how people explore and respond to uncertainty. *Scientific Reports*, *12*(1), 4122. Advance online publication. DOI: 10.1038/s41598-022-07901-1 PMID: 35260717

Young, D. L., Goodie, A. S., Hall, D. B., & Wu, E. (2012). Decision making under time pressure, modeled in a prospect theory framework. *Organizational Behavior and Human Decision Processes, 118*(2), 179–188. DOI: 10.1016/j.obhdp.2012.03.005 PMID: 22711977

Yuan, S., & Wu, X. (2020). *Deep Learning for Insider Threat Detection: Review, Challenges and Opportunities.* Cornell University. https://doi.org//arxiv.2005.12433DOI: 10.48550

Zandesh, Z. (2024). Privacy, Security, and Legal Issues in the Health Cloud: Structured Review for Taxonomy Development. *JMIR Formative Research, 8*(1), e38372. DOI: 10.2196/38372 PMID: 38345858

Zoppi, T., Bondavalli, A., Capecchi, T., & Ceccarelli, A. (2021). Unsupervised Anomaly Detectors to Detect Intrusions in the Current Threat Landscape. *ACM/IMS Transactions on Data Science, 2*(2), 1–26. DOI: 10.1145/3441140

Chapter 3
Data Sensitivity and Privacy in Connected Health Ecosystems

Olatunde Ayomide Olasehan
https://orcid.org/0009-0004-3069-7168
GOSH, UK

ABSTRACT

Digital technologies in healthcare have created connected health ecosystems using IoT devices and cloud computing. While enabling real-time monitoring and personalized care, these systems raise data privacy challenges. This chapter examines health information protection in interconnected environments. Electronic records, wearable data, and genomic information face risks of breaches and unauthorized access. The chapter explores consequences of data exposure, including identity theft and legal issues, along with patient consent and bias concerns. It analyzes medical device threats from ransomware and weak security, discussing data lifecycle management. Regulatory frameworks like HIPAA and GDPR are reviewed, alongside cloud trust models and privacy-preserving techniques. The chapter examines emerging solutions like post-quantum cryptography and self-sovereign identity, emphasizing stakeholder collaboration for data security in connected health ecosystems.

1.0. INTRODUCTION

1.1. Background and Context

Connected health ecosystems represent a transformative integration of digital technologies that enable seamless data exchange and real-time monitoring to en-

DOI: 10.4018/979-8-3373-4918-3.ch003

hance patient care, relying heavily on Internet of Things (IoT) devices and cloud computing infrastructures. These ecosystems encompass wearable sensors, remote monitoring systems, and interconnected platforms that collect physiological data, facilitating proactive interventions and shifting from traditional clinical settings to patient-centric models. IoT enables continuous data acquisition from devices like heart rate monitors and smart implants, while cloud technologies provide scalable storage, analytics, and accessibility, supporting applications such as telemedicine and predictive health management. This synergy drives efficiency in healthcare delivery but introduces complexities in managing vast data volumes across distributed networks.

Data Sensitivity

Data sensitivity in healthcare pertains to the intrinsic vulnerability of personal health information (PHI), encompassing medical records, genomic data, and real-time biometrics. Such information can disclose intimate details regarding individuals' physical and mental conditions, thereby posing risks of misuse if compromised. Privacy concerns emerge from potential breaches, unauthorized access, and secondary uses of data, such as in analytics or sharing with third parties, which may lead to identity theft, discrimination, or erosion of trust. The proliferation of connected devices exacerbates these issues, as sensitive data traverses insecure networks, rendering it susceptible to cyber threats like ransomware and phishing. Additionally, ethical dilemmas concerning consent and data ownership further intensify the stakes.

Overview of Regulatory Frameworks in Healthcare Ecosystem

Regulatory frameworks such as the General Data Protection Regulation (GDPR) in the European Union and the Health Insurance Portability and Accountability Act (HIPAA) in the United States provide foundational standards for safeguarding health data. GDPR emphasizes comprehensive protection of personal data, including consent requirements, data minimization, and rights to access or erasure, applying broadly to any entity processing EU residents' information. HIPAA focuses on securing PHI through privacy and security rules, mandating safeguards for covered entities like providers and insurers to ensure confidentiality, integrity, and availability. These frameworks intersect in global healthcare operations, requiring compliance to mitigate risks and foster accountability. In this chapter we would be exploring these regulatory framweorks and how they affect healthcare data.

1.2. Objectives of the Chapter

This chapter examines the multifaceted challenges of data sensitivity and privacy in connected health ecosystems, including vulnerabilities from IoT integration, data breaches, and ethical issues in AI-driven analytics, to highlight gaps in current protections.

It evaluates existing and emerging regulatory frameworks, such as GDPR and HIPAA, alongside state-level laws and international harmonization efforts, assessing their effectiveness in addressing modern threats like quantum computing and cross-border data flows.

The chapter discusses advanced technologies for protecting patient privacy, including post-quantum cryptography, federated learning, and anonymization techniques, to enable secure data utilization in research and care delivery.

Finally, it proposes trust-based models, such as zero trust architecture and blockchain-enabled systems, alongside AI-powered solutions for transparent data usage and accountability, aiming to build resilient ecosystems that prioritize patient autonomy and innovation.

2.0. DATA SENSITIVITY IN CONNECTED HEALTH ECOSYSTEMS

The rapid expansion of connected health ecosystems, which integrate a complex network of wearable sensors, mobile applications, and remote monitoring devices, has created unprecedented opportunities for personalized healthcare interventions and proactive disease management strategies. These technologies facilitate continuous, real-time physiological data acquisition, enabling individuals to actively participate in their healthcare management and promoting a shift from traditional hospital-centric models to patient-centric, home-based care paradigms (Tao et al., 2023). The convergence of advanced biosensor technologies, refined healthcare delivery mechanisms, and the increasing sophistication of machine learning algorithms has enhanced the impact of digital health solutions, providing continuous and cost-effective physiological data measurement and interpretation, both within and beyond conventional clinical settings (Xu et al., 2022). The integration of body-integrated electronic sensors offers clinicians the capability to remotely monitor vulnerable populations, irrespective of geographical limitations, thereby improving treatment efficacy (Rogers et al., 2018). The growing prevalence of Internet of Things devices and body area sensor networks is advancing continuous health monitoring by enabling the collection and analysis of real-time physiological data in diverse environments (Wan et al., 2018). Wearable technology, ranging from wrist-worn activity trackers to implanted monitors, is becoming an essential component of modern healthcare, facilitating ongoing monitoring and personalized treatments for chronic illnesses (Jafleh et al., 2024).

Nevertheless, the expansion of connected health ecosystems introduces significant challenges related to data sensitivity, privacy, and security, which demand rigorous attention. The growing dependence on interconnected devices and platforms heightens the risk of unauthorized access, data breaches, and potential misuse of sensitive patient information, thereby necessitating the implementation of robust security measures (Popoola et al., 2024). Although the continuous monitoring capabilities of wearable devices hold the potential to detect health risks and enhance treatment outcomes, they also raise substantial ethical and practical concerns regarding pervasive surveillance and the collection of excessive data (Mennella et al., 2024). Despite the convergence of physiological sensing modalities, advanced data analytics, and sophisticated software development technologies in advancing the wearable healthcare paradigm, critical challenges persist, including data quality assurance, algorithmic bias mitigation, and the establishment of robust data governance frameworks (W. Kim & Choi, 2016). The capacity of these devices to collect and process vast amounts of personal data necessitates a thorough examination of the ethical implications and potential risks associated with their widespread adoption (Davis Iii & Ruotsalo, 2025).

2.1. Sensitive Health Data

Within the complex framework of connected health ecosystems, a wide range of sensitive data types demands meticulous attention and robust protective measures. These ecosystems, distinguished by their extensive utilization of sensing technologies, computational resources, and communication networks, produce a substantial amount of information. While this information holds significant potential for advancing healthcare, it also poses considerable privacy risks (Thapa & Camtepe, 2020a). Data encompassing personal identification details, detailed medical histories, and comprehensive treatment plans represent only a portion of the sensitive health information circulating within these systems (Odeh et al., 2024). The consequences of unauthorized access or disclosure of such data extend beyond mere inconvenience, potentially resulting in significant financial threats, severe psychological distress, medical identity theft, and even social stigmatization or discrimination, particularly for individuals managing specific health conditions (Madanian et al., 2024). Given the intimate and personal nature of health data, maintaining its confidentiality is crucial to ensuring individuals feel secure in seeking medical care and openly sharing sensitive information with healthcare providers. The seriousness of these potential consequences underscores the necessity for implementing stringent data protection measures that safeguard individual privacy while fostering trust in connected health technologies (Griesser, 1989).

Electronic Health Records (EHRs) and Their Sensitivity

Electronic Health Records represent a pivotal advancement in healthcare, offering a centralized and readily accessible repository of patient information. Electronic health record systems have emerged as indispensable tools, fundamentally reshaping healthcare practices and serving as the cornerstone for various e-health solutions (Rhayha et al., 2025). These systems encompass a wide array of functionalities, including the storage, management, and exchange of patient data, thereby fostering enhanced communication and collaboration among healthcare providers (Alarfaj & Rahman, 2024). This transition towards digitization has revolutionized the management of patient information, enabling seamless communication between healthcare providers, improving diagnostic precision, and facilitating personalized treatment plans (Enahoro et al., 2023). The integration of Electronic Health Records into healthcare systems has led to substantial improvements in efficiency, communication, and overall quality of care (Jackson et al., 2023). However, this digital transformation also introduces significant challenges, particularly concerning data sensitivity and privacy (Odeh et al., 2024).

The transition to Electronic Health Records (EHRs), while offering numerous advantages such as enhanced communication, information exchange, and error reduction, also presents potential drawbacks if not managed effectively (Baniulyte et al., 2023). The sensitive nature of patient data within EHRs necessitates robust security measures to prevent breaches and unauthorized access (S & K R, 2025). The architecture of EHR systems, particularly when reliant on wireless communication channels for data transmission, introduces vulnerabilities that malicious actors can exploit (G. Liu et al., 2024). The increasing adoption of interconnected systems and cloud-based storage solutions, while enhancing accessibility and scalability, concomitantly broadens the attack surface, thereby rendering healthcare organizations increasingly vulnerable to sophisticated cyberattacks and potentially catastrophic data breaches (Dou et al., 2025). The inherent design of interconnected EHR networks, while promoting data fluidity and interoperability, concurrently establishes intricate webs of potential intrusion points, thereby augmenting the risk profile for unauthorized data access and exfiltration.

Wearable Device Data and Real-time Biometric Streams

The seamless integration of wearable sensor technologies with interconnected health platforms has led to an unprecedented increase in the volume and speed of personal health data, offering transformative possibilities for proactive healthcare delivery while also presenting complex challenges related to data security and individual informational autonomy. The widespread adoption of wearable devices capable of continuously monitoring a range of physiological signals, such as heart rate variability, sleep patterns, and activity levels, generates a constant stream of detailed, high-resolution data. This data can be utilized to gain novel insights into individual well-being and population health trends (W. Kim & Choi, 2016). These devices, now ubiquitous and increasingly affordable, represent a paradigm shift in healthcare, enabling continuous, real-time monitoring of patients' health status, a significant departure from traditional, episodic clinical encounters (Hughes et al., 2023). The capability to track and analyze these data streams holds immense potential for personalized interventions, early disease detection, and the optimization of treatment strategies (Mennella et al., 2024). Wearable technology facilitates the automatic collection of patient health data, eliminating the need for healthcare providers to manually gather such information (Meisami et al., 2023).

Nonetheless, the inherent characteristics of data produced by wearable technology, which give it its distinct value such as continuous collection, a high degree of personalization, and detailed resolution also heighten the risk of privacy violations and misuse. The vast amount of data these devices generate, along with the growing complexity of data analytics methods, presents opportunities to deduce sensitive information about individuals that may go well beyond the original intent of data collection (Davis & Ruotsalo, 2024). The ability to infer private lifestyle information through the analysis of daily step counts illustrates the potential for unintended disclosures (J. W. Kim et al., 2020). Moreover, combining data from various sources, such as wearable devices, electronic health records, and social media, can construct a detailed profile of an individual, making them more susceptible to identification and discrimination (Mone & Shakhlo, 2023).

Genomic Data and its Unique Privacy Concerns

Genomic data, characterized by its complex structure and extensive implications, poses distinct challenges to data sensitivity and privacy within interconnected health ecosystems. The amalgamation of clinical data, genomic information, imaging results, and data from wearable sensors to advance personalized medicine introduces considerable complexities in the management of healthcare data (Bent & Dunn, 2020). Genomic data constitutes the foundation of an individual's biological attributes, and when integrated with clinical data, it holds the potential to transform medical research and diagnostics (Subhani & Anjum, 2020).

Nevertheless, the deeply personal and predictive characteristics of genomic data demand strong protections to guard against unauthorized access, discrimination, and misuse (Thapa & Camtepe, 2020b). The probabilistic aspect of genomic data, particularly when linked with extensive datasets to identify rare occurrences, highlights the ethical and legal issues related to its application (Francis, 2014). Genomic information is unique due to its lasting nature and the potential for its interpretations to change over time, which poses long-term privacy challenges (M. S. Williams et al., 2019). The merging of large-scale datasets with individual genomic profiles heightens the necessity for rigorous ethical guidelines and data governance policies, especially given the sensitivity of medical data (B. D. Mittelstadt & Floridi, 2015). The challenge lies in skillfully navigating the complex terrain of genomic data use, balancing the quest for scientific progress with the inviolable principles of personal privacy and self-determination (Price & Cohen, 2019). Big Data research introduces ethical dilemmas such as ensuring fairness, honoring patient autonomy through proper consent, and safeguarding participants' privacy (Elenberg & Howe Iii, 2020).

2.2. Risks Associated with Health Data Exposure

The rapid expansion of connected health ecosystems presents a complex paradox: while these systems have immense potential to revolutionize healthcare delivery through personalized and proactive interventions, they also pose significant challenges related to data sensitivity and the erosion of individual privacy. The allure of leveraging big data analytics in the medical field is tempered by the stark reality that personal health information faces unprecedented threats in this digital age (N. Liu & Chen, 2022).

Identity Theft and Insurance Fraud Risks

Addressing the complexities of data sensitivity and privacy within connected health ecosystems requires a comprehensive understanding of the inherent risks, particularly those related to identity theft and insurance fraud. While the interconnected nature of these ecosystems enhances healthcare delivery, it simultaneously increases vulnerabilities to data breaches and misuse (Thapa & Camtepe, 2020b). The sensitivity of medical data, combined with its extensive distribution across diverse processing environments, presents significant security and privacy challenges (Dou et al., 2025). The proliferation of digital health data, facilitated by electronic health records, telemedicine, and mobile health applications, has rendered the protection of sensitive health information a critical concern (Odeh et al., 2024). Unauthorized access to patient records can lead to identity theft, financial fraud, and even medical fraud, where personal health information is exploited to obtain drugs or file fraudulent claims (Odeh et al., 2024). Such breaches not only compromise individual privacy but also have the potential to erode public trust in healthcare systems, possibly deterring individuals from seeking necessary medical care.

Reputational Damage To Healthcare Providers

A significant consequence of data breaches within connected health ecosystems is the potential for reputational harm to healthcare providers and affiliated organizations. In the event of such a breach, the erosion of public trust can be both profound and enduring. Patients may lose confidence in the capacity of healthcare providers to safeguard their personal information, resulting in a reluctance to disclose sensitive details essential for effective treatment. This decline in trust extends beyond individual patients, influencing the broader perception of the healthcare provider within the community and potentially diminishing their competitive advantage. It is imperative for organizations to recognize that maintaining data integrity and security is crucial for sustaining patient trust and preserving their reputation in an increasingly interconnected healthcare landscape.

Legal Repercussions For Data Breaches

The legal framework governing connected health ecosystems places significant emphasis on the principle of data minimization, which stipulates that only data essential for a specific purpose should be collected and processed. Additionally, data retention policies must be meticulously designed to ensure that health information is not stored indefinitely but is retained solely for the duration necessary to achieve the intended purpose. This principle seeks to mitigate the risk of data breaches and unauthorized access by restricting the volume of sensitive information stored and processed. Given the sensitive nature of patient data, obtaining informed consent is fundamental to ethical and legal compliance within connected health ecosystems. Patients must be comprehensively informed about the types of data being collected, the purposes for which it will be utilized, and the entities with whom it may be shared.

Moreover, individuals should have the right to access, correct, and delete their health information, as well as the right to withdraw their consent at any time. Cybercriminals often target healthcare providers because they believe the healthcare industry is an easy target, and vulnerabilities in the industry can be attributed to a number of factors, including a lack of security knowledge among care staff, a large attack surface, and a substantial reliance on unpatched legacy systems that are no longer supported (Drake & Ridder, 2022). The consequences of these cybersecurity breaches have had far-reaching effects, threatening patients' lives and disrupting healthcare systems, resulting in financial losses (Portela et al., 2022). Cybersecurity incidents can lead to legal consequences for clinicians who are custodians of patient data (Elendu et al., 2024). The escalating sophistication and frequency of cyberattacks targeting healthcare infrastructure have raised significant national security concerns, as compromised systems can disrupt critical healthcare services, endanger patient safety, and potentially expose sensitive data that could be exploited for malicious purposes (Yeng et al., 2022). Cybersecurity is essential to maintaining patient confidentiality, data integrity, and the availability of healthcare services in today's digital environment (Alanazi, 2023).

2.3. Data Lifecycle Management in Healthcare IoT

In the realm of Healthcare IoT, Data Lifecycle Management involves the thorough process of managing sensitive health data from its inception to its eventual disposal within interconnected healthcare networks. This strategy requires the implementation of strong security protocols at each phase of data management, including its collection, storage, processing, sharing, and deletion. Healthcare entities need to enforce strict access controls, utilize encryption methods for data both in transit and at rest, and conduct regular audits of data usage to ensure adherence to privacy laws. The lifecycle also encompasses data quality assurance, ensuring that information remains precise and current throughout its usage. As IoT devices in healthcare produce large volumes of real-time patient data, effective lifecycle management is essential for maintaining data integrity, safeguarding patient privacy, and facilitating secure data sharing to enhance care coordination. Organizations must also tackle challenges such as data interoperability, the long-term storage of historical health records, and the ethical considerations of data retention and deletion policies. Ultimately, a well-crafted Data Lifecycle Management strategy in Healthcare IoT not only protects sensitive information but also improves the overall efficiency and effectiveness of healthcare delivery.

2.3.1. Data Collection and Storage Processes In IoT Devices

The increasing integration of Internet of Things (IoT) devices within connected health ecosystems has fundamentally transformed healthcare delivery, facilitating continuous patient monitoring, personalized treatment plans, and remote healthcare access. These IoT devices, which include wearable sensors, medical implants, and remote monitoring systems, generate a substantial volume of patient data, encompassing physiological parameters, activity levels, and environmental factors (Ianculescu et al., 2025). This data is utilized to monitor patient symptoms in real-time (Mamdiwar et al., 2021). The shift from traditional manual recording of patient data to IoT-enabled automated data collection has markedly enhanced the efficiency and accuracy of healthcare practices (Yeole & Kalbande, 2021). IoT sensors facilitate data collection, aiding in the early detection of emergencies and alerting family members (Abdulmalek et al., 2022). This transformation is further augmented by the advancement of IoT devices, which are anticipated to revolutionize healthcare in conjunction with prevailing sociological trends (Habibzadeh et al., 2019).

The architecture of connected health ecosystems typically involves several layers, starting with data acquisition at the edge, where IoT devices directly interact with patients to capture physiological data (Meisami et al., 2023). To mitigate bandwidth limitations and latency issues, edge computing paradigms are increasingly employed, enabling local data processing and filtering directly on the IoT devices or nearby edge servers (Anjum et al., 2023). The edge devices also capture data on vital signs like blood pressure, oxygen levels, and sugar levels (Ziwei et al., 2024). These data streams are then transmitted to a central cloud infrastructure, which provides scalable storage, advanced analytics capabilities, and secure data management (Dankolo et al., 2025).

2.3.2. Data Processing and Transmission Vulnerabilities

In connected health ecosystems, the intricacies of data processing and transmission present a multifaceted landscape of vulnerabilities that demand rigorous attention. As digital healthcare services become more accessible, the industry faces external and internal attacks (Seh et al., 2020). In these interconnected environments, the sensitivity of medical data, coupled with its extensive distributed processing, introduces significant security and privacy challenges (Dou et al., 2025). Within the connected health environment, data processing vulnerabilities constitute a critical area of concern, encompassing weaknesses and potential exploits that can compromise the integrity, confidentiality, and availability of sensitive healthcare information (Odeh et al., 2024). Data aggregation, a process central to generating valuable insights from diverse sources, can inadvertently expose patient data to unauthorized access or deanonymization risks, especially when datasets are not properly anonymized or when aggregation techniques fail to adequately protect patient privacy. Furthermore, data storage vulnerabilities, such as insecure databases or inadequately protected cloud storage environments, can create opportunities for malicious actors to access and exfiltrate sensitive healthcare data.

The transmission of healthcare data across networks introduces additional vulnerabilities that must be carefully addressed to ensure the confidentiality and integrity of patient information (Odeh et al., 2024). Cyberattacks on healthcare systems can occur through multiple points of entry, with hackers commonly scanning IT systems for vulnerabilities or using phishing emails to introduce malware (Perry et al., 2022). Wireless communication channels, commonly used for transmitting data from wearable sensors or remote monitoring devices, are susceptible to eavesdropping or interception attacks, potentially exposing sensitive patient data to unauthorized parties. Data interception poses a significant risk, particularly when wearable devices rely on wireless communication protocols like Bluetooth, making them vulnerable to man-in-the-middle attacks where attackers can intercept and manipulate data transmitted between the device and the healthcare system (Elsayed et al., 2025). Inadequate authentication mechanisms or weak encryption protocols can further exacerbate these risks, allowing attackers to gain unauthorized access to sensitive data transmitted over the network (Bada & Von Solms, 2022). It is imperative to recognize that the vulnerabilities inherent in data processing and transmission within connected health ecosystems not only pose significant risks to patient privacy and data security but also undermine the trust and confidence that individuals place in healthcare providers and technology vendors (Meisami et al., 2023). Robust cybersecurity measures are essential for safeguarding the integrity of healthcare infrastructure, protecting sensitive patient data, and maintaining the trust of individuals in the digital healthcare ecosystem (Popoola et al., 2024).

2.3.3. Secure Data Disposal Methods in Healthcare

In the healthcare sector, the secure disposal of data is of utmost importance to safeguard sensitive information, including genomic data, electronic health records (EHRs), and data generated by the Internet of Things (IoT), from unauthorized access. Inadequate disposal practices can result in data breaches, thereby violating regulations such as the Health Insurance Portability and Accountability Act (HIPAA) and the General Data Protection Regulation (GDPR), and consequently undermining patient trust. Effective disposal methods ensure that data is rendered irretrievable, addressing both digital and physical media, while adhering to rigorous compliance standards.

Digital Data Destruction: Secure erasure techniques are essential for the management of electronic health records (EHRs), genomic datasets, and other digital records stored on servers, cloud platforms, or devices. The process of overwriting data with random patterns, as outlined in NIST Special Publication 800-88, ensures that data recovery is not possible. In the case of solid-state drives (SSDs), cryptographic erasure, which involves the deletion of encryption keys, effectively renders data inaccessible and offers an efficient solution. It is recommended that automated tools be employed to monitor and verify the wiping processes, with audit trails maintained to ensure compliance with regulatory standards.

Physical Media Disposal: To prevent data recovery, it is imperative to destroy physical media such as hard drives, USB drives, and backup tapes. Methods such as shredding or pulverizing these devices into small fragments ensure that data retrieval is impossible. Additionally, degaussing, which disrupts the magnetic fields on tapes or hard drives, and incineration are effective techniques for certain types of media. Healthcare organizations must collaborate with certified vendors to ensure adherence to environmental regulations and maintain a documented chain of custody to prevent mishandling.

IoT Device Decommissioning: Internet of Things (IoT) devices, including wearable health monitors and connected diagnostic equipment, frequently store sensitive data locally. Prior to disposal or repurposing, it is imperative that these devices undergo secure data wiping or factory resets to ensure complete data erasure. Manufacturers are advised to incorporate secure data removal mechanisms, while healthcare providers must ensure that no residual data remains (Kruse et al., 2017). In instances where data wiping is not feasible, physical destruction of the devices is necessary to mitigate risks.

Staff Training and Governance: Human error constitutes a considerable risk in the process of data disposal. It is imperative that regular training programs are implemented to educate healthcare personnel on secure disposal protocols, with a strong emphasis on adherence to standardized procedures (Abouelmehdi et al., 2018). Governance policies should clearly delineate responsibilities, mandate regular audits, and ensure comprehensive documentation to uphold accountability. Furthermore, collaboration with certified e-waste recyclers and disposal vendors is essential to enhance compliance and mitigate associated risks.

By implementing these secure disposal methods, healthcare organizations can safeguard sensitive data, ensure regulatory compliance, and maintain patient trust within connected health ecosystems.

2.4. Ethical Considerations in Health Data Utilization

The imperative of securing informed consent from patients concerning the collection, utilization, and dissemination of their health data is crucial for maintaining ethical standards and honoring individual autonomy. This process necessitates transparency regarding the types of data being collected, the intended purposes of its use, and the potential risks and benefits associated with data sharing (Gabarron et al., 2015). The ethical considerations within connected health ecosystems are complex, necessitating careful attention to individual privacy rights, data security protocols, and the potential for algorithmic bias (Price & Cohen, 2019). It is essential to ensure that the deployment of these technologies does not exacerbate existing health disparities or engender new forms of discrimination (Elenberg & Howe Iii, 2020)..

Patient Consent Issues in Data Collection and Usage

To effectively gather and manage patient consent for data collection, storage, and use within connected health ecosystems, transparent and efficient systems are essential. Concerns about data misuse or privacy breaches may cause individuals to hesitate in fully adopting the advantages of connected health systems. Healthcare providers are utilizing these devices as vital tools to collect significant health data directly from patients (J. W. Kim et al., 2020). The advent of telemedicine and remote patient monitoring is revolutionizing healthcare delivery, enhancing convenience and accessibility for patients (Odeh et al., 2024). Patients now have the ability to receive medical advice and manage their health conditions from the comfort of their homes. Patient autonomy, a fundamental aspect of medical ethics, is closely tied to informed consent, which necessitates that individuals clearly understand how their data will be used and the potential consequences (Elenberg & Howe Iii, 2020). This understanding enables patients to make informed healthcare decisions that align with their personal values. Patients are entitled to be informed about their diagnoses, health status, treatment processes, therapeutic outcomes, test results, costs, health insurance contributions, or other medical information. Securing informed consent from patients before collecting their medical images and ensuring the protection of their personal information are crucial components of ethical data collection (Padmapriya & Parthasarathy, 2023). Patients have the ethical right to self-determination and to participate in collaborative decision-making regarding their healthcare choices (Farmer & Lundy, 2017). In some cases, data may be collected without the individual's knowledge of its intended use, which can erode trust between patients and healthcare providers (Reddy et al., 2019). Therefore, maintaining transparency about data usage is crucial for upholding ethical standards.

The utilization of health data poses intricate ethical dilemmas, especially concerning data collection, accessibility, and potential bias (B. Mittelstadt, 2019). Establishing robust data governance frameworks is crucial to define the conditions for data access, the responsibilities of data users, and the principles of benefit sharing, ensuring ethical and equitable data use (Vayena et al., 2017). This involves implementing measures to protect patient privacy, prevent data breaches, and ensure data is used in ways that benefit both individuals and the broader healthcare system (Abujaber & Nashwan, 2024). Trust is essential for individuals to willingly share their personal data to improve healthcare services (Thapa & Camtepe, 2020b). If this trust is eroded, the potential benefits of data sharing may be outweighed by concerns over privacy breaches and misuse of personal information (Zwitter, 2014).

Transparency In Ai-Driven Health Analytics

It is necessary to incorporate ethical and philosophical principles that address issues like bias and transparency (Topcu et al., 2023). Transparency, robustness, and fairness in AI models are vital for building trust in these systems (Saw & Ng, 2022). The swift progress of AI in healthcare offers both opportunities and challenges, requiring a comprehensive understanding of the ethical implications and the establishment of strong governance frameworks (Abujaber & Nashwan, 2024). The ethical considerations in AI-driven healthcare necessitate careful attention to prevent biases and ensure fair access (Abujaber & Nashwan, 2024). The development and implementation of AI technologies in healthcare must follow ethical guidelines to promote responsible innovation.

Potential Biases In Healthcare AI Systems

Artificial intelligence technologies play a crucial role in processing the enormous volumes of data produced within these ecosystems, yet they also bring significant concerns regarding the protection and privacy of patient data (Rony et al., 2024). The lack of uniform guidelines for the ethical application of AI and machine learning in healthcare further complicates these issues (Khan et al., 2023). The intricate nature of AI algorithms, often referred to as "black boxes," poses challenges in understanding decision-making processes, potentially undermining trust and accountability in medical diagnoses and treatments (Topcu et al., 2023). It is crucial to recognize that biases in the datasets used for training AI systems can result in disparities in healthcare, especially when the data does not adequately represent various demographic groups (Uygun Ilikhan et al., 2024). Moreover, biases can emerge during data collection, model development, evaluation, deployment, and publication, impacting AI algorithms and clinical decision-making (Cross et al., 2024).

Bias in medical artificial intelligence (AI) can emerge and intensify throughout the AI lifecycle, potentially resulting in suboptimal clinical decisions and the worsening of existing healthcare disparities (Cross et al., 2024). Such biases may be introduced during data collection, where certain patient populations might be underrepresented or misrepresented, leading to AI systems that are less effective and equitable (Cross et al., 2024). It is imperative to comprehend the sources of bias inherent in AI-based algorithms (Nazer et al., 2023). Electronic health records, which serve as a rich data source for training AI models, are vulnerable to biases that mirror the implicit and unconscious biases of clinicians, the tools employed for data processing, and the methods of data collection and labeling (Perets et al., 2024). Although the application of AI in emergency medicine holds promise, it is also fraught with risks associated with biases in data and design (Chenais et al.,

2022). Inaccurate or incomplete data in electronic health records can lead to misclassifications and measurement errors, further distorting the outcomes of machine learning algorithms (Gianfrancesco et al., 2018). The potential for AI to perpetuate healthcare disparities is a significant concern, particularly if algorithms are trained on homogeneous datasets that do not reflect the diversity of the patient population (Celi et al., 2022). AI algorithms can inadvertently perpetuate and even amplify existing healthcare disparities, especially when trained on datasets that lack diversity or reflect historical biases (Li et al., 2025). Such biases can result in AI models that perform inadequately for certain demographic groups, leading to less accurate diagnoses and treatment recommendations (Marko et al., 2025).

To promote fairness and equity in AI-based healthcare, it is crucial for developers to focus on data diversity, utilize advanced statistical techniques to detect and reduce biases, and follow well-defined reporting standards (Cross et al., 2024). Additionally, the exchange of data for innovation heightens the risks to data security and privacy, necessitating strong security protocols and rigorous data governance frameworks (Nasir et al., 2025). Conducting algorithmic audits and ensuring transparency in model development are vital strategies for reducing bias and fostering an inclusive and fair healthcare AI environment (Panch et al., 2019). Moreover, it is essential to create AI models that are transparent and interpretable, enabling both clinicians and patients to comprehend decision-making processes and identify any potential biases.

3.0. PRIVACY CHALLENGES IN IOT-ENABLED HEALTHCARE

The integration of Internet of Things (IoT) devices into healthcare systems introduces novel privacy challenges, as these devices continuously collect and transmit sensitive patient data. Safeguarding this information requires robust encryption protocols, secure authentication methods, and regular security audits to prevent unauthorized access and data breaches. Additionally, healthcare providers must establish clear policies concerning data retention, usage, and sharing, ensuring compliance with regulatory frameworks such as the Health Insurance Portability and Accountability Act (HIPAA) and the General Data Protection Regulation (GDPR), while balancing the imperative for data-driven innovations in patient care.

3.1. Threat Landscape for Connected Medical Devices

The convergence of widespread connectivity and the advancement of sophisticated medical devices has created a complex ecosystem, offering both unprecedented opportunities for enhanced patient care and a significantly expanded attack surface for malicious actors. The integration of medical devices into the Internet of Things has transformed healthcare, facilitating real-time monitoring, remote diagnostics, and AI-driven decision-making (Deb et al., 2025). However, this increased connectivity has inadvertently exposed medical devices to numerous cybersecurity vulnerabilities, converting what was once a relatively isolated environment into a potential hotspot for cyberattacks (Isong et al., 2024). While the digitization of healthcare has improved treatment accessibility and convenience, it has also rendered the industry a prime target for both external and internal threats (Seh et al., 2020).

Vulnerabilities in Implantable Medical Devices

Implantable medical devices, such as pacemakers, insulin pumps, and neurostimulators, while offering substantial therapeutic advantages, present a complex array of privacy and security vulnerabilities that necessitate thorough examination. The increasing connectivity of these devices, designed to enhance patient care through remote monitoring and personalized treatment, paradoxically enlarges the attack surface for malicious actors (Machal, 2023). The vulnerabilities inherent in medical devices may originate from various sources, including insufficient security protocols during the design and development stages, the utilization of outdated software with known deficiencies, and the absence of robust authentication mechanisms (Siddiqi et al., 2020). Cybersecurity incidents are preventable if the complexities of the operational environment are recognized alongside technical vulnerabilities (P. Williams & Woodward, 2015). Addressing the cybersecurity challenges associated with medical devices necessitates a multi-faceted approach, encompassing proactive security measures, continuous monitoring, and rapid incident response capabilities (Richter & Ammenwerth, 2023).

Security Risks in Remote Monitoring Systems

Remote monitoring systems in healthcare introduce additional security risks due to their dependence on wireless communication and data transmission over networks. These systems frequently gather and transmit sensitive patient data, making them appealing targets for cybercriminals looking to exploit vulnerabilities. The distributed nature of remote monitoring setups also broadens the attack surface, potentially exposing devices to unauthorized access, data interception, and manipulation. The inherent interconnectedness of IoT ecosystems creates a complex web of potential attack vectors, where a single compromised device can serve as a strategic entry point, allowing malicious entities to spread laterally throughout the entire network (Deb et al., 2025). The convergence of IoT and cloud computing adds further layers of complexity, with data traversing multiple network domains and storage environments, thereby heightening the risk of interception, tampering, and unauthorized access. The use of IoT in healthcare necessitates a rigorous and multifaceted approach to security, encompassing robust authentication mechanisms, end-to-end data encryption, stringent access control policies, and comprehensive vulnerability management strategies to effectively mitigate the risks associated with this evolving technological landscape. Potential vulnerabilities in IoT devices, data communication, and storage techniques can be exploited by malware and ransomware, thereby hindering the progress of IoT in healthcare (Podder et al., 2020). The lack of robust security measures in IoT-enabled healthcare systems can lead to severe repercussions, including the compromise of patient privacy, disruption of clinical workflows, and potential harm to patients due to device malfunction or manipulation (Macedo et al., 2019).

3.2. Data Interception and Unauthorized Access Risks

IoT-enabled healthcare systems present considerable vulnerabilities related to data interception and unauthorized access, necessitating the implementation of robust security measures to protect sensitive patient information. The extensive deployment of interconnected medical devices, intended to facilitate remote patient monitoring and personalized treatment plans, paradoxically expands the attack surface accessible to malicious entities seeking to compromise data confidentiality and system integrity (Jiang, 2021). The convenience of continuous health supervision via connected sensors and wearable devices is counterbalanced by the increased risk of data streams being intercepted or devices being compromised, thereby exposing confidential patient data (Popoola et al., 2024). The transmission of patient data, often wirelessly, between medical devices, gateways, and cloud servers creates opportunities for eavesdropping and man-in-the-middle attacks, where unauthorized parties can intercept and potentially alter or steal sensitive information (Isong et al., 2024). These vulnerabilities underscore the necessity for implementing robust encryption protocols and secure communication channels within the IoT healthcare ecosystem. It is essential for healthcare providers and device manufacturers to prioritize the development and integration of advanced authentication mechanisms and intrusion detection systems to mitigate the risks associated with data interception and unauthorized access. Furthermore, conducting regular security audits and updates for IoT medical devices is crucial to address emerging threats and ensure the ongoing protection of patient data in an increasingly interconnected healthcare landscape.

Man-in-the-Middle Attacks in Healthcare IoT

The architecture of IoT-enabled healthcare systems, while possessing the potential to transform patient care through remote monitoring and personalized treatment regimens, presents numerous security vulnerabilities, particularly susceptible to man-in-the-middle attacks. These attacks, characterized by an unauthorized third party intercepting and potentially altering communication between two endpoints, pose a significant threat to the confidentiality, integrity, and availability of sensitive medical data. The complexity of IoMT networks, often comprising heterogeneous devices with varying security capabilities, creates multiple entry points for malicious actors to infiltrate the communication channels (Shaikh et al., 2024). Specifically, the reliance on wireless communication protocols, such as Bluetooth, Zigbee, and Wi-Fi, for data transmission between medical devices, patient wearables, and central servers, introduces inherent vulnerabilities that can be exploited by attackers within range (Jiang, 2021). The consequences of successful man-in-the-middle attacks in healthcare can be catastrophic, potentially leading to the exposure of highly sensitive patient information, the manipulation of medical device functionality, and the disruption of critical healthcare services (Elsayed et al., 2025). The lack of robust authentication and encryption mechanisms in many legacy and even contemporary IoMT devices significantly exacerbates the risk profile associated with man-in-the-middle attacks (Popoola et al., 2024). The deployment of weak or default credentials, coupled with the absence of regular security updates, renders these devices prime targets for exploitation.

The establishment of mutual authentication mechanisms, where both parties verify each other's identities before exchanging data, is crucial to prevent unauthorized access and data interception (G Lopes & Gondim, 2020). This can be achieved through certificate-based authentication, which uses digital certificates to establish trust and verify the authenticity of devices and servers. Additionally, adopting end-to-end encryption, which ensures data protection from its origin to its final destination, is essential for maintaining data confidentiality and preventing eavesdropping. The use of strong encryption algorithms, such as Advanced Encryption Standard and Transport Layer Security, is highly recommended to safeguard data both in transit and at rest. Incorporating intrusion detection systems capable of detecting and mitigating anomalous network behavior is also vital for identifying and preventing man-in-the-middle attacks in real-time (Shaikh et al., 2024).

Insecure APIs and Their Implications

In the domain of IoT-enabled healthcare, the widespread presence of insecure APIs poses a significant threat to patient data privacy and system integrity, necessitating careful attention and robust security measures. The interconnected nature of IoT devices and healthcare systems is heavily reliant on APIs for data exchange, device management, and service integration, rendering them prime targets for malicious actors seeking to exploit vulnerabilities (Macedo et al., 2019). Weak authentication mechanisms, lack of encryption, and inadequate input validation in APIs can expose sensitive patient information, including medical records, personal details, and real-time health data, to unauthorized access and manipulation (Isong et al., 2024). Compromised APIs can result in data breaches, identity theft, and even manipulation of medical devices, potentially causing severe harm to patients (Jiang, 2021). Addressing these API security vulnerabilities requires a multifaceted approach, encompassing secure coding practices, robust authentication and authorization mechanisms, encryption of data in transit and at rest, and continuous monitoring and vulnerability assessments. The absence of robust security measures in IoT-enabled healthcare creates numerous opportunities for privacy breaches and security compromises (Popoola et al., 2024). Traditional models that place control of healthcare data with third parties have proven unreliable due to their susceptibility to security breaches (Meisami et al., 2023). The security weaknesses inherent in IoT devices and networks, combined with the sensitive nature of healthcare data, create a perfect storm of privacy risks (Dou et al., 2025).

Weak Authentication Mechanisms in Medical Devices

While the Internet of Medical Things (IoMT) offers numerous benefits, its extensive use brings about notable privacy issues, mainly due to the inherent weaknesses in IoT devices and the sensitive nature of healthcare information. A major issue stems from the insufficient authentication methods used in many IoMT devices (Abbasi et al., 2024). Numerous IoMT devices still depend on default passwords or weak, easily guessed credentials, making them vulnerable to unauthorized access (Shaikh et al., 2025). The computational constraints of many IoMT devices present a significant obstacle, hindering the implementation of authentication protocols that demand substantial processing power. The diverse nature of IoMT devices, encompassing a wide range of hardware architectures, operating systems, and communication protocols, significantly complicates the establishment of uniform and effective security measures (Ahmad et al., 2024). Furthermore, the mobility of many IoMT devices, which often operate across various networks and geographical areas, poses challenges for maintaining consistent authentication and authorization policies (Ferrag et al., 2019). These authentication issues are further compounded by the limited user interfaces on many IoMT devices, which can make it challenging for users to enter complex passwords or engage in multi-factor authentication. The absence of regular software updates and patches for IoMT devices also leaves them exposed to known security vulnerabilities, as manufacturers frequently prioritize functionality over security maintenance. Additionally, the interconnected nature of IoMT ecosystems means that a single compromised device could potentially serve as a gateway for attackers to access sensitive medical data across an entire network.

3.3. Regulatory Compliance and Cross-Border Data Flows

Effectively navigating the complex landscape of regulatory compliance within connected health ecosystems requires a comprehensive understanding of both domestic and international legal frameworks that govern data privacy and security. As healthcare data increasingly crosses jurisdictional boundaries, organizations must contend with a diverse array of data protection laws, including the General Data Protection Regulation in Europe, the Health Insurance Portability and Accountability Act in the United States, and various national data protection laws worldwide (Bernier et al., 2022). A comparative analysis of these international regulations elucidates best practices and underscores areas where further harmonization is necessary to safeguard healthcare data on a global scale (Elendu et al., 2024). Understanding the distinctions among these regulations is essential for healthcare organizations operating internationally, as compliance with one regulation does not ensure compliance with others (Reis et al., 2024).

3.3.1. HIPAA Requirements For Connected Health

The Health Insurance Portability and Accountability Act (HIPAA) creates a detailed system for protecting Protected Health Information in the U.S. healthcare sector. When HIPAA was enacted in 1996, it represented a significant advancement in data security, establishing crucial guidelines to ensure the confidentiality, integrity, and accessibility of sensitive patient information (Kruse et al., 2017). Entities covered by HIPAA, which include health plans, healthcare clearinghouses, and healthcare providers involved in electronic transactions, are required to adhere to its rigorous standards (Rocchiccioli, 2003). HIPAA's reach is extensive, covering various communication methods such as electronic, paper, and oral, thus impacting a wide range of healthcare activities (Feld, 2005). Title II of the Act specifically targets the prevention of healthcare fraud and abuse and outlines the requirements for administrative simplification (Brown, 2005).

HIPAA's Privacy Rule establishes a national standard for safeguarding individually identifiable health information, commonly known as Protected Health Information (PHI). This rule regulates the use and disclosure of PHI by covered entities, granting patients substantial rights concerning their health information, including the rights to access, amend, and receive an accounting of disclosures (Kruse et al., 2017). The Security Rule complements the Privacy Rule by setting national standards for securing electronic Protected Health Information (e-PHI). It requires covered entities to implement administrative, physical, and technical safeguards to ensure the confidentiality, integrity, and availability of e-PHI. These safeguards are designed to protect against reasonably anticipated threats and hazards to the security or integrity of e-PHI, as well as unauthorized uses or disclosures (Andriole, 2014). HIPAA also underscores the importance of information integrity, guiding healthcare administrators in identifying vulnerabilities within their stored information and data-sharing practices (Fedorowicz & Ray, 2004). The Enforcement Rule delineates the procedures for investigating and enforcing HIPAA violations, including potential civil and criminal penalties for non-compliance. Furthermore, the Breach Notification Rule mandates that covered entities and their business associates notify affected individuals, the Secretary of Health and Human Services, and, in certain cases, the media, following a breach of unsecured PHI. These comprehensive regulations collectively form a robust framework for protecting patient privacy and data security in the healthcare sector, necessitating ongoing vigilance and adaptation from healthcare organizations to maintain compliance.

3.3.2. GDPR Implications for Global Health Data

The General Data Protection Regulation (GDPR) exerts a substantial influence on the connected health ecosystem by enforcing rigorous requirements for the processing of personal data, particularly sensitive health data. Enacted by the European Union, the GDPR seeks to safeguard the fundamental rights and freedoms of individuals concerning their personal data (Georgiou & Lambrinoudakis, 2020). It establishes a harmonized legal framework for data protection across EU member states (Georgiou & Lambrinoudakis, 2020). Organizations operating within the connected health domain, irrespective of their geographical location, are required to comply with the GDPR if they process the personal data of EU residents (Biswal & Kulkarni, 2021). This encompasses healthcare providers, manufacturers of wearable devices, developers of mobile health applications, and research institutions. The core principles of the GDPR, such as data minimization, purpose limitation, and storage limitation, necessitate a paradigm shift in the collection, utilization, and retention of health data within connected health ecosystems (Torre et al., 2020). The principle of accountability obliges data controllers to demonstrate compliance with the GDPR, necessitating the implementation of appropriate technical and organizational measures to ensure data protection (Becker et al., 2024). The importance of data privacy has escalated with the advent of big data and the ensuing regulations (Klymenko et al., 2023). The impact of the GDPR extends beyond mere compliance, influencing the design and implementation of connected health technologies from inception. Organizations must adopt a "privacy by design" approach, integrating data protection measures into their products and services from the earliest stages of development. This proactive stance not only facilitates regulatory compliance but also fosters trust with users, potentially leading to increased adoption and engagement with connected health solutions.

4.0. CLOUD TRUST MODELS FOR HEALTHCARE DATA PRIVACY

Cloud trust models are essential for ensuring the security and privacy of sensitive healthcare information in cloud settings. An effective cloud trust model should include several critical components, such as strong access control systems, data encryption methods, audit logs, and compliance certifications (Elmogazy & Bamasag, 2016). Access control systems must adhere to the principle of least privilege, allowing users only the necessary access to fulfill their roles, while data encryption should safeguard information both during transmission and when stored, making it unreadable to unauthorized individuals (Gholami & Laure, 2016). Audit logs offer a comprehensive account of all data access and modification activities, helping organizations identify and examine potential security incidents, and compliance certifications, like HIPAA and GDPR, reflect an organization's dedication to following industry standards for data security. The adoption of cloud computing brings about security and privacy challenges, such as multi-tenancy, trust, loss of control, and accountability (Gholami & Laure, 2015, 2016). While storing patient data in the cloud can speed up clinical processes, it is crucial to prioritize security and privacy concerns (Jpc Rodrigues et al., 2013). One notable strategy is the adoption of attribute-based access control, which facilitates precise regulation of data access by considering a combination of user attributes, resource attributes, and environmental conditions. The integration of cloud computing within the healthcare sector enhances accessibility in a cost-effective manner by merging medical data with cloud computing capabilities, thereby offering patients and industries legitimate solutions (Banimfreg, 2023).

4.1. Secure Cloud Architectures for Health Data

Cloud computing has become a game-changing approach in the healthcare sector, providing scalability, cost savings, and easy access to medical data and applications. This technology enables smooth information sharing among healthcare participants, such as patients, physicians, and pharmacists, which is especially advantageous in remote or underserved regions where medical facilities might be scarce (Banimfreg, 2023). While cloud computing itself is not a novel technology, it represents a new way of delivering computing resources (Kuo, 2011). Cloud solutions offer the potential to transform health information technology, improve healthcare services, and drive progress in medical research (Kuo, 2011).

4.1.1. Zero-Trust Models in Healthcare Cloud Systems

The migration of healthcare data to cloud environments represents a significant paradigm shift, offering improved accessibility, scalability, and cost-effectiveness. Nevertheless, this transition poses substantial challenges related to data privacy and security, necessitating the development of robust trust models to protect sensitive patient information (Banimfreg, 2023). Traditional security perimeters, which assume trust within a network, are increasingly insufficient in the face of sophisticated cyber threats and the inherent complexities of cloud infrastructure (Ajish, 2024). The Zero Trust architecture emerges as a promising alternative, fundamentally rejecting the notion of implicit trust and advocating for continuous verification of every user, device, and application attempting to access resources (Ghasemshirazi et al., 2023). Zero Trust operates on the principle of "never trust, always verify," requiring strict identity verification for every individual and device attempting to access network resources, regardless of their location (Chandramouli, 2023). This approach mandates that every access request, both internal and external, is rigorously authenticated, authorized, and encrypted before granting access to protected health information (Dhiman et al., 2024). Addressing the complexities of integrating a Zero Trust model involves identifying the data requiring protection, classifying it, and delineating its traffic flows, which then clarifies how the access policy should be structured.

Adopting Zero Trust in the healthcare sector requires a thorough approach that integrates several essential components, such as microsegmentation, multi-factor authentication, least privilege access, and ongoing monitoring.

Microsegmentation: This involves breaking the network into separate segments to restrict attackers' lateral movement and contain any breaches.

Multi-factor authentication: This enhances security by demanding multiple forms of identification from users, like passwords, biometric scans, or one-time codes, before access is granted.

Least privilege access: It ensures that users and applications have only the necessary level of access to perform their specific tasks, thereby minimizing the risk associated with compromised accounts.

Continuous monitoring: This entails the real-time analysis of network traffic and user behavior to identify and address unusual activities (Chandramouli, 2023).

A fundamental principle is the dynamic evaluation of trust for each access request, ensuring that authorization is based on real-time assessments rather than static permissions (Ramezanpour & Jagannath, 2022). Zero Trust Architecture also emphasizes the importance of encryption for data both in transit and at rest. This approach ensures that even if an attacker gains access to the network, they cannot easily read or manipulate sensitive information. Additionally, Zero Trust models often incorporate automated threat detection and response systems, which can quickly identify and mitigate potential security breaches without human intervention.

4.1.2. Confidential Computing Techniques

The intrinsic weaknesses found in cloud environments, such as data breaches, unauthorized access, and insider threats, highlight the urgent need for innovative strategies to enhance healthcare data privacy. Confidential computing emerges as a promising paradigm, offering a range of techniques aimed at protecting data while it is being used, thus reducing the risks linked to traditional encryption methods that only secure data when it is at rest or in transit (Zobaed & Salehi, 2023). Conventional security measures often fail to address the dynamic nature of cloud environments, where data is continuously processed and accessed, making it susceptible to attacks during runtime. Confidential computing establishes a trusted execution environment, also known as an enclave, where sensitive data and code can be processed in isolation, protected from the underlying operating system, hypervisor, and other potentially harmful entities (Lamptey & Zhou, 2020). This isolation is typically achieved through hardware-based security features, such as Intel SGX or AMD SEV, which provide a secure enclave for executing sensitive operations. Encryption is crucial in ensuring data confidentiality by converting data into an unreadable format, thereby safeguarding it from unauthorized disclosure (Dawson et al., 2023).

However, even with encryption, data remains vulnerable during processing, as it must be decrypted within the cloud environment, exposing it to potential attacks. By processing data within a secure enclave, confidential computing minimizes the attack surface and reduces the risk of data compromise. Homomorphic encryption, a cryptographic technique that enables computations to be performed on encrypted data without the need for decryption, represents a significant advancement in data privacy (Udendhran, 2017). By allowing computations to be performed directly on encrypted files without decryption, sensitive user information remains protected within the cloud (Loyka et al., 2018). The cloud server can process encrypted data and return encrypted results without ever gaining access to the underlying plaintext (Brännvall et al., 2023). The data owner can then decrypt the results locally, ensuring end-to-end data privacy. Cloud computing has emerged as an efficient system for storing and accessing data . Encryption serves as a safety measure to prevent sensitive information from being exposed (Shi, 2018).

4.2. Auditability and Transparency in Cloud Health Systems

Auditability is crucial for maintaining the accountability and trustworthiness of cloud-based healthcare systems. Audit trails create a clear record of all data access and changes, which helps in identifying unauthorized actions and potential security threats (Tong et al., 2013). By documenting every interaction with patient data, such as its creation, access, modification, and deletion, audit trails provide a detailed overview of data management practices within the cloud setting (Elmogazy & Bamasag, 2016).

4.2.1. Immutable Logs for Healthcare Data Tracking

Immutable logs, characterized by their append-only and tamper-evident nature, present a compelling solution for fortifying data integrity and auditability in healthcare environments. By employing cryptographic techniques, immutable logs ensure that once data is written, it cannot be altered or deleted without detection (Islam & Rahman, 2025). Blockchain technology, with its decentralized and distributed ledger, has emerged as a promising platform for implementing immutable logs in healthcare (X. Liu et al., 2024). The technology offers decentralized architecture which ensures robustness against single points of failure and enhances security against attacks and data loss (Mandarino et al., 2024). Each transaction or data entry is recorded as a block, cryptographically linked to the previous block, forming a chain of records that is virtually impossible to tamper with (Pokharel et al., 2025). Blockchain's inherent characteristics of decentralization, verifiability, and immutability render it suitable for securely storing personal medical data (Chen et al., 2018). The rise of blockchain technology presents opportunities to address critical data privacy, security, and integrity challenges in healthcare. Audit trails that leverage blockchain technology track transactions and modifications to patient records and notify all users on the network (Chang & Chen, 2020). Its decentralized architecture enables secure data sharing, while its cryptographic underpinnings ensure patient data integrity and privacy (Pokharel et al., 2025). The technology's ability to maintain data integrity and provide secure data sharing among healthcare providers and patients makes it a fundamental tool for modernizing healthcare systems (Tahir et al., 2024).

4.2.2. Compliance Reporting Requirements and Solutions

Ensuring the privacy of healthcare data within cloud environments requires a comprehensive understanding of compliance reporting requirements and the implementation of effective solutions to meet these mandates. The adoption of cloud computing for data storage and access has gained significant attention, particularly with the proliferation of electronic health records and the exchange of health information for research and other purposes (Elmogazy & Bamasag, 2016). However, the highly sensitive nature of healthcare data, coupled with stringent regulatory frameworks such as HIPAA, GDPR, and other regional and national laws, presents considerable challenges in maintaining confidentiality, ensuring data integrity, and guaranteeing availability (Seth et al., 2024). Compliance reporting is not merely a procedural formality but a critical mechanism for demonstrating adherence to these regulations, assuring stakeholders of the security posture of the cloud environment, and maintaining trust in the healthcare ecosystem.

The legal consequences for clinicians and healthcare entities following cybersecurity breaches are significant, potentially resulting in harsh penalties, damage to reputation, and loss of patient trust (Elendu et al., 2024). Therefore, healthcare organizations must focus not only on technical measures for safeguarding data but also on administrative and procedural systems to demonstrate compliance and accountability. This involves establishing comprehensive audit trails, access controls, encryption protocols, and data loss prevention strategies, all of which need to be thoroughly documented and regularly assessed. The increasing dependence on electronic health records, along with the vulnerability of digital platforms to cyberattacks, makes the protection of patient information a critical priority (Odeh et al., 2024). Cloud service providers must enforce strong security measures to prevent unauthorized access and data breaches, while healthcare organizations must maintain transparency in data management practices, ensuring patients are informed about how their information is managed (Jpc Rodrigues et al., 2013).

Cloud trust models are integral to safeguarding healthcare data privacy, offering a framework for assessing the reliability of cloud service providers and the security of their services (Thapa & Camtepe, 2020a). The integration of medical data with cloud computing enhances accessibility in a cost-effective manner, providing viable solutions for patients and industries (Banimfreg, 2023). These models typically include various components, such as security certifications, compliance attestations, data governance policies, and incident response capabilities. Moreover, healthcare organizations must perform comprehensive due diligence assessments of cloud providers, examining their security infrastructure, data handling practices, and adherence to relevant regulations. This evaluation should go beyond contractual assurances, incorporating independent audits, penetration testing, and vulnerability assessments to verify the provider's security posture.

5.0. CASE STUDIES AND REAL-WORLD APPLICATIONS

Analyzing real-world applications reveals the intricacies involved in protecting sensitive health information within interconnected ecosystems. The efficacy of these connected health ecosystems is largely dependent on the seamless and secure exchange of data among various stakeholders, highlighting the essential requirement for robust privacy-enhancing technologies. Through the examination of real-world applications, healthcare providers and technology developers can acquire valuable insights into best practices for balancing data utility with privacy protection in connected health environments.

5.1. Lessons from Major Health Data Breaches

Ransomware attacks targeting hospitals have increased markedly, resulting in significant disruptions to patient care and the exposure of sensitive data. The ransomware attack on Change Healthcare in February 2024, executed by the ALPHV/BlackCat group, compromised the protected health information of up to 100 million individuals. This incident caused extensive disruptions in claims processing, prescriptions, and payments across U.S. healthcare providers, with financial repercussions exceeding $2.4 billion. In 2023, the U.S. healthcare sector experienced a 128% increase in ransomware incidents, affecting 258 victims, including 46 hospital systems comprising 141 hospitals. These attacks frequently targeted vulnerable rural facilities, with groups such as LockBit exploiting third-party vendors and legacy systems. Consequently, these breaches led to operational downtime, delayed treatments, and increased emergency diversions to unaffected hospitals.

Internet of Things (IoT) devices in healthcare, encompassing implantable medical devices and monitoring equipment, are susceptible to exploitation due to inadequate security protocols. In 2017, vulnerabilities in cardiac devices manufactured by St. Jude Medical (now Abbott), such as pacemakers and defibrillators, permitted potential remote access via transmitters. This vulnerability enabled attackers to deplete batteries or modify pacing, necessitating a recall of nearly 500,000 units. The 2016 Mirai botnet attack compromised numerous IoT devices, including hospital cameras and monitors, to execute large-scale Distributed Denial of Service (DDoS) attacks, thereby underscoring risks to network stability within healthcare settings. Similarly, Medtronic insulin pumps have encountered cybersecurity challenges, with vulnerabilities permitting unauthorized wireless access to modify dosages, posing risks of insulin over- or under-delivery, as identified in recalls and alerts issued by the FDA from 2019 onward. These exploits highlight the expanded attack surface resulting from unpatched firmware and default credentials in devices such as infusion pumps and remote monitors.

Significant breaches in healthcare cybersecurity have exposed critical deficiencies, including the lack of regular risk assessments, insufficient encryption, and inadequate oversight of third-party vendors, frequently resulting in violations of HIPAA Security Rule requirements. The consequences of these breaches encompass financial penalties, patient harm due to delayed care, and class-action lawsuits, underscoring the necessity for proactive strategies rather than reactive responses. Preventive measures should include the implementation of multifactor authentication, encryption of protected health information (PHI), comprehensive risk analyses, and the promotion of workforce training on cybersecurity awareness. Additionally, updating HIPAA regulations to address contemporary threats, enhancing supply chain security, and fostering collaboration on threat intelligence can further mitigate risks.

5.2. Best Practices in Privacy-Preserving Health Analytics

Anonymization techniques facilitate the utilization of health data for research purposes while mitigating the risks of re-identification. Common methodologies include data masking, which involves substituting identifiers with pseudonyms; suppression, which entails the removal of high-risk data elements; perturbation, which adds noise to values; and aggregation, which groups data, such as age ranges. Advanced strategies, such as k-anonymity, ensure that individuals remain indistinguishable within groups, whereas differential privacy introduces statistical noise to large datasets in genomic or public health studies. These techniques, often automated through artificial intelligence tools, strike a balance between data utility and privacy, as evidenced in clinical trials and collaborative platforms where synthetic data generation maintains analytical value without compromising confidentiality.

Under the Health Insurance Portability and Accountability Act (HIPAA), the de-identification of medical records can be accomplished through two primary methods. The Safe Harbor method necessitates the removal of 18 specific identifiers, such as names, precise dates (retaining only the year), geographic details more specific than the state level, contact information, Social Security numbers, medical record numbers, and any unique codes or biometric data. Alternatively, the Expert Determination method involves a qualified statistician evaluating the risk of re-identification as "very small" using scientific methodologies, thereby offering flexibility for complex datasets while requiring thorough documentation. Both methods are applicable to electronic health records, with the Safe Harbor method providing a prescriptive approach for compliance, and the Expert Determination method allowing for the tailored preservation of data elements in research contexts.

Privacy-preserving initiatives in healthcare facilitate secure data collaboration through federated learning and specialized platforms. GIFT-Cloud enables the anonymized sharing of medical imaging across institutions, while Sync for Science (S4S) permits patient-controlled data sharing with electronic health record vendors for research purposes, as exemplified by the NIH's All of Us program. Federated learning frameworks, such as those employed in Health-FedNet and VANTAGE6, allow for model training on decentralized data without the transfer of raw data, thereby enhancing privacy in the analysis of electronic health records for tasks such as medical image classification. These approaches, compliant with GDPR and HIPAA regulations, support initiatives like collaborative medical diagnosis and transfusion medicine research, effectively addressing data silos while prioritizing patient consent and security.

6.0. FUTURE DIRECTIONS AND EMERGING SOLUTIONS

6.1. Post-Quantum Cryptography for Healthcare Security

Quantum computing presents substantial challenges to existing encryption standards within the healthcare sector, where sensitive patient data is safeguarded by cryptographic protocols that may be compromised. Algorithms such as Shor's, developed in 1994, possess the capability to efficiently factor large integers, thereby compromising widely utilized systems like RSA and threatening the confidentiality and integrity of electronic health records (EHRs). As quantum technologies progress, they pose risks of decrypting stored medical data, potentially resulting in breaches of patient privacy and unauthorized access to critical health information. This vulnerability extends to real-time data exchanges within connected health ecosystems, where classical encryption is inadequate against quantum-enhanced attacks, necessitating a proactive transition to more resilient alternatives.

Post-quantum cryptographic methods offer promising defenses by relying on mathematical problems resistant to quantum attacks. Lattice-based cryptography, such as CRYSTALS-KYBER, uses hard lattice problems for key encapsulation and has been standardized by NIST for its efficiency and security. Code-based approaches, like those derived from error-correcting codes (e.g., McEliece), provide robust encryption, while hash-based signatures (e.g., SPHINCS+) ensure integrity without vulnerability to factorization. Multivariate polynomial cryptography and supersingular isogeny-based systems further diversify options, with NIST's ongoing standardization process selecting algorithms like KYBER and Dilithium for broad deployment. These methods maintain security even against large-scale quantum computers, supporting applications from secure EHR transmission to telemedicine.

Implementing post-quantum cryptography in healthcare systems presents several challenges, such as ensuring compatibility with existing infrastructure and managing resource constraints. The larger key sizes required by lattice-based methods increase computational demands, which can strain low-power devices in IoMT environments and necessitate hardware upgrades. Integration issues also emerge from the need for hybrid systems during transition periods, compounded by budget limitations for staff training and protocol updates. Additionally, regulatory compliance, including alignment with HIPAA, adds complexity. Ensuring minimal disruption to clinical workflows requires careful migration strategies to prevent downtime in critical care settings.

6.2. AI for Transparent Health Data Usage

Transparency in AI-driven healthcare is crucial for building trust among clinicians and patients, as opaque "black-box" models can create uncertainty in decision-making and lead to potential errors with significant consequences. This necessity stems from ethical imperatives for accountability, where AI systems must justify their recommendations to align with evidence-based practices and address biases in diverse patient populations. In connected health ecosystems, transparency allows for the verification of AI outputs, reducing risks such as misdiagnosis and supporting informed consent by clarifying how patient data influences outcomes. Without transparency, adoption is hindered by concerns over liability and fairness, highlighting the importance of explainable AI (XAI) in developing reliable, patient-centric systems.

Explainable AI techniques for medical diagnostics enhance interpretability by revealing model reasoning, categorized into methods like feature-oriented, local, and global explanations. Local Interpretable Model-agnostic Explanations (LIME) and SHapley Additive exPlanations (SHAP) attribute importance to input features, such as highlighting key pixels in imaging for tumor detection. Gradient-weighted Class Activation Mapping (Grad-CAM) visualizes heatmaps on medical images to show decision foci, while concept-based models like Training calibration-based explainers (TraCE) provide high-level interpretations for diagnostics. These techniques, often applied to deep learning models, improve diagnostic accuracy in areas like radiology and pathology by making predictions traceable and verifiable.

Accountability measures in AI-based treatments involve interdisciplinary frameworks that integrate legal, ethical, and technical safeguards. Regulatory oversight, such as FDA guidelines for AI transparency, mandates auditable decision logs and bias audits to ensure equitable outcomes. Ethical evaluations stress the importance of informed consent and clinician oversight, with tools like datasheets for datasets enhancing traceability. Continuous monitoring through explainable models fosters responsibility, allowing for post-deployment reviews to address adverse events and incorporate human judgment for personalized care.

6.3. Self-Sovereign Identity (SSI) for Patient-Centric *Privacy*

Self-sovereign identity (SSI) enables users to manage their digital identities independently, without relying on intermediaries, by utilizing decentralized identifiers (DIDs) and verifiable credentials (VCs) stored in personal wallets. In the healthcare sector, SSI transitions from centralized systems to patient-centric models, facilitating selective disclosure of health data while preserving privacy through zero-knowledge proofs. Its significance lies in addressing fragmented electronic health records (EHRs), promoting secure, interoperable data sharing among providers, and enhancing patient autonomy within connected ecosystems.

Implementing SSI in health systems faces challenges such as scalability, key management, and compatibility with existing infrastructures. The limitations of blockchain storage and the necessity for user-friendly recovery mechanisms for lost credentials complicate adoption, while ensuring compliance with regulations like GDPR introduces governance hurdles. Additionally, establishing emergency access protocols for unconscious patients and addressing risks posed by non-technical users further complicate deployment in diverse healthcare settings.

Potential benefits of SSI include enhanced patient data control, reducing breaches by minimizing centralized repositories and enabling granular consent for sharing. It promotes interoperability, lowers administrative costs through streamlined verification, and supports privacy-preserving exchanges, ultimately fostering trust and empowering patients in personalized care.

7.0. CONCLUSION

7.1. Summary of Key Findings

The investigation into data sensitivity and privacy within connected health ecosystems uncovers a landscape filled with significant challenges that jeopardize patient confidentiality, system integrity, and overall trust in healthcare delivery. Key challenges include the susceptibility of sensitive data types, such as electronic health records (EHRs), wearable-generated data, and genomic information, to breaches, unauthorized access, and misuse, as highlighted in discussions on identity theft, insurance fraud, and reputational damage. Cybersecurity threats further intensify these issues, with ransomware attacks, IoT device exploits, man-in-the-middle attacks, and insecure APIs posing risks to data interception and manipulation (Popoola et al., 2024). Ethical concerns, including informed consent, algorithmic bias in AI, and compliance with regulations like HIPAA and GDPR, add complexity to the environment, potentially leading to disparities, discrimination, and legal repercussions (Price & Cohen, 2019). The data lifecycle from collection and transmission to disposal presents ongoing vulnerabilities, exacerbated by the interconnected nature of IoT ecosystems and the proliferation of digital platforms (Abouelmehdi et al., 2018).

The chapter proposes a range of solutions and best practices to mitigate these risks while encouraging innovation. Implementing robust security measures, such as zero trust architecture, confidential computing, and blockchain-based immutable logs, enhances data protection in cloud environments (Chandramouli, 2023). Privacy-preserving techniques, including anonymization, differential privacy, and federated learning, enable health analytics without compromising individual data (Cross et al., 2024). Emerging solutions like post-quantum cryptography, explainable AI, and self-sovereign identity (SSI) provide forward-looking defenses against evolving threats, promoting patient-centric control and interoperability (Thapa & Camtepe, 2020b).

7.2. Future Outlook

Recent advancements in healthcare cybersecurity highlight a growing focus on integrating artificial intelligence, implementing quantum-resilient defenses, and adopting proactive threat intelligence strategies to counter the increasing frequency of cyberattacks. Ransomware continues to be a major threat, with incidents in the United States expected to rise by 128% from 2023 to 2025, particularly impacting legacy systems and third-party vendors. Simultaneously, AI-driven threats like deepfakes and automated phishing demand the use of advanced endpoint encryption and zero trust segmentation. Regulatory updates, such as proposed amendments to the HIPAA Security Rule and the Health Infrastructure Security and Accountability Act, emphasize the need for accountability and supply chain security. Additionally, the growing prevalence of Internet of Medical Things (IoMT) devices and telehealth services intensifies the need for edge computing security and the formation of collaborative public-private partnerships for sharing threat data.

The long-term implications for connected health ecosystems present a dual-edged transformation. On one hand, enhanced security through decentralized models like blockchain and SSI could reduce centralized vulnerabilities and promote equitable access. On the other hand, persistent gaps in privacy protections might undermine patient autonomy, enabling behavioral control and exacerbating disparities if not addressed. As digital health expands, inadequate regulations could stifle innovation, leading to increased data silos and a loss of trust. Conversely, robust frameworks such as GDPR harmonization and AI governance could foster sustainable, patient-centered ecosystems with improved interoperability and resilience against global threats. Ultimately, these ecosystems could evolve into more secure, efficient networks, but only if privacy-by-design principles are integrated to mitigate risks like re-identification in big data analytics.

7.3. Call to Action

In the domains of healthcare, technology, and policy, stakeholders must prioritize collaborative initiatives to enhance data privacy and security. Healthcare providers are advised to conduct comprehensive risk assessments, adopt zero trust models, and invest in staff training on cybersecurity protocols (Elendu et al., 2024). Technology developers should integrate privacy-enhancing technologies, such as explainable AI and post-quantum encryption, from the design phase, ensuring compatibility with legacy systems (Mennella et al., 2024). Policymakers are encouraged to advance harmonized regulations, including updates to HIPAA and GDPR, to address AI and IoT-specific risks, while promoting public-private partnerships for threat intelligence sharing (Bernier et al., 2022). Emphasis should be placed on ongoing research into emerging threats and innovative solutions, alongside interdisciplinary collaboration to balance data utility with ethical protections, ultimately fostering resilient and trustworthy connected health ecosystems for the future.

REFERENCES

Abbasi, I. A., Jan, S. U., Alqahtani, A. S., Khan, A. S., Algarni, F., Nyangaresi, V. O., Nyangaresi, V. O., Nyangaresi, V. O., & Nyangaresi, V. O. (2024). A lightweight and robust authentication scheme for the healthcare system using public cloud server. *PLoS One*, *19*(1), e0294429. Advance online publication. DOI: 10.1371/journal.pone.0294429 PMID: 38289970

Abdulmalek, S., Nasir, A., Jabbar, W. A., Almuhaya, M. A. M., Bairagi, A. K., Khan, M. A.-M., & Kee, S.-H. (2022). IoT-Based Healthcare-Monitoring System towards Improving Quality of Life: A Review. *Healthcare (Basel)*, *10*(10), 1993. DOI: 10.3390/healthcare10101993 PMID: 36292441

Abouelmehdi, K., Khaloufi, H., & Beni-Hessane, A. (2018). Big healthcare data: Preserving security and privacy. *Journal of Big Data*, *5*(1), 1. Advance online publication. DOI: 10.1186/s40537-017-0110-7

Abujaber, A. A., & Nashwan, A. J. (2024). Ethical framework for artificial intelligence in healthcare research: A path to integrity. *World Journal of Methodology*, *14*(3). Advance online publication. DOI: 10.5662/wjm.v14.i3.94071 PMID: 39310239

Ahmad, I., Shahid, F., Islam, J., Haque, K., & Harjula, E. (2024). *Adaptive Lightweight Security for Performance Efficiency in Critical Healthcare Monitoring*. / arxiv.2406.03786DOI: 10.1109/ISMICT61996.2024.10738175

Ajish, D. (2024). The significance of artificial intelligence in zero trust technologies: A comprehensive review. *Journal of Electrical Systems and Information Technology*, *11*(1), 30. Advance online publication. DOI: 10.1186/s43067-024-00155-z

Alanazi, A. T. (2023). Clinicians' Perspectives on Healthcare Cybersecurity and Cyber Threats. *Cureus*, *15*(10). Advance online publication. DOI: 10.7759/cureus.47026 PMID: 37965389

Alarfaj, K. A., & Rahman, M. M. H. (2024). The Risk Assessment of the Security of Electronic Health Records Using Risk Matrix. *Applied Sciences (Basel, Switzerland)*, *14*(13), 5785. DOI: 10.3390/app14135785

Andriole, K. P. (2014). Security of Electronic Medical Information and Patient Privacy: What You Need to Know. *Journal of the American College of Radiology*, *11*(12, 12 Pt B), 1212–1216. DOI: 10.1016/j.jacr.2014.09.011 PMID: 25467897

Anjum, M., Shahab, S., Whangbo, T., & Ahmad, S. (2023). Preventing overloaded dissemination in healthcare applications using NonDelay tolerant dissemination technique. *Heliyon, 9*(8), e18783. DOI: 10.1016/j.heliyon.2023.e18783 PMID: 37576207

Bada, M., & Von Solms, B. (2022). *A Cybersecurity Guide for Using Fitness Devices*. Springer., DOI: 10.1007/978-3-030-94285-4_3

Banimfreg, B. H. (2023). A comprehensive review and conceptual framework for cloud computing adoption in bioinformatics. *Healthcare Analytics, 3*, 100190. DOI: 10.1016/j.health.2023.100190

Baniulyte, G., Rogerson, N., & Bowden, J. (2023). Evolution – removing paper and digitising the hospital. *Health and Technology, 13*(2), 263–271. DOI: 10.1007/s12553-023-00740-8 PMID: 36846741

Becker, R., Ziaka, A., Tzortzatou-Nanopoulou, O., Comandè, G., Thorogood, A., Dove, E. S., Molnár-Gábor, F., & Chokoshvili, D. (2024). Purpose definition as a crucial step for determining the legal basis under the GDPR: Implications for scientific research. *Journal of Law and the Biosciences, 11*(1), lsae001. Advance online publication. DOI: 10.1093/jlb/lsae001 PMID: 38313429

Bent, B., & Dunn, J. P. (2020). Optimizing sampling rate of wrist-worn optical sensors for physiologic monitoring. *Journal of Clinical and Translational Science, 5*(1), e34. Advance online publication. DOI: 10.1017/cts.2020.526 PMID: 33948257

Bernier, A., Molnár-Gábor, F., & Knoppers, B. M. (2022). The international data governance landscape. *Journal of Law and the Biosciences, 9*(1), lsac005. Advance online publication. DOI: 10.1093/jlb/lsac005 PMID: 35382430

Biswal, S. P., & Kulkarni, M. S. (2021). Implications of GDPR on Emerging Technologies. *Revista Gestão Inovação e Tecnologias, 11*(4), 4898–4912. DOI: 10.47059/revistageintec.v11i4.2512

Brännvall, R., Linge, H., & Forsgren, H. (2023). *HEIDA: Software Examples for Rapid Introduction of Homomorphic Encryption for Privacy Preservation of Health Data* (Vol. 302). Institut F R Ost Und S Dosteuropaforschung., DOI: 10.3233/SHTI230116

Brown, C. (2005). HIPAA Programs: Design and Implementation. *Information Systems Security : ... International Conference, ICISS ... : Proceedings, 14*(1), 10–20. DOI: 10.1201/1086/45098.14.1.20050301/87267.3

Celi, L. A., Dee, E. C., Yao, S., Eber, R., Mitchell, W. G., Moukheiber, L., Schirmer, J., Charpignon, M.-L., Park, J., Paguio, J., Dernoncourt, F., Situ, J., Wawira, J. G., & Cellini, J. (2022). Sources of bias in artificial intelligence that perpetuate healthcare disparities-A global review. *PLOS Digital Health, 1*(3), e0000022. DOI: 10.1371/journal.pdig.0000022 PMID: 36812532

Chandramouli, R. (2023). *A Zero Trust Architecture Model for Access Control in Cloud Native Applications in Multi-Cloud Environments*. DOI: 10.6028/NIST.SP.800-207A.ipd

Chang, S. E., & Chen, Y. (2020). Blockchain in Health Care Innovation: Literature Review and Case Study From a Business Ecosystem Perspective. *Journal of Medical Internet Research, 22*(8), e19480. DOI: 10.2196/19480 PMID: 32865501

Chen, Y., Yang, S., Xu, Z., Ding, S., & Zheng, H. (2018). Blockchain-Based Medical Records Secure Storage and Medical Service Framework. *Journal of Medical Systems, 43*(1), 5. Advance online publication. DOI: 10.1007/s10916-018-1121-4 PMID: 30467604

Chenais, G., Gil-Jardiné, C., & Lagarde, E. (2022). *Artificial Intelligence in Emergency Medicine: Viewpoint of Current Applications and Foreseeable Opportunities and Challenges (Preprint)*. Jmir. DOI: 10.2196/preprints.40031

Cross, J. L., Choma, M. A., & Onofrey, J. A. (2024). Bias in medical AI: Implications for clinical decision-making. *PLOS Digital Health, 3*(11), e0000651. DOI: 10.1371/journal.pdig.0000651 PMID: 39509461

Dankolo, N. M., Radzi, N. H. M., Mustaffa, N. H., Arshad, N. I., Nasser, M., Gabi, D., & Yusuf, M. N. (2025). Optimizing resource allocation for IoT applications in the edge cloud continuum using hybrid metaheuristic algorithms. *Scientific Reports, 15*(1), 14409. Advance online publication. DOI: 10.1038/s41598-025-97648-2 PMID: 40274877

Davis, K., & Ruotsalo, T. (2024). *Physiological Data: Challenges for Privacy and Ethics*. https://doi.org//arxiv.2405.15272DOI: 10.48550

Davis Iii, K. M., & Ruotsalo, T. (2025). Physiological Data: Challenges for Privacy and Ethics. *Computer, 58*(1), 33–44. DOI: 10.1109/MC.2024.3404994

Dawson, J. K., Missah, Y. M., Frimpong, T., & Hayfron Acquah, J. B. (2023). Ensuring privacy and confidentiality of cloud data: A comparative analysis of diverse cryptographic solutions based on run time trend. *PLoS One, 18*(9), e0290831. DOI: 10.1371/journal.pone.0290831 PMID: 37676866

Deb, S., Lupu, E., Drakakis, E., Bharath, A., Leung, Z., Ma, G., & Chattopadhyay, A. (2025). *Securing the Internet of Medical Things (IoMT): Real-World Attack Taxonomy and Practical Security Measures*. https://doi.org//arxiv.2507.19609DOI: 10.48550

Dhiman, P., Hamid, Y., Kaur, A., Turaev, S., Nisa, K. U., Gulzar, Y., & Saini, N. (2024). A Review and Comparative Analysis of Relevant Approaches of Zero Trust Network Model. *Sensors (Basel)*, *24*(4), 1328. DOI: 10.3390/s24041328 PMID: 38400486

Dou, T., Zheng, Z., Qiu, W., & Ge, C. (2025). A Secure Medical Data Framework Integrating Blockchain and Edge Computing: An Attribute-Based Signcryption Approach. *Sensors (Basel)*, *25*(9), 2859. DOI: 10.3390/s25092859 PMID: 40363296

Drake, R., & Ridder, E. (2022). *Healthcare Cybersecurity Vulnerabilities*. 49–56. DOI: 10.19107/CYBERCON.2022.06

Elenberg, F., & Howe Iii, E. G. (2020). Ethical Challenges Posed by Big Data. *Innovations in Clinical Neuroscience*, *17*(10–12), 24–30. PMID: 33898098

Elendu, C., Omeludike, E. K., Oloyede, P. O., Obidigbo, B. T., & Omeludike, J. C. (2024). Legal implications for clinicians in cybersecurity incidents. *Revista de Medicina (São Paulo)*, *103*(39), e39887. DOI: 10.1097/MD.0000000000039887 PMID: 39331908

Elmogazy, H., & Bamasag, O. (2016). Securing Healthcare Records in the Cloud Using Attribute-Based Encryption. *Computer and Information Science*, *9*(4), 60. DOI: 10.5539/cis.v9n4p60

Elsayed, Z., Abdelgawad, A., & Elsayed, N. (2025). *Cybersecurity and Frequent Cyber Attacks on IoT Devices in Healthcare: Issues and Solutions*. /arxiv.2501.11250DOI: 10.1109/ICMI65310.2025.11141075

Enahoro, Q., Daraojimba, A., Anyanwu, E., Odilibe, I., Ogugua, J., & Akomolafe, O. (2023). The impact of electronic health records on healthcare delivery and patient outcomes: A review. *World Journal of Advanced Research and Reviews*, *21*(2), 451–460. DOI: 10.30574/wjarr.2024.21.2.0478

Farmer, L., & Lundy, A. (2017). Informed Consent: Ethical and Legal Considerations for Advanced Practice Nurses. *The Journal for Nurse Practitioners*, *13*(2), 124–130. DOI: 10.1016/j.nurpra.2016.08.011

Fedorowicz, J., & Ray, A. W. (2004). Impact of HIPAA on the integrity of healthcare information. *International Journal of Healthcare Technology and Management*, *6*(2), 142. DOI: 10.1504/IJHTM.2004.004954

Feld, A. D. (2005). The Health Insurance Portability and Accountability Act (HIPAA): Its Broad Effect on Practice. *The American Journal of Gastroenterology, 100*(7), 1440–1443. DOI: 10.1111/j.1572-0241.2005.50621.x PMID: 15984962

Ferrag, M., Μαγλαράς, Λ., & Derhab, A. (2019). *Authentication and Authorization for Mobile IoT Devices using Bio-features: Recent Advances and Future Trends*. Cornell University. https://doi.org//arxiv.1901.09374DOI: 10.48550

Francis, L. P. (2014). Genomic knowledge sharing: A review of the ethical and legal issues. *Applied & Translational Genomics, 3*(4), 111–115. DOI: 10.1016/j.atg.2014.09.003 PMID: 27294025

Gabarron, E., Househ, M., Bond, C., Lau, A. Y. S., Mayer, M. A., Hansen, M., Merolli, M., Bamidis, P., & Denecke, K. (2015). Ethical Issues of Social Media Usage in Healthcare. *Yearbook of Medical Informatics, 10*(1), 137–147. DOI: 10.15265/IY-2015-001 PMID: 26293861

Georgiou, D., & Lambrinoudakis, C. (2020). Compatibility of a Security Policy for a Cloud-Based Healthcare System with the EU General Data Protection Regulation (GDPR). *Information (Basel), 11*(12), 586. DOI: 10.3390/info11120586

Ghasemshirazi, S., Shirvani, G., & Alipour, M. (2023). *Zero Trust: Applications, Challenges, and Opportunities*. https://doi.org//arxiv.2309.03582DOI: 10.48550

Gholami, A., & Laure, E. (2015). *Security and Privacy of Sensitive Data in Cloud Computing : A Survey of Recent Developments*. 131–150. DOI: 10.5121/csit.2015.51611

Gholami, A., & Laure, E. (2016). *Security and Privacy of Sensitive Data in Cloud Computing: A Survey of Recent Developments*. https://doi.org//arxiv.1601.01498DOI: 10.48550

Gianfrancesco, M. A., Yazdany, J., Schmajuk, G., & Tamang, S. (2018). Potential Biases in Machine Learning Algorithms Using Electronic Health Record Data. *JAMA Internal Medicine, 178*(11), 1544. DOI: 10.1001/jamainternmed.2018.3763 PMID: 30128552

Griesser, G. (1989). Data protection in health information systems (HIS). *Biomedizinische Technik. Biomedical Engineering. Biomedizinische Technik. Biomedical Engineering, 34*(s1), 16–19. DOI: 10.1515/bmte.1989.34.s1.16 PMID: 2819143

Habibzadeh, H., Sharma, G., Dinesh, K., Soyata, T., Rajabi Shishvan, O., & Boggio-Dandry, A. (2019). A Survey of Healthcare Internet-of-Things (HIoT): A Clinical Perspective. *IEEE Internet of Things Journal, 7*(1), 53–71. DOI: 10.1109/JIOT.2019.2946359 PMID: 33748312

Hughes, A., Shandhi, M. M. H., Master, H., Dunn, J., & Brittain, E. (2023). Wearable Devices in Cardiovascular Medicine. *Circulation Research, 132*(5), 652–670. DOI: 10.1161/CIRCRESAHA.122.322389 PMID: 36862812

Ianculescu, M., Constantin, V.- ., Gu atu, A.-M., Petrache, M.-C., Mihăescu, A.-G., Bica, O., & Alexandru, A. (2025). Enhancing Connected Health Ecosystems Through IoT-Enabled Monitoring Technologies: A Case Study of the Monit4Healthy System. *Sensors (Basel), 25*(7), 2292. DOI: 10.3390/s25072292 PMID: 40218804

Islam, M., & Rahman, M. (2025). *LogStamping: A blockchain-based log auditing approach for large-scale systems*. https://doi.org//arxiv.2505.17236DOI: 10.48550

Isong, B., Kgote, O., & Abu-Mahfouz, A. (2024). Insights into Modern Intrusion Detection Strategies for Internet of Things Ecosystems. *Electronics (Basel), 13*(12), 2370. DOI: 10.3390/electronics13122370

Jackson, N., Woods, J., Watkinson, P., Brent, A., Peto, T. E. A., Walker, A. S., & Eyre, D. W. (2023). The quality of vital signs measurements and value preferences in electronic medical records varies by hospital, specialty, and patient demographics. *Scientific Reports, 13*(1), 3858. Advance online publication. DOI: 10.1038/s41598-023-30691-z PMID: 36890179

Jaflch, E. A., Alnaqbi, F. A., Almaccni, H. A., Faqcch, S., Alzaabi, M. A., & Al Zaman, K. (2024). The Role of Wearable Devices in Chronic Disease Monitoring and Patient Care: A Comprehensive Review. *Cureus, 16*(9). Advance online publication. DOI: 10.7759/cureus.68921 PMID: 39381470

Jiang, L. (2021). IoT Sensors for Smart Health Devices and Data security in Healthcare. *Journal of Biomedical and Sustainable Healthcare Applications*, 105–112. DOI: 10.53759/0088/JBSHA202101013

Jpc Rodrigues, J., De La Torre, I., Fernández, G., & López-Coronado, M. (2013). Analysis of the Security and Privacy Requirements of Cloud-Based Electronic Health Records Systems. *Journal of Medical Internet Research, 15*(8), e186. DOI: 10.2196/jmir.2494 PMID: 23965254

Khan, B., Hussain, J., Hanan, A., Qureshi, A., Abdullah, S., Kumar, S., & Fatima, H. (2023). Drawbacks of Artificial Intelligence and Their Potential Solutions in the Healthcare Sector. *Biomedical Materials &amp. Biomedical Materials & Devices, 1*(2), 731–738. DOI: 10.1007/s44174-023-00063-2 PMID: 36785697

Kim, J. W., Moon, S.-M., Jang, B., & Kang, S.-U. (2020). Effective Privacy-Preserving Collection of Health Data from a User's Wearable Device. *Applied Sciences (Basel, Switzerland), 10*(18), 6396. DOI: 10.3390/app10186396

Kim, W., & Choi, J. (2016). Challenges for wearable healthcare services. *International Journal of Web and Grid Services*, *12*(4), 407. DOI: 10.1504/IJWGS.2016.080141

Klymenko, O., Meisenbacher, S., & Matthes, F. (2023). *Identifying Practical Challenges in the Implementation of Technical Measures for Data Privacy Compliance.* https://doi.org//arxiv.2306.15497DOI: 10.48550

Kruse, C. S., Frederick, B., Jacobson, T., & Monticone, D. K. (2017). Cybersecurity in healthcare: A systematic review of modern threats and trends. *Technology and Health Care*, *25*(1), 1–10. DOI: 10.3233/THC-161263 PMID: 27689562

Kuo, A. M.-H. (2011). Opportunities and Challenges of Cloud Computing to Improve Health Care Services. *Journal of Medical Internet Research*, *13*(3), e67. DOI: 10.2196/jmir.1867 PMID: 21937354

Lamptey, M., & Zhou, G. (2020). Survey of Data Confidentiality and Privacy in the Cloud Computing Environment. *Computer Engineering and Intelligent Systems*, *11*(5). Advance online publication. DOI: 10.7176/CEIS/11-5-03

Li, D. M., Parikh, S., & Costa, A. (2025). A critical look into artificial intelligence and healthcare disparities. *Frontiers in Artificial Intelligence*, *8*, 1545869. Advance online publication. DOI: 10.3389/frai.2025.1545869 PMID: 40115119

Liu, G., Xie, H., Wang, W., & Huang, H. (2024). A secure and efficient electronic medical record data sharing scheme based on blockchain and proxy re-encryption. *Journal of Cloud Computing (Heidelberg, Germany)*, *13*(1), 44. Advance online publication. DOI: 10.1186/s13677-024-00608-w

Liu, N., & Chen, S. (2022). The Protection Mechanism of Personal Health Information in the Digital Economy Environment. *Journal of Environmental and Public Health*, *2022*(10), 1–17. DOI: 10.1155/2022/2314468 PMID: 35733982

Liu, X., Shah, R., Shandilya, A., Shah, M., & Pandya, A. (2024). A systematic study on integrating blockchain in healthcare for electronic health record management and tracking medical supplies. *Journal of Cleaner Production*, *447*, 141371. DOI: 10.1016/j.jclepro.2024.141371

Lopes, , A. P., & Gondim, P. R. L. (2020). Mutual Authentication Protocol for D2D Communications in a Cloud-Based E-Health System. *Sensors (Basel)*, *20*(7), 2072. DOI: 10.3390/s20072072 PMID: 32272675

Loyka, K., Zhou, H., & Khatri, S. P. (2018). *A Homomorphic Encryption Scheme Based on Affine Transforms*. 51–56. DOI: 10.1145/3194554.3194585

Macedo, E. L. C., De Rezende, J. F., Delicato, F. C., De Oliveira, E. A. R., Silva, F. H., Mello, R. R., Franca, F. M. G., & De Moraes, L. F. M. (2019). On the security aspects of Internet of Things: A systematic literature review. *Journal of Communications and Networks (Seoul), 21*(5), 444–457. DOI: 10.1109/JCN.2019.000048

Machal, M. L. (2023). *An Overview About Connected Medical Devices and Their Risks*. Institut F R Ost Und S Dosteuropaforschung., DOI: 10.3233/SHTI230438

Madanian, S., Airehrour, D., Subasinghage, M., Chinbat, T., Yongchareon, S., & Hassandoust, F. (2024). Health IoT Threats: Survey of Risks and Vulnerabilities. *Future Internet, 16*(11), 389. DOI: 10.3390/fi16110389

Mamdiwar, S. D., & Srinivasan, K. (2021). Recent Advances on IoT-Assisted Wearable Sensor Systems for Healthcare Monitoring. *Biosensors (Basel), 11*(10), 372. DOI: 10.3390/bios11100372 PMID: 34677328

Mandarino, V., Pappalardo, G., & Tramontana, E. (2024). A Blockchain-Based Electronic Health Record (EHR) System for Edge Computing Enhancing Security and Cost Efficiency. *Computers, 13*(6), 132. DOI: 10.3390/computers13060132

Marko, J. G. O., Neagu, C. D., & Anand, P. B. (2025). Examining inclusivity: the use of AI and diverse populations in health and social care: a systematic review. *BMC Medical Informatics and Decision Making, 25*(1), 57. Advance online publication. DOI: 10.1186/s12911-025-02884-1 PMID: 39910518

Meisami, S., Meisami, S., Yousefi, M., & Aref, M. (2023). *Combining Blockchain and IOT for Decentralized Healthcare Data Management*. https://doi.org//arxiv.2304.00127DOI: 10.48550

Mennella, C., Maniscalco, U., De Pietro, G., & Esposito, M. (2024). Ethical and regulatory challenges of AI technologies in healthcare: A narrative review. *Heliyon, 10*(4), e26297. DOI: 10.1016/j.heliyon.2024.e26297 PMID: 38384518

Mittelstadt, B. (2019). The Ethics of Biomedical 'Big Data' Analytics. *Philosophy &amp. Philosophy & Technology, 32*(1), 17–21. DOI: 10.1007/s13347-019-00344-z

Mittelstadt, B. D., & Floridi, L. (2015). The Ethics of Big Data: Current and Foreseeable Issues in Biomedical Contexts. *Science and Engineering Ethics, 22*(2), 303–341. DOI: 10.1007/s11948-015-9652-2 PMID: 26002496

Mone, V., & Shakhlo, F. (2023). Health Data on the Go: Navigating Privacy Concerns with Wearable Technologies. *Legal Information Management, 23*(3), 179–188. DOI: 10.1017/S1472669623000427

Nasir, M., Siddiqui, K., & Ahmed, S. (2025). Ethical-legal implications of AI-powered healthcare in critical perspective. *Frontiers in Artificial Intelligence*, *8*, 1619463. Advance online publication. DOI: 10.3389/frai.2025.1619463 PMID: 40673212

Nazer, L. H., Ma, H., Mathur, P., Khanna, A. K., Zatarah, R., Moukheiber, L., Moukheiber, M., Moukheiber, D., Hicklen, R. S., Waldrip, S., & Ke, J. X. C. (2023). Bias in artificial intelligence algorithms and recommendations for mitigation. *PLOS Digital Health*, *2*(6), e0000278. DOI: 10.1371/journal.pdig.0000278 PMID: 37347721

Odeh, A., Abdelfattah, E., & Salameh, W. (2024). Privacy-Preserving Data Sharing in Telehealth Services. *Applied Sciences (Basel, Switzerland)*, *14*(23), 10808. DOI: 10.3390/app142310808

Padmapriya, S. T., & Parthasarathy, S. (2023). Ethical Data Collection for Medical Image Analysis: A Structured Approach. *Asian Bioethics Review*, *16*(1), 95–108. DOI: 10.1007/s41649-023-00250-9 PMID: 37361687

Panch, T., Mattie, H., & Atun, R. (2019). Artificial intelligence and algorithmic bias: Implications for health systems. *Journal of Global Health*, *9*(2), 010318. Advance online publication. DOI: 10.7189/jogh.09.020318 PMID: 31788229

Perets, O., Stagno, E., Yehuda, E. B., Mcnichol, M., Anthony Celi, L., Rappoport, N., & Dorotic, M. (2024). Inherent Bias in Electronic Health Records: A Scoping Review of Sources of Bias. In medRxiv *: the preprint server for health sciences*. Cold Spring Harbor Laboratory. DOI: 10.1101/2024.04.09.24305594

Perry, H., Tsai, E. M., Perusse, K., Herschorn, S. D., & Watson, E. J. (2022). Breast Imaging During a Cyberattack and Global Pandemic: What We Did to Pick Up the Pieces. *Seminars in Ultrasound. Seminars in Ultrasound, CT, and MR*, *44*(1), 18–22. DOI: 10.1053/j.sult.2022.10.001 PMID: 36792269

Podder, P., Mondal, M. R. H., Bharati, S., & Paul, P. K. (2020). Review on the Security Threats of Internet of Things. *International Journal of Computer Applications*, *176*(41), 37–45. DOI: 10.5120/ijca2020920548

Pokharel, B. P., Paudel, S., Kshetri, N., & Sharma, S. R. (2025). blockHealthSecure: Integrating Blockchain and Cybersecurity in Post-Pandemic Healthcare Systems. *Information (Basel)*, *16*(2), 133. DOI: 10.3390/info16020133

Popoola, O., Rodrigues, M. A., Marchang, J., Shenfield, A., Ikpehai, A., & Popoola, J. (2024). An optimized hybrid encryption framework for smart home healthcare: Ensuring data confidentiality and security. *Internet of Things : Engineering Cyber Physical Human Systems*, *27*, 101314. DOI: 10.1016/j.iot.2024.101314

Portela, D., Almeida, R., Nogueira-Leite, D., & Cruz-Correia, R. (2022). *Economic Impact of a Hospital Cyberattack in a National Health System: Descriptive Case Study (Preprint)*. Jmir. DOI: 10.2196/preprints.41738

Price, W. N.II, & Cohen, I. G. (2019). Privacy in the age of medical big data. *Nature Medicine, 25*(1), 37–43. DOI: 10.1038/s41591-018-0272-7 PMID: 30617331

Ramezanpour, K., & Jagannath, J. (2022). Intelligent zero trust architecture for 5G/6G networks: Principles, challenges, and the role of machine learning in the context of O-RAN. *Computer Networks, 217*, 109358. DOI: 10.1016/j.comnet.2022.109358

Reddy, S., Cooper, P., Allan, S., & Coghlan, S. (2019). A governance model for the application of AI in health care. *Journal of the American Medical Informatics Association : JAMIA, 27*(3), 491–497. DOI: 10.1093/jamia/ocz192 PMID: 31682262

Reis, O., Abrahams, T., Ehimuan, B., Olorunsogo, T., Eneh, N., & Anyanwu, A. (2024). PRIVACY LAW CHALLENGES IN THE DIGITAL AGE: A GLOBAL REVIEW OF LEGISLATION AND ENFORCEMENT. *International Journal of Applied Research in Social Sciences, 6*(1), 73–88. DOI: 10.51594/ijarss.v6i1.733

Rhayha, R., El Ouali Lalami, A., El Malki, H., Merabti, A., El Hilaly, J., Mahla, T., Bahli, B., & Alaoui Ismaili, A. (2025). Factors influencing clinician performance post-electronic health record implementation: An empirical analysis in Moroccan hospitals. *BMC Health Services Research, 25*(1), 324. Advance online publication. DOI: 10.1186/s12913-025-12438-w PMID: 40016779

Richter, S., & Ammenwerth, E. (2023). IT risk management for medical devices in hospital IT networks: A catalogue of measures and indicators. *BMJ Health & Care Informatics, 30*(1), e100639. DOI: 10.1136/bmjhci-2022-100639 PMID: 36724909

Rocchiccioli, J. (2003). Health Insurance Portability and Accountability Act: Administrative Simplification to Understand the Revised Proposed Privacy Standards—A Policy Update. *The Journal of the Association of Nurses in AIDS Care: JANAC, 14*(2), 63–66. DOI: 10.1177/1055329002251000 PMID: 12698767

Rogers, J., Someya, T., & Malliaras, G. (2018). Biomedical devices go wild. *Science Advances, 4*(9), eaav1889. Advance online publication. DOI: 10.1126/sciadv.aav1889 PMID: 30255157

Rony, M. K. K., Akter, F., Tushar, H., Johra, F. T., Numan, S. M., Akter, K., Mondal, S., Parvin, M. R., Uddin, M. J., Das, M., Debnath, M., & Begum, J. (2024). Nurses' perspectives on privacy and ethical concerns regarding artificial intelligence adoption in healthcare. *Heliyon, 10*(17), e36702. DOI: 10.1016/j.heliyon.2024.e36702 PMID: 39281626

S, M., & K R, J. (2025). Blockchain-enabled federated learning with edge analytics for secure and efficient electronic health records management. *Scientific Reports, 15*(1). DOI: 10.1038/s41598-025-12225-x

Seh, A. H., Zarour, M., Alenezi, M., Sarkar, A. K., Agrawal, A., Kumar, R., & Ahmad Khan, R. (2020). Healthcare Data Breaches: Insights and Implications. *Health Care, 8*(2), 133. DOI: 10.3390/healthcare8020133 PMID: 32414183

Seth, D., Ranjan, P., & Najana, M. (2024). Compliance and Regulatory Challenges in Cloud Computing: A Sector-Wise Analysis. *International Journal of Global Innovations and Solutions (IJGIS)*. DOI: 10.21428/e90189c8.68b5dea5

Shaikh, J. A., Wang, C., Muhammad, W. U. S., Arshad, M., Owais, M., Alnashwan, R. O., Chelloug, S. A., & Muthanna, M. S. A. (2024). RCLNet: An effective anomaly-based intrusion detection for securing the IoMT system. *Frontiers in Digital Health, 6*, 1467241. Advance online publication. DOI: 10.3389/fdgth.2024.1467241 PMID: 39421756

Shaikh, J. A., Wang, C., Sima, M. W. U., Arshad, M., Owais, M., Hassan, D. S. M., Alkanhel, R., & Muthanna, M. S. A. (2025). A deep Reinforcement learning-based robust Intrusion Detection System for securing IoMT Healthcare Networks. *Frontiers in Medicine, 12*, 1524286. Advance online publication. DOI: 10.3389/fmed.2025.1524286 PMID: 40309737

Shi, Y. (2018). *Data Security and Privacy Protection Data Security and Privacy Protection in Public Cloud*. https://doi.org//arxiv.1812.05745DOI: 10.48550

Siddiqi, M. A., Doerr, C., & Strydis, C. (2020). IMDfence: Architecting a Secure Protocol for Implantable Medical Devices. *IEEE Access : Practical Innovations, Open Solutions, 8*, 147948–147964. DOI: 10.1109/ACCESS.2020.3015686

Subhani, M., & Anjum, A. (2020). *Multiclass Disease Predictions Based on Integrated Clinical and Genomics Datasets*. https://doi.org//arxiv.2006.07879DOI: 10.48550

Tahir, N. U. A., Alshara, M. A., Javed, Y., Cao, Y., Rashid, U., Ahmad, N., & Hadi, H. J. (2024). Blockchain-Based Healthcare Records Management Framework: Enhancing Security, Privacy, and Interoperability. *Technologies, 12*(9), 168. DOI: 10.3390/technologies12090168

Tao, Q., Liu, S., Zhang, J., Jiang, J., Jin, Z., Huang, Y., Liu, X., Lin, S., Zeng, X., Li, X., Tao, G., & Chen, H. (2023). Clinical applications of smart wearable sensors. *iScience, 26*(9), 107485. DOI: 10.1016/j.isci.2023.107485 PMID: 37636055

Thapa, C., & Camtepe, S. (2020a). Precision health data: Requirements, challenges and existing techniques for data security and privacy. *Computers in Biology and Medicine, 129*, 104130. DOI: 10.1016/j.compbiomed.2020.104130 PMID: 33271399

Thapa, C., & Camtepe, S. (2020b). *Precision Health Data: Requirements, Challenges and Existing Techniques for Data Security and Privacy*. https://doi.org//arxiv.2008.10733DOI: 10.48550

Tong, Y., Li, P., Sun, J., & Chow, S. S. M. (2013, October 1). *Towards auditable cloud-assisted access of encrypted health data*. DOI: 10.1109/CNS.2013.6682769

Topcu, A., Tomar, N., Demir, U., Zhang, Z., Keles, E., Jha, D., Håakegård, J., Yazidi, A., Hagos, D., Srivastava, A., Sharma, V., Rauniyar, A., & Bagci, U. (2023). *Ensuring Trustworthy Medical Artificial Intelligence through Ethical and Philosophical Principles*. https://doi.org//arxiv.2304.11530DOI: 10.48550

Torre, D., Sabetzadeh, M., Soltana, G., Alférez, M., & Briand, L. (2020). *Model Driven Engineering for Data Protection and Privacy: Application and Experience with GDPR*. Cornell University. https://doi.org//arxiv.2007.12046DOI: 10.48550

Udendhran, R. (2017). *A hybrid approach to enhance data security in cloud storage*. 1–6. DOI: 10.1145/3018896.3025138

Uygun Ilikhan, S., Özer, M., Tanberkan, H., & Bozkurt, V. (2024). How to mitigate the risks of deployment of artificial intelligence in medicine? *Turkish Journal of Medical Sciences, 54*(3), 483–492. DOI: 10.55730/1300-0144.5814 PMID: 39050000

Vayena, E., Brownstein, J. S., Dzenowagis, J., & Sheikh, A. (2017). Policy implications of big data in the health sector. *Bulletin of the World Health Organization, 96*(1), 66–68. DOI: 10.2471/BLT.17.197426 PMID: 29403102

Wan, J., O'Grady, M., Cao, N., Li, M., & Al-Awlaqi, A A H. (2018). M., Gu, X., & Wang, J. (2018). Wearable IoT enabled real-time health monitoring system. *EURASIP Journal on Wireless Communications and Networking*, (1). Advance online publication. DOI: 10.1186/s13638-018-1308-x

Williams, M. S., Taylor, C. O., Walton, N. A., Goehringer, S. R., Aronson, S., Freimuth, R. R., Rasmussen, L. V., Hall, E. S., Prows, C. A., Chung, W. K., Fedotov, A., Nestor, J., Weng, C., Rowley, R. K., Wiesner, G. L., Jarvik, G. P., & Del Fiol, G. (2019). Genomic Information for Clinicians in the Electronic Health Record: Lessons Learned From the Clinical Genome Resource Project and the Electronic Medical Records and Genomics Network. *Frontiers in Genetics, 10*(146), 1059. DOI: 10.3389/fgene.2019.01059 PMID: 31737042

Williams, P., & Woodward, A. (2015). Cybersecurity vulnerabilities in medical devices: A complex environment and multifaceted problem. *Medical Devices (Auckland, N.Z.)*, *8*(10), 305. DOI: 10.2147/MDER.S50048 PMID: 26229513

Xu, S., Rogers, J. A., Ghaffari, R., Walter, J. R., & Kim, J. (2022). Translational gaps and opportunities for medical wearables in digital health. *Science Translational Medicine*, *14*(666), eabn6036. Advance online publication. DOI: 10.1126/scitranslmed.abn6036 PMID: 36223451

Yeng, P. K., Fauzi, M. A., Sun, L., & Yang, B. (2022). Assessing the Legal Aspects of Information Security Requirements for Health Care in 3 Countries: Scoping Review and Framework Development. *JMIR Human Factors*, *9*(2), e30050. DOI: 10.2196/30050 PMID: 35612891

Yeole, A., & Kalbande, D. R. (2021). *Ensuring Security and Privacy in IoT for Healthcare Applications*. 299–314. DOI: 10.1002/9781119711308.ch11

Ziwei, H., Dongni, Z., Man, Z., Yixin, D., Shuanghui, Z., Chao, Y., & Chunfeng, C. (2024). The applications of internet of things in smart healthcare sectors: A bibliometric and deep study. *Heliyon*, *10*(3), e25392. DOI: 10.1016/j.heliyon.2024.e25392 PMID: 38356528

Zobaed, S., & Salehi, M. (2023). *Confidential Computing across Edge-to-Cloud for Machine Learning: A Survey Study*. https://doi.org//arxiv.2307.16447DOI: 10.48550

Zwitter, A. (2014). Big Data ethics. *Big Data &amp. Big Data & Society*, *1*(2), 205395171455925. DOI: 10.1177/2053951714559253

Chapter 4
Lessons From Real-World Data Breaches in Healthcare:
Toward Stronger Digital Safeguards

Indumathi Srinivasan
https://orcid.org/0009-0009-6035-471X
Saveetha School of Management, India & Saveetha Institute of Medical and Technical Sciences, India

A. K. Subramani
https://orcid.org/0000-0003-0783-7113
Saveetha School of Management, India & Saveetha Institute of Medical and Technical Sciences, India

ABSTRACT

The expeditious digitization of healthcare has intended to enhance service delivery, operational efficacy, and patient involvement. Also, it suffers from unprecedented cybersecurity limitations. Data breaches in healthcare industry are considered to be regulatory indicators of insufficient knowledge, systematic inadequacies, and developing threat landscapes. This chapter explores real-time data breaches from a multidisciplinary lens, emphasizing institutional education, digital ethics, and policy reform. Under the application of six intensive case studies from Anthem to Medibankit examines how breaches evolved, what went wrong, and how they can be prevented. As a result, a brief resilience framework has been developed, helping

DOI: 10.4018/979-8-3373-4918-3.ch004

healthcare firms towards a human-based digital ecosystem. Recommendations are deployed for providers, policymakers, technical developers, and scholars to arrange cyber-security principle with patient security, belief, and dignity.

1. INTRODUCTION

In ancient times, information is one of the major aspects of modern healthcare systems. From medical decision-making to population health monitoring, digital data and inter-linked industries have been changed the way of delivered, estimated, and financed. However, some of the models activate this transformation are highly under siege. Globally, healthcare firms have been suffering from a surge in data breaches, ransomware outbreaks, as well as cyber-intrusions which affects data security and patient trust.

This technical deployment and increasing vulnerability has been considered as one of the common problem in digital health. According to U.S. Department of Health and Human Services (2023), more than 700 records were reported breaches in 2022; as a result it has impacted over 50 million peoples. Consequently, the survey of this incident is outstanding, and results are far-reaching: financial loss, operational interruption, reputational disruption, and at times, physical illness could be developed to patients because of delayed medical examination (Choi et al., 2019; McLeod & Dolezel, 2018).

In contrast to breaches in other fields, medical data breaches mostly involves in highly sensitive and longitudinal data which cannot be modified or revoked like healthcare details, genetic information, as well as mental health data. This enhancement makes medical data highly valid on black market and particularly while it is exposed for any virtual damage (Ozair et al., 2015). Despite of this high validity, healthcare has been suffering from various other factors like cyber-security preparedness (Martin et al., 2017).

This chapter intends to show the space involved when a data breach has been examined as isolated as feature, but as systemic assaults with legal, ethical, operational, and technological directions. Instead of concentrating on technical factors of breaches, it applies a brief-cased model. In addition, it tracks the how this method has been applied in real-time applications as unfolded, what are the vulnerabilities has been exploited, and what broader lessons could be retrieved for institutional resilience and welfare.

Key questions addressed in this chapter include:

- What are the major aspects involved in medical data breaches?

- How the academic institutions have replied, and what challenges are evolved while retrieving the data?
- What policy, governance, and human aspects are involved in breach prevention?
- How can healthcare models adopt effective digital securities with unauthorized features and new evolution?

In this chapter, examination of various case studies and thematic reviews has intended to show academic discourse as well as the real time modification of healthcare breaching. Also, it is considered to be an alarm for healthcare professionals, examiners, technicians, and medical representatives to transform cyber-security not only as a technological input, but also as a major aspect of ethical, patient-based care.

2. THE EXPANDING DIGITAL SURFACE IN HEALTHCARE

Recently, digital transformation of healthcare has made a drastic change in some of the elements like precision, personalization as well as patient empowerment. Electronic Health Records (EHRs), telemedicine industries, mobile health apps, portable devices, cloud-based analysis, and Internet of Medical Things (IoMT) has re-modified the boundaries of clinical delivery. But, these developments have made a digital expansion in digital attack surface as tedious, inter-linked endpoints, databases, and networks where more number of cybercriminals exist.

2.1 The Acceleration of Digital Adoption

Before the pandemic period (COVID-19), digital transformation in healthcare has been progressed by incentives like Health Information Technology for Economic and Clinical Health (HITECH) Act present in U.S. and some of the relevant reforms around the world (Adler-Milstein & Jha, 2017). Unfortunately, Covid-19 was one of the deadliest parts where it enforced the medical systems to work in over time. Under the application of Telehealth, US has surged from less than 1% of outpatient presence in 2019 to around 50% at the time of pandemic (Koonin et al., 2020). Globally, healthcare leaders have developed convolutional digital architecture with maximal pressure and focus in speed when compared to security.

This immense pressure gas intended to spread application of video conferencing devices, cloud storage, mobile data access, as well as digital communication broadcasts without effective vetting processes. Consequently, many of the hospitals have become more vulnerable with unauthorized remote access points, disrupted databases, as well as expired protocols to be followed by medical systems (Alshamrani et al., 2021).

2.2 Growth of Cloud-Based Systems and IoMT

In general, Cloud computing is one of the commonly used technology which is considered to be integral portion for new era of healthcare structure, which is capable to provide scalability, cost effective, and data sharing facilities. But, most of the providers have poor knowledge in developing secure cloud platforms, which may result breaches, which is also because of public-based storage buckets, vulnerable access points, and lost encryption modules (Zhou et al., 2019). In addition, third-party vendors try to use these services where it may have stringent healthcare-based standards such as HIPAA or GDPR.

The emergence of Internet of Medical Things (IoMT) like infusion pumps, modern monitors, and inter-linked diagnostic tools has developed the threat landscape globally. Maximum tools are working on legacy firmware or older operating systems, which would make them delicate and leads to ransomware attacks (Radanliev et al., 2020). In contrast to classical IT models, connecting or changing clinical tools is highly difficult because of regulatory obstacles, operational attacks, or proprietary software conflicts.

2.3 Bring Your Own Device (BYOD) and Mobile Health

The evolution of mobile health (mHealth) as well as Bring Your Own Device (BYOD) applications aims in improving patient involvement for treatment and medical flexibility. Unnecessary usage of mobile phones, tablets, and laptops tends to enhance the vulnerability of withdrawing sensitive data from medical records (McLeod & Dolezel, 2018). A study done by the Ponemon Institute (2022) has stated that, over 68% of medical IT officers have raised a complaint regarding information leakage from mobile device illegally without their own concern.

In general, mHealth application is employed to accumulate and save information with minimum security and some of them are subjected to similar regulatory oversight as formal health modules. Also, these frameworks are mostly applied to transfer data to third parties for data analytics or data marketing, amplify risks to patient integrity (Dehling et al., 2015). Hence, this problem is been expanded in low-resource settings, while informal digital devices replace formal structure.

2.4 Fragmentation and Integration Challenges

Healthcare ecosystems are highly considered as tedious, decentralized systems which include clinics, hospitals, medical insurers, laboratory, pharmacies, and third-party professionals. Inter-connecting these vendors using Health Information Exchanges (HIEs) or Application Programming Interfaces (APIs) is considered to be one of the important processes at care coordination, however it is ensured to suffer with few challenges when interoperability is considered as supreme when compared to security.

For instance, weakly secured APIs are highly prone to provide data to unauthorized users. A survey at 2021 has stated that around 30% of APIs in medical apps are poor because of ineffective security or poor data masking (Kritikos et al., 2021). Such technological problems can be resolved by organizational silos, in which IT, agreement, and medical departments should be functioned independently, delayed response to cyber incidents.

2.5 Lack of Proportional Cybersecurity Investment

Even though the digital surge is applied, the financial state of cybersecurity in healthcare is still considered to be lower. Basically, medical firms afford less than 6% of their IT budgets on security, when compared to 10–15% in the financial industries (HHS, 2023). Small and medium-sized schemes, especially, it is very hard to allocate resources for cybersecurity devices, audits, and to train the employees.

As a result, it provides a unauthenticated data retrieval. A 2023 HIMSS survey has reported that over 60% of healthcare cybersecurity officers trusted that there are minimum budget to meet the fundamental security standards. Most of the organizations prefer to work at traditional networks because of minimal cost, despite of well-documented vulnerabilities (Alotaibi & Federico, 2017).

Table 1. Common Digital Transformation Drivers and Their Associated Cybersecurity Risks

Digital Transformation Component	Description	Primary Cybersecurity Risks
Electronic Health Records (EHR)	Centralized digital patient records	Unauthorized access, misconfigured authority
Telemedicine Platforms	Remote consultations and monitoring	Weak authentication, unencrypted communications
Cloud Storage and Services	Scalable data hosting and analytics	Insecure cloud configurations, vendor risk
IoMT Devices	Network-connected medical equipment	Firmware vulnerabilities, lack of updates
mHealth Apps and BYOD	Patient and clinician mobile tools	Data leakage, weak app security, device theft
Health APIs and HIEs	System-to-system data exchange	API exposure, interoperability over security

Sources: Dehling et al. (2015); Radanliev et al. (2020); HIMSS (2023); Ponemon Institute (2022)

Here, the digital acceleration in medical fields —while beneficial—is not mapping with proportional advances in cybersecurity performance. The upcoming section will transform focus to real-time data breaches, which implies how such vulnerabilities are exploited and the consequences applied.

3. ANATOMY OF REAL-WORLD HEALTHCARE DATA BREACHES

Learning healthcare data breaches needs data security when compared to technical scrutiny—it also requires a holistic review of how institutional weakness, manual behaviors, and governance failures link with developing cyber threats. This section rebuilds the anatomy of breaches by examining the models used by cyber-criminals, the criteria applied for diverse incidents, as well as the regulatory vulnerabilities which lead to exploitation.

3.1 Common Breach Vectors in Healthcare

Here, diverse models have been applied in healthcare breaching; however there are few constraints involved with alarming consistency. Based on the statement of Verizon Data Breach Investigations Report (DBIR, 2023), the commonly used breach vectors in healthcare are:

- **Phishing and Social Engineering Attacks**

In order to acquire the system accessibility, cyber criminals often exploit manual behaviour. Phishing emails is one of the generalized method used in masquerading legitimate communications—and trigger the users to reveal secret credentials or download them in an illegal manner. In most of the reported cases, phishing is considered to be initial access vector (IBM, 2023).

- **Ransomware**

Ransomware is highly a disruptive type of attack. It is defined as malicious software where data encryption take place and make them inaccessible unless a ransom is paid. Healthcare industries are subsequent targets because of maximum range as well as emergency of patient information (Coventry & Branley, 2018).

- **Exploitation of Unpatched Systems**

Most of the healthcare firms make use of classical software networks. Also, attackers exploit well-known liabilities in legacy structure and apply computerized devices for scanning infiltrate such vulnerabilities (Martin et al., 2017).

- **Third-Party and Vendor Compromise**

External service providers like billing firms, cloud storage vendors, or clinical tools manufacturers, often holds system access but vulnerable security criteria. Most of the high-profile breaches, cyber-criminals might gain the access through via third-party networks (Ponemon Institute, 2022).

- **Insider Threats and Misuse**

Staffs having authentic access might compromise data without their concern. Followed by, insider threats like unauthenticated access, interfering in medical records, or falling attacker to phishing which implies internal credentials (Choi et al., 2019).

3.2 Breach Impact Typology

Healthcare data breaches vary based on few criteria including, scale, intent, and final result. The following typology categories breaches which is relied on impact and inspiration:

Table 2. Breach Impact Typology

Breach Type	Description	Examples
Opportunistic Attacks	Randomly targeted, often automated, attacks looking for known vulnerabilities	WannaCry (2017)
Targeted Attacks	Deliberate efforts to access specific institutions or individuals	SingHealth (2018)
Financially Motivated	Attacks aimed at selling data or demanding ransom	Medibank (2022), Vastaamo (2020)
Political/Espionage	State-sponsored actors targeting high-value data for geopolitical reasons	SingHealth (2018), Anthem (2015)
Insider Breaches	Caused by negligent or malicious employees	Numerous local hospital incidents

Sources: DBIR (2023); IBM (2023); Choi et al. (2019)

3.3 The Human Element: Weakest Link or Greatest Defense?

Even under enormous financial support for cyber-security models, human mistakes are still considered to be a major reason for breaches. Frail passwords, reused identities, and failure to find phishing attempts have been registered as major incidents (Ponemon Institute, 2022).

For instance:

- In case of Anthem breach (2015), attackers have employed spear-phishing emails to withdraw administrator passwords and secured information.
- In the Vastaamo case (2020), weaker access control as well as unencrypted databases has implied mental health data to public blackmail.

Employee training is a complicated task where it is defined to be a frontline defense process. However, many medical firms do not offer compulsory, role-centered cyber-security awareness (Martin et al., 2017).

3.4 Institutional Blind Spots

A framework over breach case studies are defined as lack of well-documented incident response protocols. Even well-refined health models often lack at the following factors:

- **Real-time breach prediction mechanisms**
- **Clear lines of communication during crises**
- **Legal and psychological preparedness for patient disclosures**
- **Post-incident analysis and systemic reform**

For instance, the University of Vermont Medical Center (2020) has inadequate isolated backup network, which delays the data recovery from a ransomware attack for prolonged duration. Additionally, hospitals were enforced to offer the medical history paper-based systems, that delays medical examination and lower patient trust (HHS, 2023).

3.5 Breach Disclosure and Accountability Gaps

In most of the reported cases, data breach notification ethics are considered to be non-existent, or weakly enforced. Only few industries provide late response to prevent the reputational harm or regulatory penalties which leaves patients information illegally.

For instance, the Medibank (2022) breach in Australia tends outrage when it was known that sensitive reproductive health and dependent information were used in prior before it was revealed to public forum (Australian Cyber Security Centre, 2023). But, this delay has reduced emotional impact and degraded the trust of an institution.

Figure 1. Typical Healthcare Breach Lifecycle

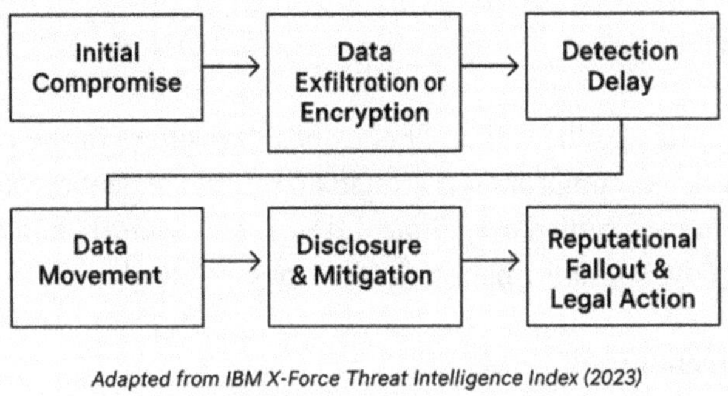

3.6 Compounding Effects in Healthcare

What differentiates healthcare breaches from these sectors from **compounding effect**:

- **Clinical Disruption** – Surgery ignorance, missed treatment, and ER closures
- **Ethical Harm** – Violation of patient respect and confidentiality
- **Legal Liability** – Lawsuits and regulatory platforms
- **Public Distrust** – prolonged degradation of institutional trust

The combination of personal damage, public disclosure, as well as digital exposure tends to make healthcare breaches highly susceptible.

Followed by, healthcare data breaches adopt familiar patterns which are intended to develop regulatory weaknesses: minimal investment, insufficient educational awareness, third-party interference, as well as lack of maintenance. Such vulnerabilities tend to explore **real-time breach case studies**, where it provides particular awareness for better improvement.

4. CASE STUDIES OF MAJOR HEALTHCARE DATA BREACHES

In order to transform generalizations and abstract risks, this section exhibits six real-time case studies of healthcare data breaches. In every single study, it implies diverse fact of systemic weakness, from technical space and manual mistakes to ethical catastrophes and geopolitical failures. Moreover, a brief, manual-based cyber-security principle in healthcare is essential globally.

4.1 Anthem (2015) – A Wake-Up Call for Insurance Giants

Incident Overview:

In February 2015, Anthem Inc., famous health insurers in the U.S., has stated that a cyber-attack has compromised around 80 million patient records. The breach records include names, birth dates, clinical IDs, Social Security numbers, residence details, and employment information (Office for Civil Rights, 2016).

Breach Mechanics:

Attackers have applied spear-phishing emails to provide authority to the credentials of a healthcare system leader. Followed by, they have performed undefined data extraction from unencrypted databases (Choi et al., 2019).

Key Vulnerabilities:

- Absence of multi-factor authorization
- Lack of encrypting significant information
- Non-feasible intrusion prediction

Consequences:

- $115 million class-action settlement (maximum number in healthcare history)
- Major degradation as well as customer dissatisfaction
- Regulatory scrutiny by U.S. Department of Health and Human Services (HHS)

Lesson Learned:

Well-equipped attackers exploit fundamental security oversights. Mostly, sensitive information should not be unencrypted, and proper authentication has to be tailored and protected with multi-factor authorization.

4.2 NHS & WannaCry (2017) – Legacy System Vulnerabilities

Incident Overview:

The WannaCry ransomware outbreak in May 2017 impacted around 200,000 systems more than 150 countries. Additionally, UK's National Health Service (NHS) was one of the hardest hit, with around 80 hospitals that was impacted including cancelled surgeries, rerouted ambulances (Department of Health, 2018).

Breach Mechanics:

The ransomware leveraged EternalBlue exploit—weaker device in traditional Microsoft systems. Most of the NHS skipped the process of using a critical security patch which was invented by Microsoft (Martin et al., 2017).

Key Vulnerabilities:

- Application of classical operating systems (Windows XP)
- Insufficient timely patch management
- Lack of effective backup as well as isolation frameworks

Consequences:

- Improper functioning of hospitals for prolonged duration
- Around £92 million disruptions (UK Parliament, 2018)
- Public outcry and parliamentary inquiry

Lesson Learned:

Cybersecurity hygiene like time to time updates as well as patching is considered to be a major aspect. Even well-trained systems become weaker when legacy technique is undefended.

4.3 SingHealth (2018) – A National Security Threat

Incident Overview:

Between the period of June–July 2018, Singapore's largest healthcare firm, SingHealth, has gone through a cyberattack which had lost sensible information of 1.5 million patients. Even, Prime Minister Lee Hsien Loong, medical record has been lost, which was the main aim of attackers to retrieve (Singapore Ministry of Health, 2018).

Breach Mechanics:

The cyber-criminals infiltrated the system through a front-end workstation and attained privileged access via vulnerable segmentation as well as credential management. Hence, breach was concerned to be state-sponsored.

Key Vulnerabilities:

- Lack of network segmentation
- Inadequate access controls
- Vulnerable breach prediction

Consequences:

- National cyber-security examination and reforms
- Compulsory breach reporting laws introduced
- High investment in national digital health resilience

Lesson Learned:

Even technically enhanced systems become ineffective. Political targeting increases the stakes and demands for national-level response for digital health threats.

4.4 University of Vermont Medical Center (2020) – The Cost of Disruption

Incident Overview:

In October 2020, a ransomware attack stopped the University of Vermont Medical Center (UVM), by impacting the EHR systems, scheduling, finance as well as cancer treatment management devices (HHS, 2021).

Breach Mechanics:

Attackers exploit remote access vulnerabilities to develop ransomware. Also, recovery function takes longer time duration because of using segmented backup systems.

Key Vulnerabilities:

- Unauthenticated remote access
- Lack of offline or immutable backup networks
- Lack of cyber-security investment in mid-range clinics

Consequences:

- Postponed cancer treatments and surgeries
- Employees enforced to apply paper-centered workflows
- Critical budget planning as well as reputational degradation

Lesson Learned:

Operational continuity has to be listed in breach management. Also, healthcare organizations should check for business continuity and monitor the problem solving plans regularly.

4.5 Vastaamo, Finland (2020) – The Ethical Crisis of Psychotherapy Breaches

Incident Overview:

Recently, hackers perform healthcare breach at Finnish psychotherapy center Vastaamo and exfiltrated sensitive therapist notes of around 33,000 patients. Moreover, attackers would threaten patients and bargain for money so that they would not release their sensible credentials and information (Yle News, 2020).

Breach Mechanics:

The network had inadequate fundamental cyber-security management: data would be saved in plain text format, without encryption. Hence, breach remains still unpredicted for prolonged duration.

Key Vulnerabilities:

- No encryption process for sensible psychological data
- No logging or audit trail
- Late public disclosure

Consequences:

- Increasing suicidal reports because of stressful lifestyle
- Bankruptcy of the therapy provider
- Public backlash as well as national trauma

Lesson Learned:

Sensitive mental health information requires special security. Legal considerations like trauma-based response protocols which are decided to be a portion of incident management.

4.6 Medibank, Australia (2022) – Sensitive Data in the Spotlight

Incident Overview:

In October 2022, Australian health insurer Medibank publicized a breach which affected 9.7 million new and old customers. The lost information includes names, addresses, clinical numbers, and details relevant to addiction, abortion, as well as chronic attack (Australian Cyber Security Centre, 2023).

Breach Mechanics:

The attack contributes with stolen data which can access production networks. Information which has been exfiltrated for longer days could be stored through online process.

Key Vulnerabilities:

- Vulnerable password integrity and credential theft
- No zero-trust structure
- Late breach prediction as well as communication

Consequences:

- Public outrage and class-based lawsuits
- Data related in media and dark web platforms
- Regulatory security and calls for novel cyber-security legislation

Lesson Learned:

The social effect of data breaches are increased while involving sensible topics like reproductive or addiction. Significant breach notification timelines and empathy-based communication principles are highly required.

Table 3. Summary of Case Studies and Their Lessons

Case	Year	Key Weakness	Primary Impact	Key Takeaway
Anthem	2015	Vulnerable authentication and encryption	Largest U.S. breach in healthcare	Harden credential systems and encrypt data
NHS (WannaCry)	2017	Outdated systems, no patching	Service disruption and public inquiry	Patch management is critical
SingHealth	2018	Weaker access segmentation	Political fallout and policy reform	Isolating systems and strengthen monitoring
UVM Medical Center	2020	No backup isolation	Treatment delays and high costs	Assure disaster recovery readiness
Vastaamo	2020	No encryption, unethical handling	Patient trauma, provider collapse	save mental health data ethically
Medibank	2022	Credential theft, delayed disclosure	Social harm, lawsuits, legislation	Secure access and act immediately

Each cases present in above table shows diverse fact of cybersecurity loss and it underscores the significance of institutional awareness in technical updates.

5. CROSS-CUTTING THEMES AND LESSONS LEARNED

Even though every breach case is explored as defined in previous section, it has unique reasons and results with tremendous recurring ideas which are being familiar globally in healthcare cybersecurity system. Such themes explain a deep-rooted structural weakness, persistent human aspects, as well as regulatory management failures which has to be monitored briefly; so that upcoming disaster can be prevented at earlier state.

5.1 The Human Factor: Persistent Vulnerability and Untapped Potential

Here, one of the common and persistent healthcare data breaches is considered to be human error or manual mistake. Starting from phishing emails to misleading the access points, it often ends up with failure (Ponemon Institute, 2022). Unfortunately, human abilities become unemployed in defense at some cost.

Key Issues:

- **Credential Management:** older or reused passwords would be exploited in the Anthem, SingHealth, and Medibank breaches.
- **Phishing Susceptibility:** Staffs working in different fields have fallen for social engineering scams and frauds because of insufficient knowledge in cyber-attack.

- **Training Gaps:** Most of the employees have inadequate knowledge in cybersecurity to find risk and threats.

Lesson:

The process of Cybersecurity should be developed with bounded, role-based, and proper updated training schemes. Also, human beings should be considered as primary source of defense and not as a liable property (Choi et al., 2019).

5.2 Third-Party Risks: The Extended Attack Surface

In general, healthcare is based on external vendors only for cloud services, IT architecture, billing, as well as data processing. But, third-party vendors are considered to be vulnerable link in case of security chain where data integrity cannot be assured (Verizon DBIR, 2023).

Examples:

- Most of the breaches raised from weaker APIs or data exposed on interrupted cloud services.
- Absence of strong vendor risk management leaves healthcare leaders to underscore the vulnerabilities.

Lesson:

Healthcare firms should implement vendor risk management schemes, like:

- Due diligence before onboarding
- Contractual security standards
- Periodic audits as well as certification needs (e.g., SOC 2, ISO/IEC 27001)

5.3 Outdated and Fragmented Infrastructure

Here, legacy systems used in public sector hospitals or low budget rural centers have been operated without any important notes or support from the government. The WannaCry attack examined the reason for suspending software systems using massive number of NHS that make use of Windows XP in 2017 (Martin et al., 2017).

Challenges:

- Software updates might interfere with medical workflows.
- Clinical tools are operated under closed, un-patchable networks.
- Data is distributed over siloed databases, by minimizing the transparency and responding ability.

Lesson:

Infrastructure modernization should be considered as major aspect with dedicated cybersecurity funding, especially for medium firms. Investment in interoperable, secure-by-design modules are defined as a prerequisite for resilience.

5.4 Insufficient Incident Response Preparedness

Many of the healthcare organizations suffer from lack of proper infrastructure, verified incident response plans (IRPs). In case of UVM Medical Center case, assimilated backups and insufficient chain of command tends to make longer downtime and ambiguity.

Common Failures:

- No verified response protocols
- Absence of communication principles with patients and social network
- Postponed contribution with law enforcement and regulatory ethics

Lesson:

Every clinical firms are forced to prepare isolated room, effectively updated Incident Response Plan, including:

- Designated response teams (technical, legal, PR, clinical)
- Planned breach drills
- Unambiguous breach notification schemes

5.5 Regulatory and Jurisdictional Inconsistencies

Globally, healthcare is considered to be a significant tool; however the cybersecurity standards and breach statement laws might be different dramatically based on jurisdiction.

Examples:

- In Vastaamo case, there was an ambiguous breach response for mental health officers.
- Medibank's suspension in disclosure leads to legal quires based on Australian data protection ethics.

Lesson:

Consequently, there is a requirement for harmonized international policies for health data integrity and breach disclosure. Regulatory bodies should have limited cybersecurity standards, assured timelines for breach notifications, and expose useful penalties for non-compliance (Ozair et al., 2015).

5.6 Ethics and Empathy in Breach Response

Systematic recovery reduces the effects of human impact in breach process. In Vastaamo, patients who undergo psychotherapy have separate records including trauma, stigma, and coercion. Identically, Medibank's breach of reproductive health as well as addiction information has shown the degradation enacted by digital form at weaker groups.

Failures:

- No psychological support or trauma-based communication
- Breach letters written in legal jargon without empathy
- Media releases exacerbating stigma as well as public controversies

Lesson:

Breaches with sensitive or stigmatized information (e.g., mental health, multiplicative care, HIV status) need trauma-informed response protocols, such as:

- Patient-based communication
- Authority to provide counselling and crisis maintenance
- Safeguards over subordinate exposure (e.g., media release)

Table 4. Cross-Cutting Themes and Organizational Implications

Theme	Observed in Cases	Required Response
Human error	Anthem, UVM, Medibank	Compulsory training and simulations
Third-party vulnerability	Anthem, SingHealth	Contractual vendor risk management
Outdated infrastructure	NHS (WannaCry), UVM	Legacy system upgrades, dedicated cybersecurity funding
Incident unpreparedness	UVM, Vastaamo	Active Incident Response Plan and regular testing

continued on following page

Table 4. Continued

Theme	Observed in Cases	Required Response
Regulatory inconsistency	Vastaamo, Medibank	Harmonized global data defence and enforcement policies
Ethical response failure	Vastaamo, Medibank	Trauma-informed communication and patient support systems

Sources: Compiled from case studies and industry reports (Choi et al., 2019; Ponemon, 2022; HHS, 2023)

As a result, the overall point from above data breaches states a singular truth (i.e.) cyber-security in healthcare is technical limitation as well as it is related to organizational, law, and governance imperative. The upcoming section moves to **policy and practice recommendations** transformed to healthcare leaders, policy-makers, technical developers, as well as proffers.

5.7 Future Trends and Emerging Threats

While traditional breaches offer valid lessons, the healthcare field has to be ready to generate emerging cybersecurity threats which helps in developing digital health for future. Most of the converging methods have been deployed to enhance both the scale as well as complexity of data security.

1. AI-Driven Cyberattacks and Defenses

Artificial intelligence (AI) is highly employed by attackers to systematize phishing, develop real-time deepfakes, as well as to find the vulnerabilities rapidly when compared to historical models. Simultaneously, AI helps in opposing major activities like anomaly prediction as well as predictive risk modeling. Some of the systematic explorations supports both the advantages and threats involved in AI by means of cybersecurity, also it shows the emergency requirement for promising maintenance of AI-based defense modules (Khairuddin et al., 2023; Roopesh, Nishat, & Rasetti, 2024).

2. Exploitation of Expanding IoMT Ecosystems

The Internet of Medical Things (IoMT) is still developed along with connected diagnostic tools, portable monitors, as well as implantable methods that is being considered mainstream. Hence, this extension results in enormous attack surface. Vulnerable patching, irregular communication protocols, as well as device interoperability limitations are defined to be major threats unless regulations are processed (Chen & Wald, 2025).

3. Cloud and Blockchain Integration

Since health data transforms to the cloud, by protecting multi-tenant and cross-border structures that tends to be highly complicated. Furthermore, blockchain has been deployed as additional method for securing the patient's identity, and assure auditability, mitigate the dependence on weaker databases (Agbo, Mahmoud, & Eklund, 2022). Hence, blockchain proposes scalability and energy-requirement which has to be reported before widespread adoption.

4. Global Policy Fragmentation and Governance Gaps

Even though regulations like HIPAA and GDPR are considered to be significant precedents, gaps are still named in low- and middle-income countries, while there is minimal harmonization over jurisdictions. Here, few reports from the World Health Organization (2021) and OECD (2023) explains the requirement for international data maintenance to prevent additional segmentation, especially in terms of tele-medicine and AI diagnosis transcend borders.

5. Ethical and Patient-Centered Risks

New advanced threats are not technical but it is ethical-based. Breaches of mental health or reproductive information could affect the marginalized populations, by exacerbating inequalities. Most of the researchers discuss that privacy as well as equity should be restructured as major pillars of digital health ethics, by expanding over compliance-driven frameworks (Lupton, 2023; Véliz, 2022).

6. Resilience in a Post-Quantum Era

Consequently, the enhancement of quantum computing implies massive threats in recently developed encryption techniques. But, it is not defined as major issue, while healthcare firms have to be prepared for upcoming responsibilities in which quantum-safe cryptography is required to save crucial details (Alshaikh & Maynard, 2023).

Developing the **future-based risks** needs a proactive and reactive posture. Unification of AI with IoMT security, using blockchain becomes highly possible, harmonizing global maintenance, and encompassing equity along with cybersecurity planning that builds resilience in future digital transformation.

6. REGULATORY AND ETHICAL GAPS IN GLOBAL CONTEXT

Inspite of increasing cyberattacks on health care globally, systematic responses are diversified, reactive, as well as inconsistent. The combined global policy for healthcare cybersecurity is considered to be subtle, enforces every firm to hold complicated ethics and standards. Followed by, this section examines the limitations involved in governance: from suspended breach notifications to cross-border data examination as well as the law of saving weaker group of people.

6.1 Fragmented Global Legal Landscape

Generally, preHealthcare is a vital tool in public medical centers—but cybersecurity needs are increased in various modules over the jurisdictions. For instance, when Health Insurance Portability and Accountability Act (HIPAA) in the US makes a compulsion for breach notification within 3 months, General Data Protection Regulation (GDPR) in Europe is in need for a prior notification before 72 hours of prediction (European Commission, 2016; U.S. HHS, 2023). Unlike, Asian countries or African countries support medium number of breach disclosures.

This irregularity tends to create an ambiguous and underscored situation at public. Some of the firms working in abroad like multinational insurers or telehealth highly suffer to reduce the cyber-attack activity with limited protocols, data localization needs as well as enforcement devices used in safeguarding the sensible information.

Figure 2. Timeline Comparison of Breach Notification Laws by Region

Region	Mandatory Notification	Deadline After Discovery
United States	Yes (HIPAA)	Within 60 days
European Union	Yes (GDPR)	Within 72 hours
Australia	Yes (NDB Scheme)	As soon as practicable
India	Yes (PDPA)	Within 3 days
Africa (varies)	Proposed	Undefined
Africa (varies)	Inconsistent	Undefined or no requirement

Sources: *U.S. HHS (2023); GDPR (2016); OAIC Australia (2022); Singapore PDPC (2021)*

6.2 Weak Enforcement and Lenient Penalties

Despite of proposing breach laws and ethics, enforcement mechanism becomes highly vulnerable. Regulatory teams suffer from improper authentication, reliable sources, or even famous political parties would execute substantial fine amounts. For instance, before launching GDPR, data protection fine in Europe has been extended to additional amount of thousand euros. Post-GDPR, fine was increased; however it still remains to be contradiction (Tikkinen-Piri et al., 2018).

Also, in the U.S., when HHS Office for Civil Rights (OCR) assures HIPAA, penalties lightly differ in size that is from $100,000 for mid-range clinics to $16 million in Anthem case. This difference tends to develop tedious atmosphere for healthcare organizations to learn the threats involved in non-compliance.

6.3 Jurisdictional Gaps in Cross-Border Healthcare

In general, digital healthcare delivery particularly telemedicine as well as AI-relied diagnostics are highly implied as blurred national boundaries. An officer from Germany might have a consultation with a patient from India under the application of cloud platforms which was deployed in U.S. Unfortunately, when breach takes place, there are few queries raised, some of them are:

- Which jurisdiction governs the breach?
- Who is in-charge for notifying the patient?
- Whose law implies penalties and remediation?

Hence, the above jurisdictional challenges are highly sensible in multinational health insurance, international medical trials, as well as pandemic response aspects. When there is absence of international agreements, cybersecurity protocols for healthcare where patients are exposed and regulators have minimum awareness regarding the whole process.

6.4 Ethical Gaps: Beyond Compliance

Compliance policies mostly fail to report the ethical direction of breaches especially while a sensible data in contributed. Based on the rule of Vastaamo and Medibank breaches, data relied in mental health, reproductive care, or substance application would be exploited, which leads to psychological illness.

Some of the ethical failings are listed below:

- Failure to indicate affected individuals regularly

- Absence of psychological support for victims
- Disclosure letters developed in technical language without any empathy
- Lack of security for weaker populations

Moreover, there are inadequate ethical guidelines that enclose breach disclosure with minors, LGBTQ+ individuals, or patients with physical injury.

Figure 3. Dimensions of Healthcare Breach Impact

Dimension	Example of Breach Impact
Legal	Fines, lawsuits, penalties
Operational	System downtime, delays
Psychological	Patient trauma, anxiety
Social	Stigma, reputational harm
Ethical	Violation of dignity/trust
Ethical	Undefined

Sources: U.S. HHS (2023); GDPR (2016); OAIC Australia (2022); Singapore PDPC

6.5 The Case for International Standards

Based on these challenges, a healthcare organization opted for coordinated international standards immediately similar to aviation or finance sectors. Some of the effective policies are:

- A Global Healthcare Cybersecurity Charter, developed by WHO, OECD, and ITU
- An International Breach Registry, anonymized but visible, for compulting foster learning
- A UN Convention on Digital Health Ethics, aimed in rights and communication data protection

These initiatives are useful for below factors:

- To harmonize breach notification timelines
- Explain limited cybersecurity controls for healthcare networks

- Activate cross-border enforcement by mutual recognition parties

Table 5. Comparison of Breach Notification Requirements by Country

Country/ Region	Mandate Type	Notification Deadline	Enforcement Agency	Max Penalty
United States	HIPAA Breach Rule	60 days	HHS OCR	$1.5 million per violation
European Union	GDPR	72 hours	National Data Protection Authorities	Up to €20 million or 4% global turnover
Australia	Notifiable Data Breaches	As soon as practicable	OAIC	Up to AU$2.2 million
Singapore	PDPA	Within 3 days	PDPC	Up to SGD 1 million
Canada	PIPEDA	Without undue delay	OPC	CAD 100,000 per violation
India	Draft DPDP Act (2022)	TBD	Proposed Data Protection Board	Undefined
South Africa	POPIA	Reasonable time	Information Regulator	ZAR 10 million

Sources: National regulatory authorities and data protection agencies (2022–2024)

6.6 Call to Ethical Action

More than the regulation, healthcare officers mandate to use ethics-first mindset while it is ready to prepare and respond to breach, which defines as following:

- Integrating patient notes in disclosure principles
- Listing psychological integrity along legal objections
- Developing digital dignity in every healthcare system

Healthcare information is one of the significant aspect which holds complete history of an individual which is not just a random data. Safeguarding these kinds of sensible data is a mandatory option and moral duty of a national citizen.

In summary, regulatory space as well as ethical oversights makes healthcare systems transparent and unsafe. With no harmonized global support as well as empathy-based protocols, the secondary breaches become highly degraded.

7. POLICY AND PRACTICE RECOMMENDATIONS

The complication involved in healthcare cybersecurity expands over technical solutions, enclosing organizational, manual, and systematic aspects. Group of stakeholders encompassed with healthcare ecosystem is considered to be important part in providing trusted cybersecurity. Frontline medical officers should be trained with fundamental cybersecurity policies including recognizing phishing timelines and maintain robust password. Followed by, it is compulsory for IT officers to maintain robust data and well-equipped security systems, such as firewalls, Intrusion Detection Systems (IDS), and encryption schemes. Hence, software developers are allocated with a task to create secured applications which should meet the industry protocols so that data protection could be carried out in a better process. Policymakers are responsible to develop regulations which should be equally balanced between security and imperative of seamless healthcare delivery.

The prevention, detection, and response to data breaches need a combined effect over these stakeholder members. Initially, prevention process is carried out with proper security monitoring, staff training schemes, and implementation of zero-trust structure. Secondly, detection mechanism has modern threat intelligence systems as well as real-world management of network traffic. Finally, response protocols should be well-documented and implemented regularly, with vibrant communication channels among IT teams, management, as well as related regulatory systems. Followed by, a healthcare forum should cultivate a culture of frequent enhancement in cyber-security practices, tends to deploy new threats and reduce the newly developing techniques like artificial intelligence (AI) as well as machine learning (ML) for improved security protocols.

7.1 For Healthcare Providers: Strengthening Frontline Defenses

Healthcare sectors like hospitals, medical centres, insurance organization, as well as public health teams which is compulsory to view cybersecurity, not as IT issue; however, it prioritizes patient information as a primary concern. Followed by, cybersecurity in healthcare expands by saving digital assets which affects the patient data security as well as robustness. Furthermore, it should be capable to examine that cyber threats which is involved in medical tools, interrupted critical networks, and exhibit sensible patient information, that tends to malfunction in disease analysis, and physical harm. The inter-linked form of recent healthcare network defines that a breach in single region holds cascading effects at overall format, which impacts electronic health data to life-based devices.

In order to report this issue, healthcare organization should have a holistic approach to cybersecurity which combines IT security metrics along with medical workflows and patient delivery care protocols. Followed by, it contributes in consistent risk management, employee training on cybersecurity, and execution of trusted IRP. Moreover, healthcare professionals should prefer the funding in cybersecurity structure and expertise, making it as useful aspect to retain the efficiency of patient hospital records, well-qualified care. While estimating cybersecurity, healthcare sectors could perform better with high-quality records and data from the ever-evolving landscape of digital risks. Some of the major recommendations are:

Implement Zero Trust Architecture (ZTA)

- Approve the strategy of "never trust, always verify."
- Control lateral transformation within networks.
- Application of identity-relied access control for users and tools (Rose et al., 2020).

Enforce Multi-Factor Authentication (MFA)

- Application of MFA for user accounts, particularly for privileged users.
- Avoid credential-relied attacks using biometrics or one-time tokens.

Conduct Regular Cyber Hygiene Audits

- Use quarterly security assessments of endpoints, cloud assets, as well as APIs.
- Retain maximum logs of access as well as incident efforts.
- Develop internal audit trail for every critical networks.

Develop a Live Incident Response Plan

- Allocate particular roles (e.g., IT officer, legal advisor, patient care taker).
- Verify breach drills yearly once inclusive of simulations in ransomware attempts.
- Establish pre-approved patient message formats for breach disclosure.

Invest in Employee Cyber Literacy

- Deliver interactive, scenario-relied training.
- Tailor the content by role (e.g., clinical vs. admin vs. IT staff).
- Reinforce training with systematic phishing simulations.

7.2 For Governments and Regulators: Mandating and Supporting Compliance

Public-sector members play a vital role in assigning standards, funding agreement, and assure the accountability.

Set Minimum Cybersecurity Standards

- Deploy robust national baseline standards for each licensed health aspects.
- Needs ISO/IEC 27001 certification for reputed firms.

Create National Cybersecurity Funds

- Command the subsidies to develop well-equipped ambience for mid and small hospitals.
- Offer enough funding for vulnerable assets, interference verification as well as staff training.

Mandate Prompt Breach Notification

- Mandate to breach reporting deadlines (e.g., 72 hours or less).
- Make a note of real-time incidents in a central health breach registry.

Incentivize Compliance

- Develop financial or strong incentives for proactive cybersecurity funds.
- Penalize negligence with fine amount as well as limits on public reimbursement (e.g., Medicare/Medicaid in the U.S.).

Figure 4. Government Levers for Cybersecurity Reform in Healthcare

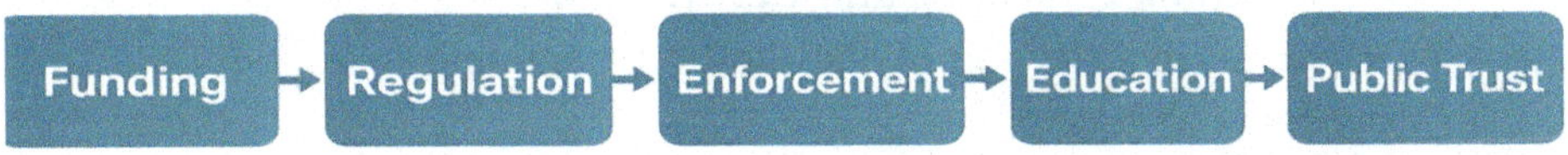

7.3 For Technology Developers and Vendors: Building Security by Design

In general, software developers, cloud providers, and device manufacturers should encompass security from initial stages of deployment.

Adopt Privacy and Security by Design

- Make use of encryption technology, access management, and anonymization schemes developed.

- Include audit logs, automated timeouts, and breach alarm systems in applications.

Secure APIs and Cloud Interfaces

- It necciates secured tokens and TLS/SSL for each and every data transaction.
- Hosting third-party penetration before deployment.

Comply with Interoperability Standards Securely

- Allocate using HL7 FHIR, SMART on FHIR, and IHE standards.
- Prefer data reduction and masking while sharing health data.

Build with the End User in Mind

- Assure these systems are intuitive and prevent security workarounds.
- It contributes in healthcare employee training in UX testing to allocate medical workflows.

7.4 For Educators and Public Health Institutions: Cultivating Cyber-Awareness Culture

Sustainable transformation in healthcare cybersecurity should be initiated with education as well as workforce deployment.

Integrate Cybersecurity into Health Curricula

- Clinical, nursing, and public health policies must have cybersecurity frameworks.
- Emphasize ethical responsibilities over digital confidentiality and patient information.

Offer Continuing Education and Certification

- People in industry to provide short-term training in digital health and cyber resilience.
- Incentivize healthcare leads to adopt for certifications like HCISPP, CIPP/US.

Host Public Awareness Campaigns

- Convey to patients regarding their data rights as well as privacy shields.
- Enforce personal cyber hygiene including secure patient websites, password protection.

Table 6. Stakeholder-Specific Recommendations for Healthcare Cybersecurity

Stakeholder	Key Actions
Healthcare Providers	No Trusted structure, MFA, breach response plans, staff training
Governments & Regulators	Lower standards, breach ethics, financial empowerment, enforcement
Technology Developers	Security by structure, API hardening, UX alignment, compliance certifications
Educators & Institutions	Curriculum inclusion, training schemes, public awareness camps

7.5 Prioritizing Trauma-Informed Breach Response

A superior governance must be provided to patients affected by data breaches—especially people who suffers from mental health, generative care, and stigmatized state.

Recommendations:

- Involve in behavioral health doctors in post-breach planning.
- Provide anonymous counselling services to affected members.
- The communication should be in plain text with empathy.
- Prevent excess technical justifications in disclosure notices.

Figure 5. Components of a Trauma-Informed Breach Response

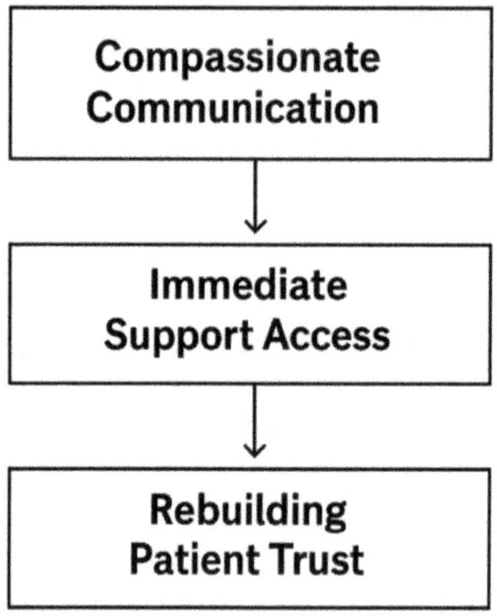

Adapted from principles outlined by the U.S. Substance Abuse and Mental Health Services Administration (SAMHSA), "Trauma-Informed Care in Behavioral Health Services," Treatment Improvement Protocol Series 57, 2014.

The above recommendations involve in changing the paradigm from reactive crisis management to proactive digital care ethics. By changing the policies to roles and responsibilities of significant stakeholders, the healthcare network could change cybersecurity from key point into basic patient-relied digital health.

8. RESILIENCE FRAMEWORK FOR HEALTHCARE CYBERSECURITY

Cybersecurity in healthcare is highly recommended to prevent the risk involved in data protection which indirectly speaks about resilience i.e. the capability to anticipate, tolerate, respond, and recover data from digital flaws at the time of retaining trust and data flexibility. Here, it defines the practical resilience scheme 14structured with 4 key star points including:

The following are:

- **Readiness**
- **Response**
- **Recovery**
- **Redesign**

The above points are considered as "4R Model" which has been changed particularly for healthcare atmosphere.

8.1 Overview of the 4R Model

Figure 6. The 4R Healthcare Cybersecurity Resilience Model

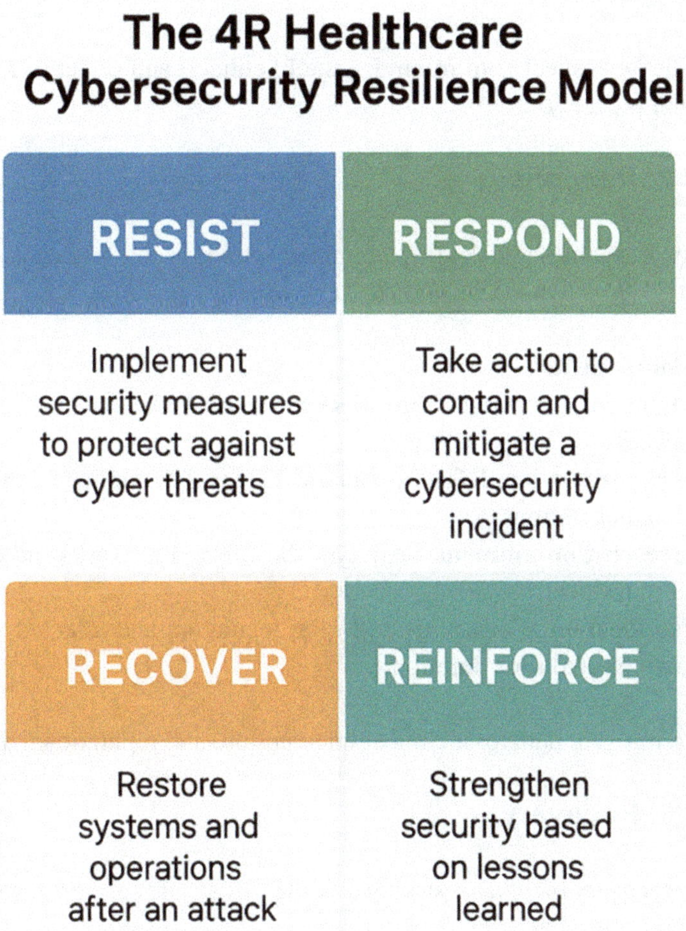

The 4R Healthcare Cybersecurity Resilience Model
RESIST
RESPOND
Implement security measures to protect against cyber threats
Take action to contain and mitigate a cybersecurity incident
RECOVER
REINFORCE
Restore systems and operations after an attack
Strengthen security based on lessons learned

8.2 Pillar 1: Readiness/Resist

Initially, Readiness contributes in proactive steps to find and mitigate the threats involved in data protection before any disaster occurs.

Key Components:

- **Risk Management**: Annual vulnerability monitoring and threat tailoring.
- **Cybersecurity Policy**: Verified roles, protocols, and responsibilities.
- **Training and Simulations**: Role-based and scenario-based simulations like phishing drills.
- **Technology Baseline**: Patch assessment, endpoint safety, as well as encrypted data.

Goal: The key aspect is to minimize the likelihood and effect of a breach via education and prevention.

8.3 Pillar 2: Response

Secondly, Response holds quick, combined actions is conducted when a breach is predicted.

Key Components:

- **Incident Response Plan (IRP)**: Enabled due to pressurized data severity.
- **Cross-Functional Team**: contains IT, legal, compliance, medical, and communications.
- **Breach Containment**: Segregate the affected networks and avoid lateral movement.
- **Notification**: Communicate to the regulators and affected individuals with limited time duration.

Goal: To mitigate data loss, clinical interruption, and reputational damage.

8.4 Pillar 3: Recovery

Thirdly, Recovery includes restoring modules, trust, and services once the threat is detected and neutralized.

Key Components:

- **System Restoration**: Apply clean backups to recover data and applications.
- **Business Continuity**: Change-over from paper to digital workflows.
- **Patient Communication**: Offer updates, reassurance, and psychological support.
- **Reputation Management**: Visible public context as well as media management.

Goal: To stop common functions while stakeholder's confidence is retained globally.

8.5 Pillar 4: Redesign

Redesign emphasizes institutional learning and systems enhancements after the occurrence of incident.

Key Components:

- **Postmortem Analysis**: Find the major causes and procedural threats.
- **Policy Revisions**: Develop new IRPs, accessible protocols, and training curricula.
- **Technology Upgrades**: Report technical debt and weakness involved in the architecture.
- **Culture Change**: Advertise cyber-laws and accountability over every staff levels.

Goal: Aims to be highly resilient with every breach inclusive of robustness and restore data.

8.6 The Cybersecurity Maturity Self-Assessment Toolkit

To operate the 4R model, few sectors make use of self-assessment toolkit. Also, it estimates the readiness over 10 domains, scores maturity, and leads to upcoming procedure.

Table 7. Sample Cybersecurity Maturity Self-Assessment Domains

Domain	Key Indicators	Maturity Levels (1–5)
1. Governance & Policy	Cyber policy, board oversight, designated roles	1 = Absent, 5 = Fully embedded
2. Risk Management	Regular risk assessments, third-party evaluations	1 = Ad hoc, 5 = Continuous
3. Access Controls	MFA, role-based access, privileged access management	1 = Basic, 5 = Automated
4. Training & Awareness	Frequency, content relevance, phishing tests	1 = Annual only, 5 = Monthly
5. Threat Detection	Monitoring tools, anomaly detection, alert responsiveness	1 = Manual logs, 5 = Real-time AI
6. Incident Response	Formal IRP, breach simulation, escalation matrix	1 = Informal, 5 = Tested & refined
7. Recovery Capabilities	Isolated backups, recovery drills, downtime thresholds	1 = Undefined, 5 = Fully mapped
8. Vendor Risk Management	Contracts, SLAs, periodic reviews	1 = None, 5 = Formal program
9. Patient Communication	Templates, transparency, trauma-informed messages	1 = None, 5 = Preapproved & tested
10. Learning & Improvement	Postmortems, reporting loops, dashboard KPIs	1 = Sporadic, 5 = Data-driven

Scoring Guidance:

- Overall possible score = 50
- 0–20 = Maximum vulnerability
- 21–35 = Medium readiness
- 36–45 = Effective foundational maturity
- 46–50 = Modern resilience

Use Case: Most of the firms are capable to perform self-examination quarterly, verify scores annually, and unify the findings as board-level reporting.

8.7 Embedding Resilience into Healthcare Culture

Organizational culture should be developed to reduce the conflicts present in cybersecurity and it is a shared responsibility for both IT and healthcare.

Some of them are:

- Allocating a **Chief Information Security Officer (CISO)** with medical contacts.

- Retaining **cybersecurity town halls** as well as cross-disciplinary training modules.
- Encouraging teams that **finds threats** or enhance processes pre-emptively.

Here, Resilience is a not a constant aim and it is defined to be a frequent journey used in identifying novel threats, techniques, and ethical procedures.

Above resilience technique provides a real-time outline of cyber-security in order to guide the academics and prevent the frequent errors which happened in past years, also to regain robust data transfer, and finally to save the patients details with increasing threats in digital world.

9. TOWARD A HUMAN-CENTERED DIGITAL HEALTH ETHIC

Since healthcare is becoming more familiar in recent times, cybersecurity cannot always remain as effective method. It should be considered as moral support where it concentrates in trust, responsibility, equity, and basic rights provided for patients. Hence, it debates for a change which is from compliance-based methods to an ethical policy developed for the purpose of patient safety as well as digital justice.

9.1 Digital Vulnerability as Human Vulnerability

Generally, healthcare information is considered to be detail description which describes about the patient and it is not an abstract. It exhibits clinical analysis, treatments, reproductive diagnosis, mental health difficulties, genetic status, and some of the personal history of a human being. While an healthcare information is lost, then the incident which occurs would be considered as informational as well as emotional, psychological, and social (Ozair et al., 2015).

Real-WorldExample:

In the Vastaamo breach, victims were imposed for data theft and blackmail. Since there was a maximum feasibility of publishing sensitive psychotherapy records which includes suicide cases, family issue, and career loss cases (Yle News, 2020). Hence, it is not only a security threat it is also defined as an ethical failure.

Key Ethical Question:

What does it mean to save an individual when their identity and dignity are saved in digital format?

9.2 Trust as a Cornerstone of Digital Care

Basically, patient provides sensitive information to healthcare leaders using implicit expectation where information will be secured with high security. Breaches violate the trust and reduce the confidence from overall healthcare network.

Trust is fragile in three ways:

- **Relational**: Patients might carry sensitive data after a breach and impairing care.
- **Institutional**: Public point of healthcare organization declines.
- **Interpersonal**: Providers suffers from moral distress for not saving the patient information.

Ethical Principle:
"First, do no harm" should expand to digital domains.

9.3 Equity and the Uneven Impact of Breaches

In general, cybersecurity failures do not show any impact every patient. People from marginalized group like racial minorities, LGBTQ+ populations, and some of them with stigmatized status where they struggles from major threats.

Disparities Include:

- Maximum social consequences when sensitive information is leaked.
- Limited resources to pursue legal action.
- Minimal access to save digital tools for care coordination.

Case in Point:

In the Medibank breach, data which is relevant to addiction and reproduction care has been leaked suspiciously, where a women affects and vulnerable populations (Australian Cyber Security Centre, 2023).

Ethical Imperative:

In general, digital health systems should be developed with equity and prefer the data protection for people struggle at greatest threats.

9.4 From Compliance to Conscience

Many of cybersecurity schemes are developed over compliance: what is legally needed, which is not morally right. But, most resilient firms go beyond regulation to list out:

"What is our duty of care to the people behind the information?"

Features of a Human-Centered Cybersecurity Ethic:

- **Empathy in design**: Develop systems which assimilate users who suffered from stress, not as rational actors.
- **Transparency in practice**: Encompass breaches early, regularly, and compassionately.
- **Inclusivity in governance**: Disclose patients, medical officers, and ethicists in cybersecurity decisions.

Figure 7. Layers of a Human-Centered Cybersecurity Approach

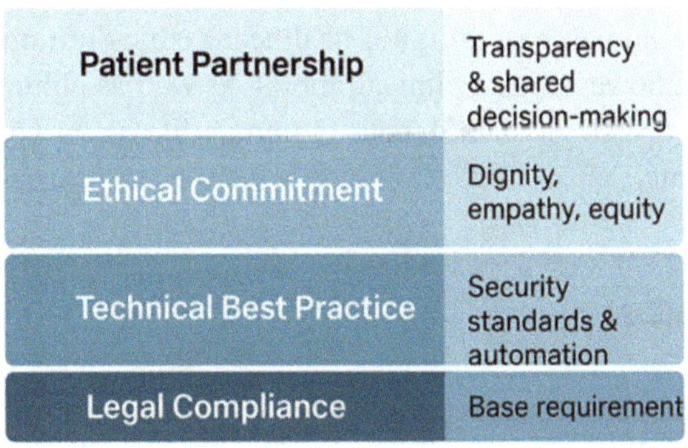

Source: Woods (2022)

9.5 Building Ethical Digital Cultures in Healthcare

Here, culture becomes blind for resilience. However, some of the firms prioritize ethics as:

- Define ethical whistleblowing if vulnerabilities are identified.
- Contains data ethics in onboarding as well as leadership deployment.
- Examine and encourage employees who consider security concerns as major protections.

Suggested Practice:

Develop a Digital Ethics Committee with cross-functional illustration along with clinicians, patients, as well as legal advisors. This group contains:

- Explore high-risk digital projects.
- Establish ethical response for breaches.
- Guide technology procurement via values lens.

9.6 Reframing Breaches as Catalysts for Moral Innovation

Even though breaches are agonizing, it has inflection points and opportunities to reflect, reform, and recommit to first strategy.

Instead of returning to the status quo post-breach, firms may ask for queries as:

- What do we now learn regarding emotional effect on patients?
- How can our novel systems better embody compassion and care?
- How can we develop digital trust as a lasting legacy of this event?

In summary, a human-based digital healthcare ethics reframes cybersecurity not as a checklist; however, as a clinical, moral, as well as cultural responsibility. It prompts that every single data denotes a human life along with responsibility, empathy, and dignity.

10. CONCLUSION

The overall summary of healthcare cybersecurity defines not only about firewalls, encryption, or compliance; it describes regarding the fragility as well as resilience of systems which contains sensible or important information of a human being. The breaches explored in this chapter—Anthem, WannaCry, SingHealth, Vastaamo, UVM Medical Center, and Medibank—were not only IT failure; but they are defined to be institutional wake-up calls which explains systemic blind spots from governance, laws, infrastructure, as well as preparedness.

Every reports addressed from above cases provide unique point based on vulnerability, starting from credential theft and unpatched models to trauma-stimulating public exposure of mental health information. However, these incidents imply that every threat can be resolved within limited time. Under the application of strategic funds, unambiguous regulations, interdisciplinary collaboration, as well as a reforming process created for human-based laws, clinical ecosystem that develop safe, trusted, and resilient digital atmosphere.

Followed by, newly developed 4R Resilience Framework called Readiness, Response, Recovery, and Redesign has provided a way to perform an effective transformation. While integrating with moveable recommendations, the policymakers, tech developers, as well as educators tends to activate healthcare to change from risk management to proactive digital stewardship.

Fundamentally, this chapter assures that saving medical information is a moral justification and it is about to protect a human being with massive security. Also, it tends to restore public confidence, maintains patient dignity, and assures that new updates cannot be expected from costlier service. In an era, where health as well as related information becomes highly attached, cybersecurity should be considered as cost and also as a moral responsibility with basic rights and traditional security methods which has to be followed securely.

REFERENCES

Adler-Milstein, J., & Jha, A. K. (2017). HITECH Act drove large gains in hospital electronic health record adoption. *Health Affairs, 36*(8), 1416–1422. DOI: 10.1377/hlthaff.2016.1651 PMID: 28784734

Alotaibi, Y. K., & Federico, F. (2017). The impact of health information technology on patient safety. *Saudi Medical Journal, 38*(12), 1173–1180. DOI: 10.15537/smj.2017.12.20631 PMID: 29209664

Alshamrani, A., Myneni, S., & Saddik, B. (2021). Security challenges in telemedicine and remote healthcare. *Sensors (Basel), 21*(6), 1965. DOI: 10.3390/s21061965 PMID: 33799616

Australian Cyber Security Centre. (2023). *Medibank cyber incident update*. Australian Government. https://www.cyber.gov.au

Choi, Y., Johnson, M. E., & Lehmann, C. U. (2019). Data breaches in the healthcare sector: Trends and implications. *Health Affairs, 38*(2), 206–212. DOI: 10.1377/hlthaff.2018.05072

Coventry, L., & Branley, D. (2018). Cybersecurity in healthcare: A narrative review of trends, threats and ways forward. *Maturitas, 113*, 48–52. DOI: 10.1016/j.maturitas.2018.04.008 PMID: 29903648

Dehling, T., Gao, F., Schneider, S., & Sunyaev, A. (2015). Exploring the far side of mobile health: Information security and privacy of mobile health apps on iOS and Android. *JMIR mHealth and uHealth, 3*(1), e8. DOI: 10.2196/mhealth.3672 PMID: 25599627

Department of Health. (2018). *Lessons learned review of the WannaCry ransomware cyber attack*. UK Government. https://www.gov.uk

European Commission. (2016). *General Data Protection Regulation (GDPR)*. https://eur-lex.europa.eu

HHS (U.S. Department of Health and Human Services). (2023). *Breach portal: Notice to the Secretary of HHS*. https://ocrportal.hhs.gov

IBM. (2023). *X-Force Threat Intelligence Index 2023*. https://www.ibm.com/reports/threat-intelligence

Koonin, L. M., Hoots, B., Tsang, C. A., Leroy, Z., Farris, K., Jolly, B., Antall, P., McCabe, B., Zelis, C. B. R., Tong, I., & Harris, A. M. (2020). Trends in the use of telehealth during the emergence of the COVID-19 pandemic—United States, January–March 2020. *MMWR. Morbidity and Mortality Weekly Report*, *69*(43), 1595–1599. DOI: 10.15585/mmwr.mm6943a3 PMID: 33119561

Kritikos, K., Papageorgiou, N., & Tsamoura, E. (2021). A systematic review of API security threats in healthcare applications. *Computer Standards & Interfaces*, *75*, 103513. DOI: 10.1016/j.csi.2021.103513

Martin, G., Ghafur, S., Kinross, J., Hankin, C., & Darzi, A. (2017). WannaCry—A year on. *BMJ (Clinical Research Ed.)*, *361*, k2381. DOI: 10.1136/bmj.k2381 PMID: 29866711

McLeod, A., & Dolezel, D. (2018). Cyber-analytics: Modeling factors associated with healthcare data breaches. *Decision Support Systems*, *108*, 57–68. DOI: 10.1016/j.dss.2018.02.007

OAIC (Office of the Australian Information Commissioner). (2022). *Notifiable Data Breaches Report: January–June 2022*. https://www.oaic.gov.au

Office for Civil Rights (OCR). (2016). *Anthem pays OCR $16 million in record HIPAA settlement*. U.S. Department of Health and Human Services. https://www.hhs.gov

Ozair, F. F., Jamshed, N., Sharma, A., & Aggarwal, P. (2015). Ethical issues in electronic health records: A general overview. *Perspectives in Clinical Research*, *6*(2), 73–76. DOI: 10.4103/2229-3485.153997 PMID: 25878950

Ponemon Institute. (2022). *The cost of a data breach report 2022*. IBM Security. https://www.ibm.com/security/data-breach

Radanliev, P., De Roure, D., Nurse, J. R. C., Nicolescu, R., Huth, M., Cannady, S., & Montalvo, R. M. (2020). Cyber risk at the edge: Current and future trends on cyber risk analytics and artificial intelligence in the industrial internet of things and industry 4.0 supply chains. *Cybersecurity*, *3*(13), 13. Advance online publication. DOI: 10.1186/s42400-020-00052-8

Rose, S., Borchert, O., Mitchell, S., & Connelly, S. (2020). *Zero Trust Architecture (SP 800-207)*. National Institute of Standards and Technology. https://doi.org/DOI: 10.6028/NIST.SP.800-207

Singapore Ministry of Health. (2018). *SingHealth cyberattack—Public report*. https://www.moh.gov.sg

Tikkinen-Piri, C., Rohunen, A., & Markkula, J. (2018). EU General Data Protection Regulation: Changes and implications for personal data collecting companies. *Computer Law & Security Review, 34*(1), 134–153. DOI: 10.1016/j.clsr.2017.05.015

Verizon. (2023). *Data Breach Investigations Report (DBIR)*. https://www.verizon.com/business/resources/reports/dbir/

Yle News. (2020). *Vastaamo data breach: Finnish psychotherapy scandal deepens*. https://yle.fi/news

Chapter 5
Cybersecure Healthcare in Electric Mobility

Swati Sharma
https://orcid.org/0000-0001-7517-7108
Jamia Millia Islamia, New Delhi, India

ABSTRACT

The convergence of digital healthcare and electric vehicles (EVs) helps in reshaping the delivery of medical services, by enabling mobile diagnostics, emergency care and health outreach specifically in underserved areas. This integration leads to complex cybersecurity and data discretion due to its reliance on cloud infrastructures and real-time communication. This chapter describes a novel cybersecure healthcare intersection within electric mobility network which emphasizes the role of adaptive cloud trust models and threat intelligence. This study discusses emerging use cases such as smart ambulances by analyzing the evolving cyber threat landscape and proposing a layered architectural framework that controls real-time encrypted data exchange mechanisms . The practical application of these concepts has been discussed using real-world case study of an EV-based smart ambulance system. The chapter concludes by delineating regulatory consideration and technical challenges which aimed at fostering secure, scalable and resilient mobile healthcare systems in electric mobility.

1. INTRODUCTION

The swift evolution of smart electric mobility and digital healthcare infrastructures has catalyzed a new standard in health service delivery which influences EVs as mobile, sustainable and intelligent healthcare platforms (Ronanki & Karneddi, 2023). The rural and underserved areas seek innovative delivery mechanisms while the

DOI: 10.4018/979-8-3373-4918-3.ch005

urban centers strive to reduce carbon emissions by accessing an advanced healthcare system. Thus, EVs ambulances are emerging strategic enablers which are equipped with advanced medical technologies. EV ambulances are no longer restricted to use in the form of transport; instead, they have evolved in the form of fully efficient mobile health units which can offer diagnostics, real-time patient monitoring, telemedicine consultations and en route critical care services. EV ambulances are increasingly utilized as the major platform for mobile healthcare delivery, as smart mobility and healthcare converges for mobile healthcare delivery. EVs represent a new frontier in digital health infrastructure because of ambulance fleets equipped with diagnostic systems to stationed mobile clinics in rural areas (Babu et al., 2022). For real-time communication, these evolving systems rely heavily on cloud computing for decision making and diagnostics, but they expose sensitive patient data to a range of cyber threats. In (Ye et al., 2020), the author discusses the integration of robust cloud trust models and threat intelligence in safeguarding healthcare operations within EV ecosystems. The recent EV-based healthcare applications include mobile clinics and smart ambulances which are capable of transmitting patient vitals in real time to hospitals that conduct on-site consultations and screening in remote locations. Under stringent environmental conditions, the medical logistics fleet transport sensitive biomedical materials for continuous analysis (Rathore et al., 2022). The seamless acquisition, dissemination and analysis of the medical data can be supported through the Internet of Medical Things (IoMT), vehicular communication networks (V2X) and cloud computing. Thus, the integration of these systems, however, brings with them significant cybersecurity susceptibility (Alnasser et al., 2019). The exchange of patient sensitive information across diverse platforms ranges from mobile diagnostics tools and EV edge devices specifically to centralized hospital data systems which are easily vulnerable to malware intrusions, data breaches, denial-of-service attacks and identity spoofing (Avatefipour et al., 2019). Among cloud service providers, cross-border data governance protocols and third-party applications, these risks are compounding in risk to the variability of the data. Nowadays, the protection of data confidentiality, integrity and system availability in terms of healthcare services has become increasingly mobile and cloud-reliant which is not only a technical necessity but also an ethical and legal imperative (Yang et al., 2019).

As EVs gradually become a data-centric platform, their on-board system transmits and processes highly sensitive health records, vehicular data, patient specific diagnostic information and biometric identifiers. These information sets are often processed at the edge within EVs itself before the information being forwarded to cloud-based hospital systems or health engines analytics. Particularly in high-stakes environments like critical care delivery or emergency response, the decentralized and mobile nature of such data introduces the unique challenges in maintaining reliable and secure communication channels (Sanghvi et al., 2021). Thus, any manipulation, unauthorized access and disruption to this healthcare information system can result in compromised delays in treatment, worst cases and clinical decisions which cause risk to human life.

Figure 1. Safeguards against cyber threats to EVs ecosystem

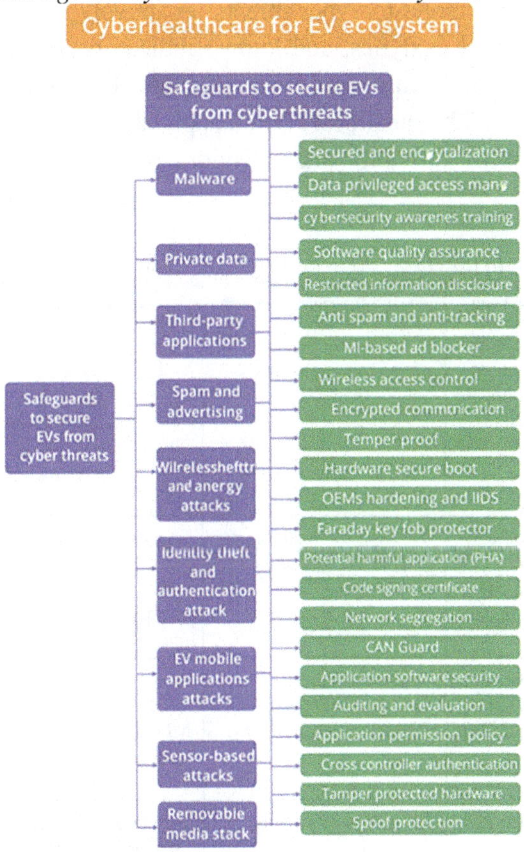

Moreover, the vehicular and healthcare systems are surrounded by the regulatory landscape which adds layers of intricacy to cybersecurity implementation (Bergies et al., 2024). Standardized compliance such as general data protection regulations (GDPR), health insurance portability and accountability act and emerging cybersecurity vehicular frameworks such as ISO/SAE 21434 are essential, yet difficult to correspond in cross-field systems. The combination of biomedical devices, cloud computing and telematics within EVs requires the development of interoperable trust frameworks that ensure legal, operational, technical resilience and ethical requirements as shown in **Figure 1**. The establishment of a secure design framework for healthcare systems and smart mobility, it becomes imperative to ensure that these novelties are not only efficient and functional but also integrally trustworthy (ElHussini et al., 2021).

In this framework, two emerging frameworks, i.e., threat intelligence and cloud trust models, offer robust mechanisms for mitigating cyber risks in EV-enabled healthcare systems. Threat intelligence equips these systems with the capability to detect, analyze, and respond to cyber threats proactively by leveraging real-time threat feeds, behavioral analytics, and known indicators of compromise (IOCs). Simultaneously, to regulate interactions and evaluate cloud trust models (Liu et al., 2014; Acharya et al., 2020), healthcare cloud applications and databases depend on data protection, identity validation and behavioral reliability as shown in **Table 1**.

Table 1. Mobile health meets electric mobility based secure systems literature review

Reference	Focus Area	Methodology/Approach	Key findings	Limitations
(Avatefipour et al., 2019)	Rechargeable ambulances with healthcare IoT	Case study on e-ambulance distribution in urban Europe	Established aids of EVs in reducing emissions and enabling telemedicine; highlighted security concerns in telematics systems	Did not offer specific security procedures
(Sanghvi and Markel, 2021)	e-health transport through cloud security	Analysis of cloud threats and HIPAA compliance	Suggested encryption-based precautions and identified main susceptibility in EV-cloud and healthcare	Validation through limited experimental data
(ElHussini et al., 2021)	VANETs through healthcare EVs	For vehicular networks an AI-based Intrusion Detection System (IDS)	Proposed AI-enhanced IDS to detect DoS, MITM attacks in V2X healthcare data and spoofing	EV healthcare settings requires real time testing
(Liu et al., 2014)	EVs based remote diagnostics	Integration of sensors and IoT in healthcare-enabled EVs	Continuous patient monitoring in transit; risks identified in wireless data transmission	In-depth study n Security framework is not properly mentioned
(Wang et al., 2024)	Mobile healthcare for Trust Models	Using edge-cloud devices designed multi-layer trust model	Introduced secure data routing via blockchain verification and TEEs	More focused on architecture instead on EVs healthcare-based application
(Sanghvi et al., 2021)	Blockchain through mobile healthcare EVs	Distributed smart contract-based privacy architecture	Ensured tamper-proof and traceability medical records in mobile health nodes	Concerns related to scalability and latency have not been addressed

continued on following page

Table 1. Continued

Reference	Focus Area	Methodology/Approach	Key findings	Limitations
(Weng et al., 2020)	Charging infrastructure of rechargeable ambulances	Risk assessment through smart grid	Vulnerabilities identified in EV charging infrastructure used for healthcare logistics	Active countermeasures have not been proposed
(Rana, 2017)	AI for cybersecurity in EV health platforms	Anomaly detection through machine learning	Real-time threat detection in rechargeable EVs	Heavily relies on large, labeled datasets
(Abedi et al., 2015)	e-healthcare vehicles using cyber-physical security	CPS integration through survey-based study	Cyberattack mapping in EVs which are used for patient monitoring	Lacks in the benchmarking performance
(Kavousi-Fard et al., 2020)	Healthcare data in transit for Privacy-preserving	Learning through rechargeable ambulances	Data privacy through multiple EV nodes without any centralized storage	Real-time use hindered because of computational modelling

The multidisciplinary intersection of healthcare informatics, cybersecurity and electric mobility in this chapter presents a comprehensive survey of cloud trust models and threat intelligence which apply to secure healthcare operations within EV ecosystems. The various real-world cases highlight the major vulnerabilities and threats which proposes a layered architectural framework for trust-aware data protection and presents a smart ambulance to illustrate practical implementation of these systems in electric mobility. Ultimately, this chapter aims to contribute to the design of cyber-resilient, intelligent and trustworthy healthcare systems in the age of electric mobility. Also, the chapter explores the intersection of cyber security, healthcare and electric mobility, focusing on how threat intelligence and cloud trust models can secure data exchange, protect infrastructure and ensure compliance in EV-based healthcare systems.

2. HEALTHCARE IN THE EV ECOSYSTEM

The integration of healthcare systems in EVs plays an important role in the delivery of medical services, particularly in the framework of decentralized, responsive care and mobile-data management. As healthcare systems evolve to meet the needs of aging populations, chronic disease management, and rural outreach, EVs serve as agile platforms capable of delivering real-time clinical interventions beyond the confines of traditional facilities as shown in **Figure 2**. By equipping EVs with diagnostic devices, communication modules and cloud-enabled interfaces, healthcare providers can offer preventive screenings, consultations and emergency care at the point of need, dramatically enhancing accessibility and patient outcomes (Wang et al., 2024; Basnet et al., 2021).

Figure 2. Healthcare in EV ecosystem

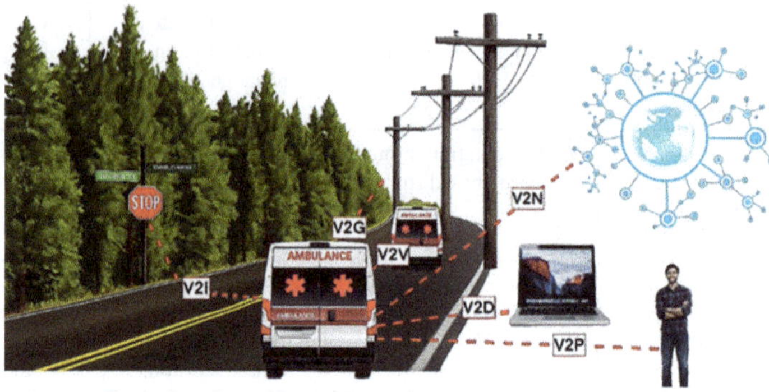

2.1 Emergency Response and Smart Ambulances

Electric mobility is powered by smart ambulances which are reshaping emergency medical services by integrating cloud computing, mobility and healthcare IoT into a single, agile platform. Smart ambulances are equipped with onboard diagnostics, real-time telemetry, high speed communication modules and AI assisted real-time telemetry with respect to conventional ambulances. These features allow emergency medical technicians (EMTs) and paramedics to collect, transmit and analyze patient vitals such as blood pressure, glucose levels, ECG data and oxygen saturation to hospitals en route. Cloud connectivity enables emergency departments to receive and prepare live patient data specialized care units (Sanghvi et al., 2021; Zhou et al., 2021; Weng et al., 2020).

These smart ambulances include telemedicine capabilities which allow remote physicians to guide paramedics during initial interventions which are perilous in high-risk situations like stroke, trauma and cardiac arrest. These services enhanced by the integration of electric mobility which further provides vibration-free environments, quite conducive to gentle medical operations. However, these innovations bring cybersecurity concerns such as unauthorized access or manipulation of patient data during emergencies which could lead to legal or incorrect liabilities. Thus, securing this ecosystem demands innovative framework for identity authentication, data encryption and integrity checks specifically for life-critical nature of such tasks.

2.2 Mobile Health Clinics for Rural and Remote Areas

For bridging the rural-urban healthcare systems can be powered by smart ambulances, which is a revolutionary solution for mobile health clinics. There are so many regions where permanent healthcare infrastructure is insufficient or absent thus, EV based clinics provide medical services such as maternal and child health, vaccinations, chronic disease management and screening of infectious diseases directly to patients. EV-based clinics are often equipped with diagnostic equipment including ultrasound devices, X-ray machines, basic surgical tools and point of care testing kits. Thus, integration of cloud connectivity helps in uploading patient data to centralized health databases which enables longitudinal follow-ups and tracking (Rana, 2017; Abedi et al., 2015).

Furthermore, EVs based clinics ensure environmental sustainability which operates on solar-charged batteries and can remain off-grid for extended periods. This feature is useful particularly in military operations, disaster relief areas and unstable electricity supply areas. However, mobile health clinics are often connected to public or low-security networks which ensure that cybersecurity is crucial for such systems. Unauthorized interception of medical data or manipulation of system software could compromise not just patient privacy, but the overall integrity of national health surveillance systems (Kavousi-Fard et al., 2020). Applying cloud trust models and secure data transfer protocols is therefore critical for maintaining confidentiality, availability and reliability of care.

2.3 EVs in Supply Chains and Medical Logistics

EVs play a pivotal role in transforming the medical logistics landscape by facilitating the timely, secure and climate-controlled transportation of critical healthcare materials. These include vaccines, blood units, diagnostic samples, surgical kits, personal protective equipment (PPE) and transplant organs. Equipped with IoT sensors, smart refrigeration units, GPS modules and tamper-evident containers, EVs ensure that medical consignments remain within the required temperature and humidity thresholds throughout the journey. Real-time telemetry allows health administrators to monitor delivery conditions continuously via cloud platforms (Li et al., 2019; Wang et al., 2020).

The integration of EVs into healthcare supply chains also aligns with green healthcare goals, reducing emissions and contributing to the overall sustainability of public health services. However, these systems are susceptible to cyber-physical threats. A targeted attack could spoof GPS data, alter temperature readings or delay deliveries intentionally, leading to severe consequences, particularly during epidemics or organ transplant logistics (Sharma and Ali, 2025; El-Rewini et al., 2020). Thus, securing these networks involves implementing cybersecurity measures like digital signatures, secure fleet management software and anomaly detection algorithms that can flag deviations in real time. Blockchain can also be leveraged to provide transparent, immutable records of shipment handling across different checkpoints (Manoj and Hasan, 2021).

2.4 Challenges in Incorporation and Interoperability

While the integration of EVs with healthcare technologies presents significant potential, it also introduces substantial technical and operational complexity. One of the key challenges lies in achieving interoperability between heterogeneous systems medical devices, EV components, telecommunication interfaces, cloud platforms and EHRs that were not originally designed to work together. For instance, a smart ambulance defibrillator may store data in a proprietary format that is not compatible with the hospital cloud-based health information system (Neaimeh and Andersen, 2020; Garofalaki et al., 2022).

Further complexity arises when multiple stakeholders such as automotive OEMs, medical equipment vendors, cloud service providers, and health institutions are involved, each with their own cybersecurity standards and compliance protocols. The various inconsistencies and absence of unified data governance frameworks applies to standards such as DICOM, ISO/IEEE 11073 and HL7 which provides wide system coordination (Hong et al., 2022). Thus, addressing these challenges requires adopting middleware platforms that facilitate secure integration of API, promoting universal healthcare interoperability standards such as fast healthcare interoperability resources (FHIR) and encouraging private-public partnerships for cybersecure EV-healthcare systems.

2.5 Cybersecurity Concerns in EV-Enabled Healthcare Systems

EV-enabled healthcare systems are surrounded by cybersecurity landscape which is highly prone to multi-vector threats. Smart ambulances connected to IoT devices, cloud infrastructure and hospital networks form a complex cyber-physical system (CPS) which is the major entry point for attackers. The threats include unsecured wireless interfaces, data interception, firmware manipulation through over-the-air (OTA) updates, denial-of serve attacks and malware injections in diagnostic modules targeting the smart ambulance cloud databases or control system.

Moreover, mobile units are often governed by processed patient data with strict privacy regulations, such as GDPR and HIPAA, making it a non-negotiable aspect of system design. Cybersecurity breaches result in financial and reputational damage which leads to legal liability and public health crises. To alleviate these risks, threat intelligence mechanisms must integrate with the system by enabling proactive identification of malevolent activities based on behavior-based anomalies or known signatures.

By dynamically assigning trust scores to entities, the cloud trust models can further enhance system resilience based on authentication strength, real-time network activity and prior behavior. Thus, this trust-based authority ensures that only verified, authenticated and personal systems are allowed to interact with patient sensitive heath data.

3. THREAT LANDSCAPE IN EV-CLOUD-HEALTHCARE SYSTEMS

The convergence of EVs, cloud computing and healthcare services introduces a complex cyber-physical environment characterized by high mobility, data sensitivity and heterogeneous device integration. While this fusion unlocks new opportunities for medical service delivery, it also significantly expands the attack surface (Kim et al., 2021).

Figure 3. EV cloud healthcare systems

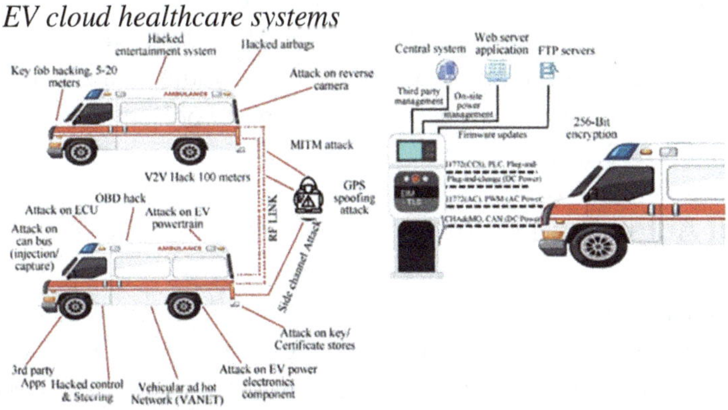

This section maps the evolving threat landscape in EV cloud, healthcare systems by categorizing key vulnerabilities, identifying adversarial actors and analyzing potential consequences of successful exploits. The intersection of these domains creates multidimensional risks that span data confidentiality, service availability, system integrity and regulatory compliance as shown in **Figure 3**.

3.1 Multi-Layered Vulnerabilities

The EV–cloud–healthcare infrastructure comprises several interconnected layers, each introducing specific threats such as-

3.1.1 Different Layers

Vehicle layer determines EVs functioning as mobile health units equipped with telematics systems, onboard diagnostics, GPS, infotainment units and wireless communication modules. Threats at this layer include CAN Bus Attacks, which is exploitation of the in-vehicle communication system to inject malicious commands. Firmware Manipulation, for unauthorized over-the-air (OTA) updates that install spyware or disable safety-critical systems. Sensor Spoofing, for manipulation of biometric or diagnostic sensors to report falsified patient data. Edge and Cloud Layer, for real-time health data from EVs is often transmitted to cloud platforms for analytics and storage. Man-in-the-Middle (MitM) Attacks, for interception and alteration of transmitted medical data during vehicular movement. Cloud Configuration Vulnerabilities, for misconfigured cloud storage buckets can expose millions of patient records Healthcare IoT Layer, for wearable devices, diagnostic equipment and telemedicine tools used inside mobile clinics are IoT-enabled and often inadequately secured. Botnet Infections, for compromised devices may be recruited into botnets, launching distributed denial-of-service (DDoS) attacks. Default Credentials Exploitation, for use of factory-set usernames and passwords, often left unchanged, leads to unauthorized access.

3.2 Threat Actors and Motives

The threat landscape is shaped by a variety of actors, each with distinct motivations such as cybercriminals which aim to monetize patient data through identity theft, ransomware and data brokerage on the dark web. Hacktivists may target mobile healthcare services to protest government policies or raise awareness about public health inequities. Nation-State Actors exploit systemic vulnerabilities for espionage, destabilization or to cripple emergency response capabilities during conflicts. Insider threats, such as disgruntled employees or negligent third-party vendors, may intentionally or inadvertently compromise system security. These actors exploit vulnerabilities across technical, operational and human layers, making proactive threat modeling essential to risk mitigation (Roopa and Venugopal, 2025).

3.3 Data Privacy and Confidentiality Breaches

Data flowing through EV–cloud healthcare systems is highly sensitive, often containing personally identifiable information (PII), diagnostic results, genetic data and real-time biometrics. Unauthorized access to such data can lead to HIPAA/G-DPR violations resulting in severe legal and financial penalties. Targeted Social Engineering Attacks, such as spear-phishing based on medical history (Algarni and Thayananthan, 2025). Reputational Damage to healthcare providers and technology vendors, eroding public trust in mobile health solutions. Furthermore, breaches in remote health monitoring systems could allow attackers to manipulate or falsify patient health records by endangering their lives.

3.4 Service Disruption and Availability Attacks

Healthcare services delivered through EVs are time-sensitive and mission-critical. Threats that impair service continuity include DDoS Attacks on Telemedicine Infrastructure, rendering mobile consultations and diagnostics unavailable during emergencies. Thus, delaying emergency transport, altering routes and remote hi-jacking of smart ambulances creates service disruption. Power system interference (PSI) disrupts the EVs' battery management or charging infrastructure which renders non-operational clinics. Such disruptions create life-threatening situations in high-risk or remote environments where EV-based units are the sole access point for care.

3.5 Emerging Threat Vectors

In healthcare EVs, the 5G technologies, edge computing and autonomous driving protect the breaching of data, recognizes the threat emerges due to edge node compromise. Thus, AI based triage algorithms helps in manipulating the autonomous decision exploits to misclassify severity among patients. Quantum Cryptography Challenges, with emerging threats from quantum computing may break current encryption standards used in EV–healthcare communications. Proactive adaptation of post-quantum cryptography, AI explainability mechanisms and zero-trust network architectures will be crucial to future proofing these systems.

Thus, the EV–cloud healthcare convergence offers transformative benefits for mobile, intelligent and equitable medical care. However, the threat landscape is rapidly expanding, dynamic and highly circumstantial. A successful security strategy must blend real-time threat intelligence, advanced trust models and ethical governance to safeguard patient data, ensuring continuous services and fostering public confidence. In this domain, the multidimensional threats anticipate the stakeholders to design a resilient system that supports both security and innovation.

4. POSITION OF THREAT INTELLIGENCE IN EV- CLOUD HEALTHCARE SYSTEMS

The merging of cloud computing, EVs and healthcare delivery introduces a dynamic cyber physical environment where outdated cybersecurity measures are insufficient. EVs evolve into healthcare platforms which are equipped with diagnostic tools, real-time communication interfaces and medical IoT devices, as they become targets and conduits to cyber threats. In this framework, threat intelligence plays a crucial role in protecting sensitive patient data for maintaining the vehicular and infrastructural integrity and ensuring healthcare delivery. It serves as a practical defense mechanism which offers malicious entities and exploitable vulnerabilities that compromise EV-healthcare systems.

4.1 Threat Intelligence in the Setting of Mobile Healthcare EVs

In EV-cloud healthcare ecosystems, threat intelligence addresses the cross-domain cyber risks emerging from the integration of medical technologies, automotive systems and cloud infrastructures. In contrast to stationary health systems, EV-based platforms operate in varied physical environments which connect intermittently to the internet and interface with numerous networks. This complexity necessitates a threat intelligence approach that captures smart ambulances telemetry anomalies, such as sudden deviations in system diagnostics or unauthorized access to EV control modules. Compromised OTA updates may install malware into smart ambulances operating system and its embedded healthcare applications. Cloud attack vectors include misconfigured APIs that bridge EVs to decision support platforms and electronic health record (EHR) systems. In EV-based clinics, malicious actors exploit mobile diagnostics, wearable medical IoT devices or onboard imaging systems. Here, threat intelligence must not only detect but prevent attacks in environments where vehicular mobility adds layers of volatility.

4.2 Types of Threat Intelligence Relevant to EV-Based Healthcare Systems

To protect this multi-layered environment, threat intelligence can be categorized into four different types:

- Deliberate threat intelligence helps in understanding the broad scale of risks such as geopolitical outbreaks on healthcare fleets or systemic susceptibility in EV software used across global ambulance services.

- Tactical threat intelligence emphases specific tactics, techniques and procedures (TTPs) used by adversaries to exploit EV communication buses, such as LIN and CAN, EV-to-cloud gateways which handle medical data and interoperability layers between healthcare diagnostic tools and the smart mobility computing environment.
- Effective threat intelligence offers real-time updates on threat campaigns, such as ransomware targeting cloud-connected hospital fleets, that may immediately affect EV-fleet services.
- Technical Threat Intelligence identifies precise indicators of compromise (IOCs), such as malicious firmware versions affecting EV battery management systems (BMS) or IP addresses associated with breaches of telemedicine services.

These types contribute exclusively to prevent data exfiltration and healthcare service disruptions in EV-based healthcare systems.

4.3 Incorporation of EV-Oriented Security Frameworks

The threat intelligence has been deeply integrated into EV fleet security operations, healthcare SOCs and vehicle telematics platforms to create an inclusive cyber defense posture. For example, a cyber-attack on an EVs' infotainment unit may be a precursor to a lateral movement targeting its medical diagnostic applications. Operational intelligence can help detect such anomalies through behavioral baselining and sensor fusion. Tactical intelligence can inform the implementation of intrusion detection systems (IDS) embedded within mobile healthcare EVs, enabling local threat detection even without a constant cloud connection. If a fleet of mobile clinics are under a coordinated phishing or malware attack, technical intelligence can trigger vehicle lockdown protocols, restrict remote access and alert nearby healthcare control centers. This layered defense model ensures that both vehicle and clinical components of the EV ecosystem are synchronized against threats. Thus, the incorporation of strategic incorporation of security protocols in EV infrastructures has various types of case study such as-

Case Study 1: Medical Response Units and EV-Based Mobile Security in Dubai, UAE

The Dubai government has initiated a program that deploys EVs as dual-purpose units which can deliver both cybersecurity operations and emergency medical care. These smart rechargeable ambulances are integrated with cutting-edge telemedicine systems, biometric patient identification tools, encrypted communication platforms and AI-powered surveillance cameras. EVs operate over a secure vehicle-to-everything (V2X) network using Transport Layer Security (TLS) and Virtual Private Networks (VPNs) to transmit incident logs and patient data to centralized control centers. Zero Trust Network Access (ZTNA) manages health and security data streams to ensure strict categorization. This cyber-physical system enables rapid response to urban smart zones incidents, specifically cardiac emergencies to physical intrusions, without compromising the integrity and privacy of sensitive data. However, any mismanagement in decryption timing or firewall rules during system audits could spread attack surfaces from healthcare domain into the security system. Thus, this initiative marks a major step toward the fusion of public safety, EV based mobility and healthcare support in real time mode.

Case Study 2: EV Healthcare Hybrids Surveillance for Disaster Area in California, USA

The department of emergency services of California collaborated with EV manufacturers to arrange smart rechargeable ambulances which are designed for post-disaster environments such as earthquakes and wildfires. Smart ambulances serve as hybrid platforms that support healthcare delivery and surveillance which are equipped with computing systems, onboard medical diagnostic equipment and satellite uplinks. EVs can launch drones for terrain monitoring during gridless operation zones, while triaging injured individuals using telemetry and smart stretchers to command centers. The EVs utilizes AES-256 encrypted mesh networks and secure boot processes from a cybersecurity standpoint with all internal devices operating under strict role-based access control (RBAC). To ensure device integrity in disconnected environments, each component is tied to a Trusted Platform Module (TPM 2.0). These rechargeable EVs function as care centers during emergencies while allowing data to be stored securely and locally at the time of restoring the connectivity. Challenges arise when high processing demand exceeds the battery capacity of rechargeable ambulances during prolonged outages which showcases the strategic advantage by integrating cybersecure healthcare operations into mobile EV platforms.

Case Study 3: AI integrated rechargeable ambulances in Seoul, South Korea

In South Korea, as per ambitious smart city initiative rechargeable ambulances are augmented with AI-powered security and healthcare technologies. These ambulances are frontier for both emergency and law enforcement medical services. They are equipped with digital medical record access, autonomous diagnostic capabilities and facial recognition systems for on-scene triage. These rechargeable ambulances maintain 5G connectivity to emergency networks with every transaction whether security related or medical related which are immutably logged on a private blockchain. This architecture ensures integrity, traceability and data transparency. Major features include intrusion detection and prevention system (IDPS) driven by machine learning (ML) which are capable of detecting anomalies in data exchange patterns and vehicular behaviors. A real-time contextual cyber risk uses these rechargeable ambulances based on environmental data and threat exposure. The implementation of real-time anonymization techniques and legal amendments based on improved multi-agency coordination, response speed and public concerns over surveillance. Despite such ethical challenges, ingenuity sets a global precedent for mixing cybersecure healthcare and security operation in urban infrastructure with smart electric mobility.

Case Study 4: Rechargeable ambulances with cybersecurity layers in Helsinki, Finland

Autonomous rechargeable ambulances function mobile clinics to support rapid-response healthcare and remote diagnostics in suburban areas. These smart ambulances are equipped with real-time video consultation capabilities, diagnostic imaging systems and AI tools for preliminary patient assessments. Helsinki's initiative to ensure cybersecurity uses end-to-end encrypted protocols (TLS 1.3), AI powered threat detection and decentralized identity management for the onboard patients in smart ambulances. When network conditions permit, the patient data is stored temporarily on encrypted SSDs within the rechargeable ambulances which are using quantum-resistant encryption protocols. The cybersecurity system incorporates blockchain based audit trials to prevent retroactive data manipulation or unauthorized access. One major advantage is that rechargeable ambulances can operate during non-peak hours by minimizing human contact and delivering care to compromised immune systems challenged populations. However, preliminary tests identify vulnerabilities in rechargeable batteries i.e., vehicle-to-infrastructure (V2I) communication during handoffs between Wi-Fi and cellular networks. Thus, using these smart electric mobility platforms, the Helsinki's model highlights the potential for scalable, secure and autonomous healthcare delivery.

Case Study 5: Secure health and bio-surveillance systems in rechargeable ambulances in Military field units in Tel Aviv, Israel

The Israeli defense forces (IDF) have begun arranging rechargeable ambulances for military health operations by combining biometric surveillance, cybersecure communications and battlefield medical response. These smart ambulances are operational with ruggedized health monitoring systems, chemical-biological threat detection tools and portable imaging. These rechargeable batteries run on encrypted and isolated military grade networks using real-time satellite and post- quantum cryptography for synchronizing the data. To detect trauma, stress and fatigue in soldiers these AI-based biometric analysis has been used. To prevent interception, these rechargeable ambulances employ strict multi-factor authentication for operators, secure firmware updates via electromagnetic shielding and blockchain. During joint drills, these rechargeable ambulances maintain mission confidentiality and data sovereignty by reducing response times. A major challenge is the intense demand for energy storage due to encrypted telemetry and high-bandwidth operations. Thus, this case provides utility to smart ambulances such as medical nodes and mobile command in cyber-prioritized, high-risk environments.

Case Study 6: Rechargeable Ambulances integrated into Urban command networks in Rotterdam, Netherlands

In Rotterdam, smart electric ambulances integrate with emergency medical services into a centralized control system and urban command. These ambulances are linked with fire, emergency dispatch centers and police through a secure data-sharing platform. Also, each smart electric ambulance is equipped with autonomous defibrillator systems, advanced on-boards diagnostics and continuous ECG monitoring which are linked directly to hospital command centers. Through the implementation of a secure multi-tenant architecture (SMTA) cybersecurity ensures that data will be segregated between medical teams and agencies. Communication is managed using a hybrid 5G/LoRa network with fallback encryption tunnels which ensure uninterrupted data flow even under infrastructure failure or cyberattack. To detect anomalies in an operator access or data traffic behavioral analytics is applied to prevent potential threats inside the smart electric ambulances. By providing hospital staff with accurate pre-arrival health metrics, the integration of cybersecure healthcare with electric mobility significantly reduces the emergency response time. Minor delays were observed during stress testing between fixed and mobile networks, but mitigation through edge computing proved to be effective. This model has been studied by other European cities as a blueprint for cyber-resilient and smart logistics.

4.4 Threat Intelligence sharing across EV–Healthcare Systems

Collaborative threat intelligence sharing is critical in scenarios where EVs function as mobile clinics, diagnostic units or emergency medical vehicles. As these platforms move between jurisdictions, networks and cloud regions, intelligence sharing ensures consistent protection. The key mechanisms include EV–Health ISACs (Information Sharing and Analysis Centers), for cross-sectoral bodies enabling automakers, healthcare providers and cybersecurity firms to share threat data. Vehicle-to-Infrastructure (V2I) Intelligence Feeds, for sharing contextual intelligence between EVs and roadside units (RSUs) or health hubs for environmental threat analysis (e.g., identifying hotspots for cyber intrusions). Secure Blockchain-Based Exchanges ensures the verifiability and immutability of shared threat intelligence, particularly useful for fleet operators managing thousands of connected EVs in real time. Such federated threat intelligence frameworks empower stakeholders to respond collectively to emerging EV-specific threats like remote engine shutdowns, medical data injection attacks or vehicular ransomware.

Case Study 1: Threat Intelligence shared through Cross-agency in Smart EV ambulances in Stockholm, Sweden

To deploy a fleet of intelligent electric ambulances in Stockholm, the regional healthcare authority is partnered with smart mobility which is connected to the IT systems and citywide hospitals. These rechargeable ambulances were integrated into a joint threat intelligence sharing framework which involves city's digital infrastructure management, hospitals and public safety networks. Each rechargeable ambulance includes onboard health telemetry, lightweight security agent and encrypted 5G communication which are capable of reporting anomalies in real-time to the National computer emergency response team (CERT). The shared intelligence such as ransomware indicators of compromise, IP-based intrusion signatures and phishing domains targeting hospital networks which are automatically disseminated across the ecosystem. To prevent a coordinated spoofing and phishing campaign, the bidirectional threat intelligence model helps hospitals to login their pages and dispatching software to rechargeable ambulances in 2022. However, the interoperability gaps emerged between public mobility interfaces and proprietary health data systems, which necessitates the adoption of standardized threat sharing formats like trusted automated exchange of intelligence information (TAXII) and structured threat information expression (STIX). This case underlines how multisector intelligence collaboration can safeguard cyber-physical system and mobile health operations.

Case Study 2: Cyber Threat Intelligence Exchange between Healthcare Cloud Providers and rechargeable ambulances in Singapore.

In Singapore smart nation initiative has piloted a cyber threat intelligence exchange system between healthcare cloud platforms and original equipment manufacturers

(OEMs) which manages mobile diagnostic rechargeable ambulances. In this model smart electric mobility integrates with real-time health record systems and cutting-edge AI modules for diagnostics which are used for healthcare screening in urban and rural zones. As cyber threats targeting mobility systems and healthcare overlap such as attacks on over-the-air (OTA) updates or Bluetooth-connected medical devices establish threat sharing protocol which allows anonymized threat logs to be exchanged between health and transport sectors. Thus, these cross-domain models allow early detection of a sophisticated MITM attack targeting both rechargeable ambulance infotainment firmware and Bluetooth sensors used for patient monitoring. This exchange informs both software patching and policy reform. The challenges involved in securing legal data-sharing agreements and cross sector trust while preserving privacy of device and patient. This case highlights cyber intelligence sharing which improves resilience in converged health mobility infrastructures.

Case Study 3: Cyber Threat Synchronization in Real-Time Emergency rechargeable ambulances in Toronto, Canada

In this case study, an emergency mobility coordination system has been implemented in Toronto where mobile clinics, hospital systems and electric ambulances can operate over a shared cyber situational awareness platform. This initiative involves cybersecurity operation centers from city's smart grid operator, electric ambulances charging stations networks and public hospitals. The core innovation is cyber synchronization gateway that disseminates and aggregates threat intelligence across all nodes which includes threats to charge smart electric ambulances, mobile health IoT devices and hospital network endpoints. In 2023, this system proved that during a coordinated malware campaign, the system vulnerability widely accesses the tool installed in hospital telemedicine servers and rechargeable ambulances fleet management software. The system uses AI-assisted prioritization of alerts, machine-readable threat formats and human-in-the-loop vetting before deploying automated countermeasures. However, the complexity in managing real-time authentication and managing trust boundaries across multiple sectors remains a significant challenge. This case demonstrates the critical role in protecting rechargeable ambulance-based healthcare operations through synchronized threat response.

Case Study 4: Distributed Threat Sharing across Smart Ambulances clinics in Bavaria, Germany

A regional healthcare mobility program in Bavaria launched smart electric mobile ambulances which are equipped with diagnostic tools and electronic health record (EHR) interfaces. The cybersecurity risks associated with Bavaria's Ministry of Health partnered with a coalition of health IT Vendors and EV manufacturers to develop a decentralized cyber threat intelligence sharing platform using blockchain. This platform logs the device vulnerabilities, firmware exploit patterns and phishing encounters through real-time mobile clinics and syncs threat logs with mobility security operations centers (SOCs) and eHealth authority. Smart contracts automatically trigger alerts and distribute remediation protocols (e.g. firewalls and patches) to all registered rechargeable ambulances. This approach mitigates the spread of malware that initially targets unsecured diagnostic apps and later attempts to lateral movement into charging station networks. The blockchain system has a major advantage that ensures data provenance and integrity, even when shared across multiple jurisdictions. However, performance blocks during large-scale updates and latency in reaching remote clinics which reveal limitations in scalability. Despite this, the initiative demonstrates the effectiveness of decentralized models for secure intelligence sharing in mixed EV-health environments.

Case Study 5: Pandemic-Response rechargeable Ambulance Through Cyber Threat Intelligence in Sao Paulo, Brazil

Sao Paulo, during COVID-19 pandemic repurposed electric buses and ambulances as vaccination units and mobile testing. These rechargeable ambulances were outfitted with cloud-synced digital patient registration tools and medical equipment. The rapid rise in cyberattacks targets pandemic infrastructure such as vaccine cold-chain tracking and COVID-19 registration APIs, the city's cybersecurity task force establishes a centralized threat intelligence hub. This hub connects cybersecurity teams, healthcare data cloud vendors and EV telematics providers via hybrid cloud security information and event management (SIEM). Through a unified dashboard, threat intelligence monitors anomalies such as DDoS attempts, phishing attacks and credential stuffing on health APIs and vehicle systems. The threat hub coordinates cyber drills with simulated attacks on vaccine-data transmission in rechargeable ambulances. Through this system, a coordinated DNS hijacking campaign to neutralize and detect the errors that occurred in smart electric ambulances while registering the names of the patient on the portals. The biggest challenge in harmonizing the data protection standards across diverse technology stacks is through cloud platforms. This case highlights the necessity of rapid coordination and real-time visibility during public health emergencies involves mobile rechargeable ambulance units.

Case Study 6: Government and Private Rechargeable ambulance operators CERTs in Bangalore, India

In this case, several private emergency service providers in Bangalore operate smart electric ambulances by integrating patient monitoring systems and telemedicine. These private rechargeable ambulances were initially isolated from public cyber defense coordination by creating vulnerabilities for both sectors. In 2023, the Indian computer emergency response team (CERT-In) initiated public-private threat intelligence partnership (PPTIP) that accesses the patient data. Through this initiative, the participated EV ambulance companies receive real-time updates on known threats, indicators of compromise (IoCs) and vulnerability disclosures related to smart electric ambulance charging software, medical IoT and remote patient monitoring. In return, the private operators report the attacked data to CERT-In using a sanitized reporting protocol that protects sensitive data while contributing to national cyber situational awareness. The early detection of an API is the key success as it manipulates vulnerability in a third-party rechargeable ambulance management application that enables mass credential theft across multiple ambulance operators. This protocol standardizes bidirectional threat intelligence sharing between fragmented mobility and health sectors. The major challenge is incentivizing small operators to join and comply with secure telemetry reporting standards. Thus, this case showcases the effectiveness of a sector spanning, national coordinates threat exchange framework.

4.5 Cybersecurity Architecture for EVs Mobile Healthcare

The modern EV–based healthcare systems require intelligent cybersecurity architectures that dynamically respond to evolve the threats such as anomaly detection engines (ADE), onboard the EV by continuously assessing the deviations in sensor readings, battery performance and patient data traffic. The dynamic access control (DAC) responds to real-time risk notches; for instance, annulling access to EHRs if the EVs' network situation is flagged as untrusted. Encrypted edge processing (EDP) ensures that medical diagnostics conducted inside EVs will remain protected even during network outages conditions. Zero-Trust vehicle networks validate every command node and data packet particularly when mobile units host life-critical equipment. These architectures allow EV-based healthcare delivery to shift from static protection to adaptive cyber resilience for optimized safety and performance.

The most important lessons emerge from the integration of threat intelligence in EV-healthcare systems by adopting standardized protocols such as TAXII and structures threat information expression (STIX). These standards ensure that cybersecurity data such as IoCs, vulnerability disclosures and attack patterns can be shared uniformly across mobility sectors and healthcare sectors, which enables timely and actionable threat responses. The use of AI models with data anonymization techniques has proven that cross-sector threat intelligence never compromises patient data and privacy. This approach allows organizations to collaborate with train cybersecurity models across multiple platforms by keeping sensitive data secure.

The integration of CERT-In into the intelligence sharing systems is one of the best practices in aggregating threat data, coordinating incident responses and issuing real-time alerts. Its involvement enhances early warning systems and ensures synchronized mitigation efforts across all entities. Furthermore, the application of secure hardware enclaves and blockchain technology offers an immutable and temper-resistant foundation for logging cyber events. These technologies strengthen the integrity of forensic data which helps in maintaining trust between stakeholders and provide transparent records of cybercrime investigations or audits. Thus, simulation exercises and cross-sector drills have emerged as a practical and necessary tool to test the willingness of smart electric ambulances against complex cyberattacks. By engaging operational teams and technical teams, the multi-vector threat scenarios help identify system weaknesses by refining response strategies and building collaborative flexibility. These practices form a robust blueprint by advancing cyber threat intelligence in the evolving intersection of healthcare and electric mobility.

4.6 Implementation Challenges

By implementing threat intelligence in EV-cloud healthcare systems involve substantial hurdles such as variability in connectivity, for EV-mobile units which operate in remote areas and may lack the bandwidth needed for real-time threat feed updates. False Positives and Sensor Noise, for intricate environments within EVs, such as heat, EM interference and vibration, can trigger non-malicious alerts that desensitize threat detection systems. The issues related to data sovereignty for cross-border operations, for EVs healthcare systems may breach national data protection laws when threat feeds or logs are shared globally. Lack of standardization for incongruent smart ambulances manufacturers, cloud service providers and healthcare IT systems often use incompatible formats for sharing and interpreting intelligence. By addressing these challenges, it may require AI-enhanced filtering, unified cybersecurity standards and edge-based caching tailored for mobile health vehicles.

Thus, in the fast-evolving domain of EV-enabled healthcare, threat intelligence acts as the guard layer which safeguards sensitive clinical operations within highly mobile and cloud-connected surroundings. It authorizes stakeholders to detect early-stage attacks on medical subsystems, EV control units and cloud infrastructures, while enabling rapid and intelligent responses. When smart mobility integrates with fleet operations, cloud APIs and healthcare platforms, the threat intelligence transforms the isolated EV units into cyber-aware entities, ensuring secure, efficient and reliable care delivery on wheels. As smart mobility increases in healthcare systems, medicine and digital security converge, the threat intelligence will remain a foundation of trustworthy and resilient healthcare networks.

5. CLOUD TRUST MODELS IN ELECTRIC HEALTHCARE

The integration of EVs into mobile healthcare bases introduces a high degree of dependency on cloud computing structure. These EVs serve as emergency medical vehicles, mobile clinics or remote diagnostic units which require real-time access to medical imaging, decision support systems, patient data and electronic health records (EHRs) which can be managed through cloud computing. In this interconnected situation, cloud trust models become indispensable to ensure reliable and secure operations. The trust models govern how data is authorized, authenticated, transmitted, encrypted and audited across diverse and dynamic EV-healthcare systems.

5.1 Need for Cloud-EV-Healthcare Convergence

The conjunction of healthcare delivery, EV mobility and cloud computing strains a multifaceted trust framework because of sensitive patient data for medical histories transmitted from EVs to hospitals or cloud databases, which are subject to strict privacy regulations, such as GDPR and HIPAA. Dynamic Network Conditions, in which EVs connect to different networks (Wi-Fi, 5G, V2X) while moving, increasing the risk of unauthorized access or data interception. Decentralized Services, for healthcare decisions may be based on AI analytics running in distributed cloud nodes, requiring trust in the computation process and the origin of medical inferences.

Figure 4. Cloud-EV-Healthcare Convergence

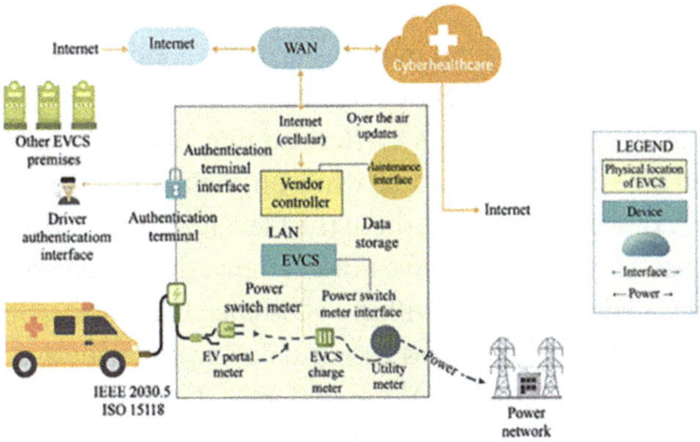

Third-Party Cloud Providers, for many healthcare services in EVs depend on external platforms such as AWS Health Lake or Azure Health Data Services, raising questions about trust, SLA enforcement and data residency (Yang et al., 2019). A comprehensive trust model must address identity verification, data provenance, confidentiality, integrity, availability and auditability across the EV-cloud-healthcare continuum as shown in **Figure 4**.

5.2 Components of Cloud Trust Models

To secure EV-enabled healthcare systems, cloud trust models encompass the following core components such as Identity and Access Management (IAM), which assign roles and privileges to users, medical devices and EV systems. For instance, only certified medical personnel should be able to access or update EHRs from within an EV. Trust Anchors and Digital Certificates, for root certificates are embedded within the EVs' onboard unit and medical subsystems to validate connections with trusted cloud services, ensuring mutual authentication. Data Integrity Assurance, for end-to-end hashing mechanisms (e.g., SHA-256 or blockchain ledgering) to ensure that patient data collected in the EV is neither altered in transit nor corrupted by cloud-side inference models (Hong et al., 2022). Confidential Computing provides trusted execution environments (TEEs) within the cloud to isolate sensitive healthcare computations (e.g., ECG anomaly detection or patient triage decisions) from potential malicious insiders or co-tenants. Provenance Tracking and Auditing, for every data access or modification from EV acquisition to cloud AI processing is logged immutably, supporting compliance and enabling forensic analysis in case of breaches. These components collectively establish a zero-trust cloud framework, ensuring that trust is not assumed but continuously verified.

5.3 Trust Models for EV-Enabled Healthcare Scenarios

Specific trust paradigms are employed based on the application context in mobile healthcare delivery such as Role-Based Trust Models, access is granted based on user roles such as doctor, technician or fleet administrator. An ambulance driver may have limited access to patient vitals, while physicians have full data interaction rights. Context-Aware Trust Models, these trust levels dynamically adjust based on location, time, risk level and behavior. For example, during emergency response, access may be elevated temporarily within a geo-fenced perimeter. Behavioral Trust Models, for AI-driven systems, assess user and device behavior over time to determine risk (Kim et al., 2021). If an EV-based diagnostic device suddenly transmits abnormal data patterns, its trust level is reduced, and access may be revoked until verified. Federated Trust Models, when EVs operate across states or countries, different healthcare systems and cloud providers must interoperate. Federated identity protocols (e.g., OAuth 2.0, SAML) allow seamless and secure access to cross-border medical data. These dynamic models support trust not only among cloud services but between the EV, its subsystems and external medical networks.

5.4 Integrating Cloud Trust Models with EV Architectures

Implementing cloud trust models within EV infrastructures requires architectural integration at multiple levels such as Telematics Gateway Security, in which the EVs' telematics control unit (TCU) serves as the main bridge to cloud platforms. Embedding cryptographic chips and secure boot processes ensures that only trusted firmware connects to healthcare clouds. Edge Cloud Interfacing, for many medical decisions are made on the edge (inside or near the EV) before cloud synchronization. Trust models must verify the integrity of edge analytics (e.g., blood pressure or glucose analysis) before data is accepted by cloud systems (Sharma and Ali, 2025). Encrypted Data Lakes, for diagnostic images, video consultations and medical history are stored in cloud data lakes. Trust models enforce encryption-at-rest and token-based decryption for authorized healthcare professionals only. Mobile VPN and Secure Tunneling, as EVs transition across different cellular or Wi-Fi networks, trust models initiate secure tunnels using IPsec or SSL/TLS to maintain session integrity without compromising latency. These integrations ensure trust continuity regardless of network variability or EV mobility conditions.

5.5 Challenges in Implementing Cloud Trust for Mobile Healthcare

Despite the potential, implementing cloud trust models in EV-based healthcare faces several obstacles such as Latency Constraints, for complex authentication or remote attestation protocols can introduce delays in emergency healthcare decisions made inside EVs. Limited Onboard Resources for embedded systems in EVs may lack the computational power to perform continuous cryptographic trust verification without draining power or reducing efficiency. Cloud Vendor Lock-In for relying on a single cloud provider may restrict flexibility, whereas multi-cloud architecture requires highly interoperable and federated trust frameworks. Patient Consent and Transparency, for dynamic trust systems must still ensure that patients remain informed about who accesses their data, even when care is delivered via an EV in a non-traditional clinical setting. Thus, by addressing these challenges demands hybrid trust architectures, combining lightweight edge trust agents with robust cloud-level enforcement mechanisms (Sanghvi and Markel, 2021; Weng et al., 2020).

Thus, cloud trust models ensure that sensitive patient data, life-critical diagnostic tools and vehicle-to-cloud (V2C) communications remain secure, verifiable and resilient. As healthcare delivery becomes increasingly mobile and cloud-dependent, these trust models serve as the invisible scaffolding that supports safe and effective care in motion. Their design must be adaptable, interoperable and transparent, balancing technological rigor with ethical responsibility. In the age of electric mobility, trust will be the currency of secure healthcare transformation.

6. THREAT-AWARE TRUST MODEL FOR EV-HEALTHCARE FRAMEWORK

The evolution of EVs into mobile healthcare units presents a transformative opportunity in improving accessibility, emergency response and patient outcomes. However, this convergence also introduces a uniquely complex cyber-physical ecosystem where trust must be established not only in cloud platforms but also across mobile, dynamic and sensitive healthcare workflows. To address this, a Threat-Aware Trust Model (TATM) specifically designed for EV-Healthcare ecosystems, integrates with real-time threat intelligence, adaptive access control and multi-tiered cloud trust management has been designed.

6.1 Framework Overview

The TATM operates as a layered framework that continuously monitors, evaluates and enforces trust across four interdependent domains such as-

- Electric Vehicle Layer
- Medical Device & Application Layer
- Cloud Infrastructure Layer
- Threat Intelligence Engine

At its core, TATM dynamically adjusts the trustworthiness of each entity, be it a user, device, cloud node or vehicular system based on contextual threat analysis, historical behavior and policy-based rules. It operates under a Zero Trust Architecture (ZTA) principle, where no entity is trusted by default and continuous verification is enforced at every communication hop.

6.2 Components of TATM Framework

The various components of TATM Framework are as follows-

6.2.1 Dynamic Trust Scoring Module (DTSM)

This module computes real-time trust scores for entities interacting within the system based on behavioral patterns (e.g., frequency of data requests, command sequences), contextual data (e.g., EV location, patient sensitivity level, emergency state), threat feed correlation (e.g., matching with known malware vectors or anomalous geolocation). Each component (EV control unit, medical application, cloud node) is tagged with a dynamic score which determines its permissions.

6.2.2 Threat Intelligence Fusion Engine (TIFE)

TIFE aggregates information from local EV-based IDS sensors (detecting anomalies in CAN bus or TCU), cloud-based SIEM platforms, national healthcare threat intelligence databases (e.g., H-ISAC, CDC alerts) and public zero-day exploit feeds. This engine contextualizes threats and pushes alerts to reconfigure trust policies in real time.

6.2.3 Context-Aware Access Control (CAAC)

Unlike traditional RBAC (Role-Based Access Control), CAAC evaluates access rights based on emergency context (e.g., code blue, trauma situation), data criticality (e.g., genomic data vs. vitals) and network trust level (e.g., secure VPN vs. public hotspot). Thus, if an EV is stationed in an insecure zone, access to sensitive data is restricted or rerouted through encrypted proxies.

6.2.4 Secure Data Orchestration Gateway (SDOG)

This component ensures trusted routing and secure orchestration between EV onboard devices (e.g., ECG, ultrasound), external healthcare clouds (e.g., EMR systems, diagnostic AI) and Third-party analytics engines (e.g., telemedicine platforms). It levers compression, data masking, policy-based key exchange and time-bound sharing.

6.3 Trust Lifecycle Management in the EV-Healthcare Framework

The TATM accomplishes trust across the subsequent lifecycle stages such as

- Loading Phase: It establishes the root-of-trust at EV boot-up using trusted platform module (TPM) which loads only verified encrypted credentials and software modules.
- Substantiation Phase: It validates the identities through digital signatures, biometrics or multifactor authentication for EV operators and medical staff.
- Unremitting Checking Phase: It updates trust scores periodically using DTSM and TIFE based on evolving settings.
- Reversal and Seclusion Phase: In case of conciliation i.e., ransomware detected, the devices are isolated, credentials are revoked and trusted backups are activated.

This development ensures continuity and resilience in both smart ambulances and healthcare delivery amenities.

6.4 System Architecture and Workflow

A simplified plan of TATM operations throughout a mobile indicative session-

- *Initiation:* EV diagnostic unit starts a session; onboard TPM verifies system integrity.
- *Authentication:* Medical staff log in; trust score is computed via DTSM using historical location awareness and patterns.
- *Threat Exposure:* TIFE detects suspicious network activity such as port scanning from unknown IP addresses.
- *Policy Implementation:* CAAC adjusts access by limiting the medical record visibility and locks the uploaded data until threat has been neutralized.
- *Transposition:* SDOG reroutes non-critical data to back up the nodes while maintaining essential services like streaming real-time vitals.
- *Audit Sorting:* All threat and trust decisions are recorded for future analysis and compliance.

6.5 Advantages of the Proposed TATM Framework

- *Threat-Response Malleability:* In static models, the TATM reacts to real-time threats with adjusted precision trust.
- *Mobility-Aware Trust Supervision:* Smart mobility is designed specifically for the high-mobility nature of EVs operating in diverse environments.
- *Integrated Secrecy and Compliance Layer:* It ensures that patient data handling respects the privacy regulations such as HIPPA and GDPR across authorities.
- *Resilience against Zero-Day Outbreaks:* TIFE combination of threat feeds allows for positive defense, even during emerging threats.

Thus, the TATM model characterizes a standard shift in managing cyber risk in EV-based healthcare systems. By merging context-aware access, behavioral analytics and integrated threat intelligence, the framework authorizes stakeholders to deliver secure healthcare on wheels. In an era where TATM ensures that trust travels with care, only when digital health must operate in motion.**Bottom of Form**

7. CONCLUSION

The combination of EVs into mobile healthcare transport has initiated a standard shift in how medical services are accessed and deployed. This alteration demands a security model that can keep pace with the mobile, dynamic and highly sensitive nature of EV-based healthcare networks. By introducing a multi-layered framework, the TATM model addresses this need by combining real-time threat intelligence, context-aware access control mechanisms and dynamic trust scoring.

The distinct conventional static trust approaches that TATM is designed to operate seamlessly within the resource-constrained and high-mobility environments that characterize EV-healthcare dispositions. By leveraging adaptive policy enforcement, threat fusion engines and secure orchestration gateways, the model provides robust cybersecurity and operational continuity in delivering life-saving care. It also aligns with global supervisory bases and enables secure, compliant data sharing across smart mobility and healthcare networks.

This chapter has demonstrated how TATM can enhance system integrity, data confidentiality and operational availability in the emerging domain of healthcare based electric mobility. In doing so, it bridges the critical gaps in interoperability, trust and threat response which ensures that digital health can safely travel where it is needed the most.

As this interdisciplinary arena progresses, several future commands emerge such as interoperability mechanisms and standardization of trust protocols which will facilitate seamless communication between medical devices, heterogeneous EV systems and cloud infrastructures. Collaborative efforts between automotive, healthcare and cybersecurity stakeholders are needed to define common APIs, encryption schemes and trust benchmarks.

Similarly, there is a pressing need for lightweight, edge-optimized trust engines which is capable of functioning under bandwidth and processing constraints common in mobile EV environments. Research into AI-driven threat intelligence, adaptive trust scoring using federated learning and privacy-preserving access controls (e.g., using zero-knowledge proofs) will shape the next generation of secure EV-healthcare platforms.

The global trust federations and policy harmonization frameworks must be established to support international EV-healthcare operations. These would enable cross-border data sharing, threat intelligence exchange and coordinated cyber incident response while respecting privacy and sovereignty. Last but not the least, as autonomous EVs and AI-powered diagnostics become more prevalent, self-evolving trust models will be critical. These systems must be capable of not only detecting threats and adapting trust policies but also learning from historical data and simulations to anticipate cyber risks before they manifest.

Thus, the convergence of electric mobility and healthcare requires a proactive, adaptive and forward-looking cybersecurity strategy. The proposed TATM lays the groundwork, but continued innovation, collaboration and policy alignment will be essential to fully realize the potential of cybersecure, intelligent and mobile healthcare delivery.

Abbreviations

The following abbreviations are used in this chapter:
EVs Electric Vehicles
V2X Vehicular communication networks
EMTs Emergency medical technicians
PPE Personal protective equipment
IoT Internet of things
CPS Cyber-physical system
OTA Over-the-air
MitM Man-in-the-Middle
PII Personally identifiable information
PSI Power System Interference
SBOM Software bill of materials
EHRs Electronic health records
TTPs Tactics, techniques and procedures
IDS Intrusion detection systems
V2I Vehicle-to-Infrastructure
ISACs Information Sharing and Analysis Centers
RSUs Roadside units
IAM Identity and Access Management
TEE Trusted execution environments
TCU Telematics control unit
V2C Vehicle-to-cloud
TATM Threat-Aware Trust Model
ZTA Zero Trust Architecture
DTSM Dynamic Trust Scoring Module
TIFE Threat Intelligence Fusion Engine
CAAC Context-Aware Access Control
SDOG Secure Data Orchestration Gateway
TPM Trusted Platform Module
HIPAA Health Insurance Portability and Accountability Act
GDPR General Data Protection Regulation
IOCs Indicators of compromise

REFERENCES

Abedi, S., Arvani, A., & Jamalzadeh, R. (2015). Cyber security of plug-in electric vehicles in smart grids: Application of intrusion detection methods. In *Plug In Electric Vehicles in Smart Grids: Integration Techniques* (pp. 129–147). Springer. DOI: 10.1007/978-3-319-22204-2_6

Acharya, S., Dvorkin, Y., & Karri, R. (2020). Public plug-in electric vehicles + grid data: Is a new cyberattack vector viable? *IEEE Transactions on Smart Grid, 11*(6), 5099–5113. DOI: 10.1109/TSG.2020.2994177

Algarni, A. M., & Thayananthan, V. (2025). Digital health: The cybersecurity for AI-based healthcare communication. *IEEE Access : Practical Innovations, Open Solutions, 13*, 5858–5870. DOI: 10.1109/ACCESS.2025.3526666

Alnasser, A., Sun, H., & Jiang, J. (2019). Cyber security challenges and solutions for V2X communications: A survey. *Computer Networks, 151*, 52–67. DOI: 10.1016/j.comnet.2018.12.018

Avatefipour, O., Al-Sumaiti, A. S., El-Sherbeeny, A. M., Awwad, E. M., Elmeligy, M. A., Mohamed, M. A., & Malik, H. (2019). An intelligent secured framework for cyberattack detection in electric vehicles' CAN bus using machine learning. *IEEE Access : Practical Innovations, Open Solutions, 7*, 127580–127592. DOI: 10.1109/ACCESS.2019.2937576

Babu, P. R., Palaniswamy, B., Reddy, A. G., Odelu, V., & Kim, H. S. (2022). A survey on security challenges and protocols of electric vehicle dynamic charging system. *Security and Privacy, 5*(3), e210. DOI: 10.1002/spy2.210

Basnet, M., & Ali, M. H. (2021). Exploring cybersecurity issues in 5G enabled electric vehicle charging station with deep learning. *IET Generation, Transmission & Distribution, 15*(24), 3435–3449. DOI: 10.1049/gtd2.12275

Bergies, S., Aljohani, T. M., Su, S.-F., & Elsisi, M. (2024). An IoT-based deep-learning architecture to secure automated electric vehicles against cyberattacks and data loss. *IEEE Transactions on Systems, Man, and Cybernetics. Systems, 54*(9), 5717–5732. Advance online publication. DOI: 10.1109/TSMC.2024.3409314

El-Rewini, Z., Sadatsharan, K., Selvaraj, D. F., Plathottam, S. J., & Ranganathan, P. (2020). Cybersecurity challenges in vehicular communications. *Vehicular Communications, 23*, 100214. DOI: 10.1016/j.vehcom.2019.100214

ElHussini, H., Assi, C., Moussa, B., Atallah, R., & Ghrayeb, A. (2021). A tale of two entities: Contextualizing the security of electric vehicle charging stations on the power grid. *ACM Transactions on the Internet of Things*, *2*(2), 1–21. DOI: 10.1145/3437258

Garofalaki, Z., Kosmanos, D., Moschoyiannis, S., Kallergis, D., & Douligeris, C. (2022). Electric vehicle charging: A survey on the security issues and challenges of the open charge point protocol (OCPP). *IEEE Communications Surveys and Tutorials*, *24*(3), 1504–1533. Advance online publication. DOI: 10.1109/COMST.2022.3184448

Hong, J., Song, T. J., Lee, H., & Zaboli, A. (2022). Automated cybersecurity tester for IEC61850-based digital substations. *Energies*, *15*(21), 7833. DOI: 10.3390/en15217833

Kavousi-Fard, A., Jin, T., Su, W., & Parsa, N. (2020). An effective anomaly detection model for securing communications in electric vehicles. *IEEE Transactions on Industry Applications*. Advance online publication. DOI: 10.1109/TIA.2020

Kim, K., Kim, J. S., Jeong, S., Park, J. H., & Kim, H. K. (2021). Cybersecurity for autonomous vehicles: Review of attacks and defense. *Computers & Security*, *103*, 102150. DOI: 10.1016/j.cose.2020.102150

Li, Y., Wang, Y., Wu, M., & Li, H. (2019). Replay attack and defense of electric vehicle charging on GB/T 27930-2015 communication protocol. *Journal of Computer and Communications*, *7*(12), 20–30. DOI: 10.4236/jcc.2019.712003

Liu, S., Chen, B., Zourntos, T., Kundur, D., & Butler-Purry, K. (2014). A coordinated multi-switch attack for cascading failures in smart grid. *IEEE Transactions on Smart Grid*, *5*(3), 1183–1195. DOI: 10.1109/TSG.2014.2302476

Manoj, B., & Hasan Ali, M. D. (2021). Exploring cybersecurity issues in 5G enabled EV charging station with deep learning. *IET Generation, Transmission & Distribution*, *15*(24), 3435–3449. DOI: 10.1049/gtd2.12275

Neaimeh, M., & Andersen, P. B. (2020). Mind the gap—Open communication protocols for vehicle grid integration. *Energy Informatics*, *3*(1), 1–17. DOI: 10.1186/s42162-020-0103-1

Rana, M. M. (2017). Attack resilient wireless sensor networks for smart electric vehicles. *IEEE Sensors Letters*, *1*(2), 1–4. DOI: 10.1109/LSENS.2017.2690907

Rathore, R. S., Hewage, C., Kaiwartya, O., & Lloret, J. (2022). In-vehicle communication cyber security: Challenges and solutions. *Sensors (Basel)*, *22*(17), 6679. DOI: 10.3390/s22176679

Ronanki, D., & Karneddi, H. (2023). Electric vehicle charging infrastructure: Review, cyber security considerations, potential impacts, countermeasures and future trends. *IEEE Journal of Emerging and Selected Topics in Power Electronics*. Advance online publication. DOI: 10.1109/JESTPE.2023

Roopa, M. S., & Venugopal, K. R. (2025). Digital twins for cyber-physical healthcare systems: Architecture, requirements, systematic analysis, and future prospects. *IEEE Access : Practical Innovations, Open Solutions*, *13*, 44963–44996. DOI: 10.1109/ACCESS.2025.3547991

Sanghvi, A., & Markel, T. (2021, June). Cybersecurity for electric vehicle fast-charging infrastructure. In *2021 IEEE Transportation Electrification Conference & Expo (ITEC)* (pp. 573–576). IEEE. DOI: 10.1109/ITEC51675.2021.9490069

Sanghvi, A., Markel, T., Granda, S., Nagarajan, A., & Jun, M. (2021). *Identification and testing of electric vehicle fast charger cybersecurity mitigations* (No. NREL/TP-5R00-80799). National Renewable Energy Laboratory. DOI: 10.2172/1786046

Sharma, S., & Ali, I. (2025). IEC 61850 communication-enabled cost optimisation for electric vehicle integration in microgrids. *International Journal of Ambient Energy*, *46*(1), 2516065. Advance online publication. DOI: 10.1080/01430750.2025.2516065

Wang, C., Song, R., & Liu, Z. (2020). Simulation of vehicle network communication security based on random geometry and data mining. *IEEE Access : Practical Innovations, Open Solutions*, *8*, 69389–69400. DOI: 10.1109/ACCESS.2020.2986338

Wang, Y., Zhao, Z., Qi, B., Cheng, Y., Tang, K., & Li, B. (2024). Vulnerability analysis of an electric vehicle fleet for car-sharing service under cyber attacks. *Sustainable Energy. Grids and Networks*, *37*, 101207. DOI: 10.1016/j.segan.2024.101207

Weng, S., Li, Y., & Ding, X. (2020). Resilient distributed coordination of plug-in electric vehicles charging under cyber-attack. *Electronics (Basel)*, *9*(5), 770. DOI: 10.3390/electronics9050770

Yang, B., Guo, L., Li, F., Ye, J., & Song, W. (2019, June). Impact analysis of data integrity attacks on power electronics and electric drives. In *2019 IEEE Transportation Electrification Conference and Expo (ITEC)* (pp. 1–6). IEEE. DOI: 10.1109/ITEC.2019.8790574

Ye, J., Guo, L., Yang, B., Li, F., Du, L., Guan, L., & Song, W. (2020). Cyber-physical security of powertrain systems in modern electric vehicles: Vulnerabilities, challenges and future visions. *IEEE Journal of Emerging and Selected Topics in Power Electronics*, *9*(4), 4639–4657. DOI: 10.1109/JESTPE.2020.3045667

Zhou, Y., Liu, W., Ma, J., Zhen, X., & Li, Y. (2021). Malicious mode attack on EV coordinated charging load and MIADRC defense strategy. *arXiv Preprint*, arXiv:2110.13681. /arXiv.2110.13681DOI: 10.48550

Chapter 6
Quantum Healthcare: Innovations, Challenges, and Ethical Frontiers

Rachana Yogesh Patil
https://orcid.org/0000-0001-9973-6998
Pimpri Chinchwad College of Engineering, India

Dipti S. Khurge
https://orcid.org/0000-0001-8475-6099
Pimpri Chinchwad College of Engineering, India

ABSTRACT

The development of quantum computing systems functions as the leader in creating technological advancements that will transform healthcare delivery. Quantum computing systems have substantial potential for healthcare facilities as the worldwide market will grow to $8.45 billion by 2027. The chapter assesses the advancement of quantum healthcare science through innovation, system challenges, and ethical limitations. It illustrates how quantum computing networks with cryptography combine to form a system that enhances healthcare through fast operations, precise medical research, drug creation, and robust data security. Two key barriers exist for quantum healthcare transformation due to resource allocation and security verification. The implementation meets substantial hurdles because data protection requirements, consent, and accessibility need proper handling. The advantages of quantum healthcare systems depend on stakeholders' ethical guidelines, multi-disciplinary partnerships, and planned investments to maintain patient equity and safety while developing systems.

DOI: 10.4018/979-8-3373-4918-3.ch006

1. INTRODUCTION

Quantum technology based on quantum mechanics principles of superposition and entanglement functions as a transformative instrument for healthcare evolution (Gruska, 1999). The process of quantum computing differs from classical computing because it handles extensive datasets in parallel rather than sequentially. The special computational power provides solutions for highly complex medical issues in healthcare systems (Horowitz & Grumbling, 2019).

Quantum computing is steadily becoming a game-changer in healthcare, offering the potential to handle complex problems like risk analysis and cost management more efficiently (Rieffel & Polak, 2000). One important focus area is optimizing system performance, guided by models like the "Triple Aim," which emphasizes better patient experience, improved population health, and reduced healthcare costs. This evolved into the "Quadruple Aim" with the addition of enhancing the clinical experience for healthcare workers (Ur Rasool et al., 2023).

Recently, a broader model called the "Pentacle Aim" has been suggested, which includes a fifth goal reducing carbon emissions. This is vital, considering that the healthcare sector contributes significantly to global emissions, indirectly harming the very lives it seeks to protect (Jayanthi et al., 2022). Quantum computing can support these goals by enabling more accurate diagnostics, efficient resource use, and better planning, helping healthcare systems move toward a more balanced, inclusive, and environmentally conscious future.

1.1 Key Applications of QC in Healthcare

1.1.1 Drug Discovery and Development

Drug development takes place through an elaborate and prolonged process. The capability of quantum computing to display molecular interactions at the quantum level speeds up drug candidate identification processes (Cao et al., 2018). The variational quantum eigensolver (VQE) represents one of the algorithms used to analyze molecular structures and determine their energy states. Pfizer and IBM along with other organizations engage in quantum simulation activities to create pharmaceutical treatments for Alzheimer's disease and cancer.

1.1.2 Genomics and Personalized Medicine

A major requirement exists for computers with great processing power to handle genomic data analysis. The analysis of genetic variations that relate to diseases becomes more efficient through quantum algorithms (Goswami & Sharma, 2024).

By analyzing individual patient genes the development of customized healthcare treatments becomes possible (Biamonte et al., 2017).

1.1.3 Medical Imaging and Diagnostics

Research indicates that quantum machine learning offers improved diagnostic precision through its applications. Quantum-enhanced algorithms serve medical imaging data in two ways: they process this data both quickly and precisely for faster condition identification such as tumors and cardiac abnormalities (Dunjko & Briegel, 2018).

1.1.4 Healthcare Logistics and Operations:

Hospital resources receive optimal distribution through quantum optimization technologies which combine with patient movement optimization to achieve better medical supply chain logistics control for essential medical stock. The approach becomes crucial in times of emergencies and pandemics because resource limitations exist (Anuradha et al., 2024).

The implementation of quantum computing for healthcare remains hindered by various substantial barriers. The implementation of quantum hardware faces three major obstacles that include quantum hardware expenses and a shortage of qualified personnel alongside ethical data security concerns. Although numerous challenges exist the advantages of quantum computing make it a revolutionary power that will transform medical practices.

1.2 Objectives

The main focus of this chapter consists of following key objectives.

- The research evaluates how quantum computing technology addresses major healthcare difficulties which include drug discovery analysis medical diagnostics and personalized medicine delivery. The chapter presents complete analysis about real-world applications that shows how quantum technology executes practical benefits in medical care.
- Researchers need to determine the technological obstacles together with funding challenges and moral complications that stand in the way of quantum computing implementation in healthcare. The chapter presents specific plans to resolve the present challenges which enable fair deployment along with security measures for quantum technologies.

- The research establishes connections which lead theory to merge with real-world applications.
- Fostering Ethical and Inclusive Practices:

The chapter works to enhance the healthcare discourse about quantum computing transformation through its examination of the identified objectives.

2. LITERATURE REVIEW

2.1 Evolution of Quantum Computing in Healthcare

Quantum computing has moved swiftly from theoretical ideas into real-world applications whose main focus is healthcare and biomedical areas. Significant technical advancements have transformed the way this technology advances through time as it finds new solutions to complex healthcare concerns (Davids et al., 2022; Jeyaraman et al., 2024). Figure 1 describes the phases of evolution of Quantum computing in healthcare.

Figure 1. Evolution of Quantum Computing in Healthcare

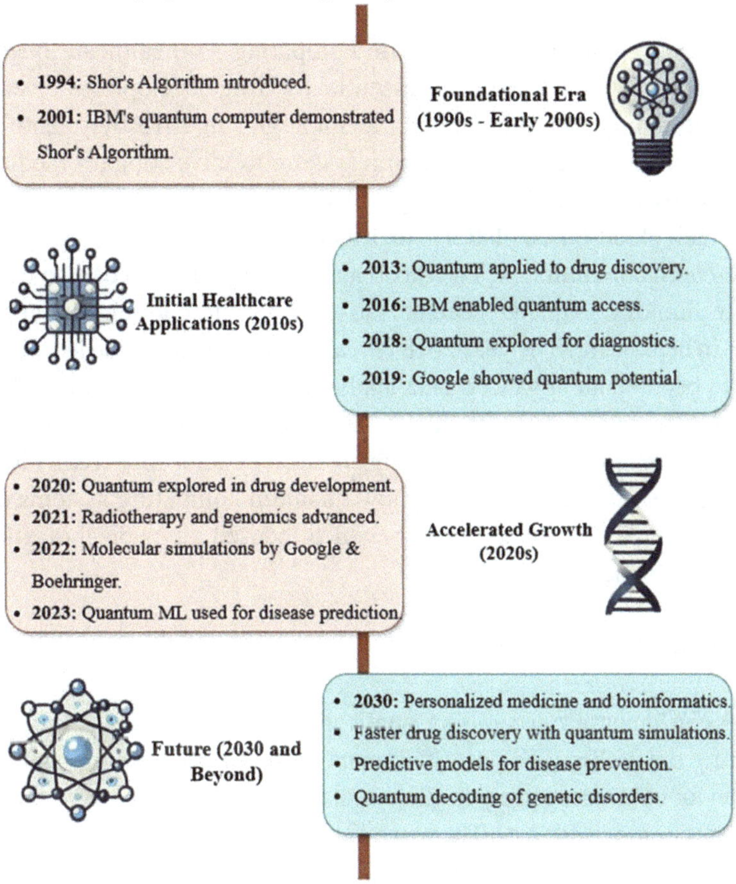

- **Foundational Era (1990s - Early 2000s)**

The first phase of quantum computing theory introduced fundamental discoveries. Research by Peter Shor in 1994 through his Algorithm allowed scientists to understand how quantum computers handle difficult problems faster than conventional computing methods. A novel breakthrough enabled scientists to identify operational advantages of quantum systems that would guide future advancements. IBM used its developed theoretical foundation to produce its initial quantum computer in 2001 which successfully ran Shor's Algorithm (Ekert & Jozsa, 1996). The procedural execution of quantum computation became feasible because scientists validated quantum operation capabilities which resulted in scientific breakthroughs and practical benefits.

- **Initial Healthcare Applications (2010s)**

The research application of quantum computing for healthcare began in the 2010s. The protein folding problems essential for drug development research were addressed through quantum computing technologies in 2013 by scientific teams. Researchers proved the ability of quantum systems to solve complex medical issues through recently achieved breakthroughs. IBM released the Quantum Experience in 2016 as their cloud-based platform to offer quantum computing resources worldwide to research communities. The broad accessibility through democratization of quantum technology enabled researchers to explore different fields for applications especially in healthcare. The year 2018 revealed quantum machine learning had the potential to become an advanced data analysis system dedicated to medical diagnostics and imaging processes. In 2019 Google demonstrated Quantum Supremacy through its achievement of outperforming classical systems for certain tasks (Arute et al., 2019). Research demonstrated how quantum computing systems delivered solutions to complex healthcare matters which focused on medical diagnostic and treatment development.

- **Accelerated Growth (2020s)**

Progress in quantum computing applications to healthcare has reached high speed during the 2020s. The year 2020 marked the beginning of quantum system exploration for optimizing drug development through promising reductions in drug development duration and costs. The year 2021 demonstrated that quantum algorithms could meet various healthcare needs because they improved radiotherapy planning while analyzing genomic data (Pakela et al., 2020). During 2022 Boehringer Ingelheim along with Google collaborated to deploy quantum computing programs that optimized molecular dynamics simulations for pharmaceutical development. The predictive quantum machine learning methodology of 2023 presents an innovative technological approach for medical diagnosis and complex health data analysis to create better therapeutic results.

- **Future (2030 and Beyond)**

Studies indicate that quantum computing will transform healthcare delivery throughout the upcoming years by bringing substantial changes to its operations. Quantum systems will deliver real-time personalized medicine to the public during 2030 through patient profiling for building customized medical approaches. New therapies will move forward quickly due to molecular interaction simulations that perform fast sophisticated simulations (Gill et al., 2022). Quantum predictive healthcare models using predictive power will spot diseases at early stages in order to reduce illnesses and achieve better medical outcomes. The technology of quantum computing serves as an essential solution for complex genetic diseases to achieve better precise medical treatments. Quantum-based solutions will optimize healthcare logistics systems as well as resource distribution and treatment delivery to establish more efficient healthcare systems. Quantum-enriched artificial intelligence systems plan to revolutionize healthcare diagnosis while improving medical choices by developing new solutions for vital medical problems affecting modern healthcare operations.

2.2 Quantum Computing vs. Classical Computing in Healthcare

Quantum and classical computing each play important roles in healthcare, but in very different ways. Standard computers excel at handling everyday work including patient information management and basic hospital operations together with data processing tasks (Arshad et al., 2023). Traditional AI tools derived from their cooperation have enhanced healthcare diagnosis methods and individualized patient care approaches. Quantum computers operate through different mechanics because they excel at resolving complicated problems such as molecule simulations for drug discovery as well as genetic data analyses for treatment customization. Medical imaging benefits from technologies which demonstrate new promise for improvement (Aggarwal et al., 2023). These technologies complement each other in advancing healthcare by providing separate functional capabilities. Table 1 summarizes the aspects of classical computing and quantum computing.

Table 1. Quantum Computing vs. Classical Computing in Healthcare

Aspect	Classical Computing	Quantum Computing
Drug Discovery	Simulates molecular interactions but limited by computational power, leading to slower processes.	Simulates molecular interactions with high precision, reducing time and cost in drug development.
Genomics	Processes genetic data sequentially, which is time-consuming for large datasets.	Analyzes genetic data faster, enabling precision medicine and understanding complex genetic disorders.
Medical Imaging	Relies on classical machine learning algorithms for image processing and pattern recognition.	Uses quantum-enhanced algorithms to improve accuracy and speed in image analysis and diagnostics.
Optimization Problems	Handles healthcare logistics and scheduling tasks but struggles with highly complex optimization problems.	Solves complex optimization problems efficiently, improving logistics and resource allocation.

continued on following page

Table 1. Continued

Aspect	Classical Computing	Quantum Computing
Data Processing	Processes data sequentially, suitable for structured and routine tasks.	Processes data in parallel using superposition, ideal for large-scale and complex challenges.
Scalability	Limited scalability when dealing with exponential growth in data and complexity.	Scales efficiently for multidimensional and unstructured problems.
Technology Maturity	Well-established and widely implemented across the healthcare sector.	Emerging technology with growing research and development efforts.
Cost and Accessibility	Relatively affordable and accessible with established infrastructure.	High costs and limited accessibility due to early-stage development and specialized requirements.

2.3 Related Work

The new quantum computing platform demonstrates its ability to transform healthcare because it helps solve complex calculations needed for drug research as well as genomic studies and customized medical solutions. Several researchers have studied the potential extent of this technology through the information presented in the table 2.

Rasool et al. (2021) present in their review the powerful effects that quantum computing can have on healthcare operations. Published research evaluation reveals rapid DNA sequencing as one of the main applications together with molecular simulations and personalized treatment approaches. The healthcare IoT benefits from quantum computing through its ability to boost Quality of Service (QoS) while delivering secure medical data processing on demand.

Jeyaraman et al. (2024) show how quantum computing enables simultaneous genomic study and image-based treatment design for better medical diagnoses. Through their work the authors show how quantum algorithms use improved data processing capabilities to enhance both diagnostic functions and personalized treatment planning methods. Quantum computing according to Arya et al. (2024) performs drug discovery operations more efficiently while handling large genomic data for precise medicine delivery.

The research by Arshad et al. (2023) investigates the wide range of healthcare applications for quantum computing which includes medical imaging and drug discovery methods. Quantum computing has proven its ability to enhance essential healthcare functions in addition to verifying its current early stage of development according to the presented study. The Chandrasekaran et al. (2023) research demonstrates how quantum systems use medical data to identify drug mechanisms for disease treatment and creates practical solutions for healthcare system development.

Quantum technology computational powers receive analysis from Malviya et al. (2021) and Aggarwal et al. (2023). Study findings from Malviya show how quantum computing operates health data in real-time with power efficiency improvements according to the research. Aggarwal applies "precision-based granular" methodology in patient diagnosis and achieves promising results in testing oxygen and heart rate monitoring.

Gupta et al. (2022) conducted research on quantum computing applications for organizational and management functions in healthcare applications. The team behind Gupta et al. (2022) generated an original methodology through professional interviews to illustrate how quantum computing contributes to healthcare system sustainability development. Durant et al. (2024) explain biomedical research and diagnostic applications of quantum computing but more research is needed to address hardware and scalability challenges.

The security aspects of quantum computing applications in healthcare environments stand out as the most important issue for analysis. Pulipeti et al. (2022) study how quantum-based healthcare systems face cryptographic problems that demonstrate the need for secure patient data systems.

Ullah et al (2024) conduct a study about integrating quantum machine learning systems into healthcare applications. The authors review 49 analytical studies to present how quantum algorithms shift data forecasting methods and individualized medical care direction while creating new healthcare approaches.

The research paper compares quantum computing healthcare applications using table 2 to review drug discovery, genomics, medical imaging and additional healthcare domains. Each research paper includes essential findings together with an analysis of encountered challenges and research approaches and possible implementation directions for the future.

Table 2. Comparison of Quantum Computing Applications in Healthcare

Reference	Focus Area	Key Contributions	Challenges	Methodology	Dataset/Tools	Future Work
(Qayyum, 2023)	Quantum IoT & medical data	DNA sequencing, molecular simulations, secure medical data	QoS, real-time processing	Quantum computing + IoT frameworks	Simulations, molecular datasets	Real-time quantum processing for healthcare
(Jeyaraman et al., 2024)	Genomics & treatment planning	Quantum diagnostics, genomics, personalized medicine	Scalability of quantum algorithms	Genomic modeling, quantum algorithms	Public datasets (1000 Genomes)	Optimize quantum for large genomic datasets
(Arya & Verma, 2024)	Drug discovery & precision med.	Genomic analysis for drug discovery, treatments	Practical system integration	Quantum ML models	Protein-ligand (PDB) datasets	Develop quantum ML for drug testing
(Arshad, Murtza, & Arshad, 2023)	Imaging & drug discovery	Improved imaging accuracy, streamlined workflows	Early-stage quantum tech	Quantum-enhanced imaging	Medical imaging (CT/ MRI) datasets	Quantum imaging in clinical practice
(Chandrasekaran, Agrawal, Dutt, & Vyas, 2023)	Drug mechanisms	Disease-specific drug analysis using quantum systems	Integration with healthcare	Quantum simulations, binding	Molecular drug datasets	Extend to disease-specific testing
(Mysore, 2022)	Real-time health data	Energy-efficient, real-time data analysis	Limited quantum hardware	Hybrid classical-quantum systems	IoT health sensor data	Hardware-software for real-time data
(Aggarwal, Sachdeva, & Goswami, 2023)	Wearable diagnostics	Heart rate/ oxygen monitoring with granular models	Clinical deployment	Granular quantum analytics	Wearable device data	Enhance wearable accuracy and usability
(Gupta, Modgil, Bhatt, Jabbour, & Kamble, 2023)	Healthcare system management	Quantum's role in sustainable systems	Transition from classical	Case studies, interviews	None (survey-based study)	Economic analysis of quantum healthcare
(Durant et al., 2024)	Biomedical research	Quantum ML for research and diagnostics	Hardware scalability	Quantum ML + hybrid neural nets	Private biomedical datasets	Scale quantum ML for diagnostics
(Pulipeti & Kumar, 2023)	Cryptographic security	Vulnerabilities in quantum healthcare applications	Secure quantum infrastructure	Cryptographic algorithms review	Public/private healthcare data	Post-quantum cryptography protocols
(Ullah & Garcia-Zapirain, 2024)	Predictive analytics	Systematic review of 49 studies on QML for healthcare	Ethical concerns, integration	Literature review	Aggregated studies	Address ethics and interoperability in QML

The existing research about quantum computing in healthcare provides essential information while ignoring crucial unresolved matters. The practical application of quantum technologies meets challenges due to their limited scalability and insufficient development of quantum infrastructure as well as barriers in integration with current healthcare operational systems. The majority of research by (Qayyum, 2023 and Jeyaraman et al., 2024) presents theoretical accomplishments without providing deployable solutions which could improve real-time healthcare systems.

The research by (Ullah & Garcia-Zapirain, 2024) identifies a crucial gap in healthcare quantum computing studies due to insufficient analysis of ethical factors and interoperability problems and economic consequences during adoption. Post-quantum cryptographic protocols require more detailed research regarding patient data protection and system resilience according to (Pulipeti & Kumar, 2023) to resolve security problems.

New experimental findings are needed since current research lacks sufficient evidence. Research heavily relies on computational simulations and theoretical frameworks while both medical imaging data from real patient evaluations together with genomic information receive little use in current studies. Studies about diagnostic tools and drug discoveries do not extend beyond their specific areas to include telemedicine infrastructure and supply chain distribution and healthcare resource utilization in healthcare systems.

Research within this field lacks sufficient frameworks to integrate artificial intelligence with quantum computing and Internet of Things and advanced analytics for developing whole healthcare solutions. Healthcare systems need future research to close gaps between theoretical quantum computing capabilities and practical implementation in order to achieve security along with ethical scalability in their quantum computing solutions.

3. INNOVATIONS IN QUANTUM MEDICINE

The health care scene undergoes gradual transformation because quantum technologies develop revolutionary approaches to processing, diagnosis, treatment planning and personalized patient care. Advanced medical research is discovering new possibilities in healthcare through decreased biological data processing times along with quantum-level molecular simulation. The figure 2 demonstrates current applications of quantum discoveries in crucial medical fields.

Figure 2. Innovations in Quantum Medicine

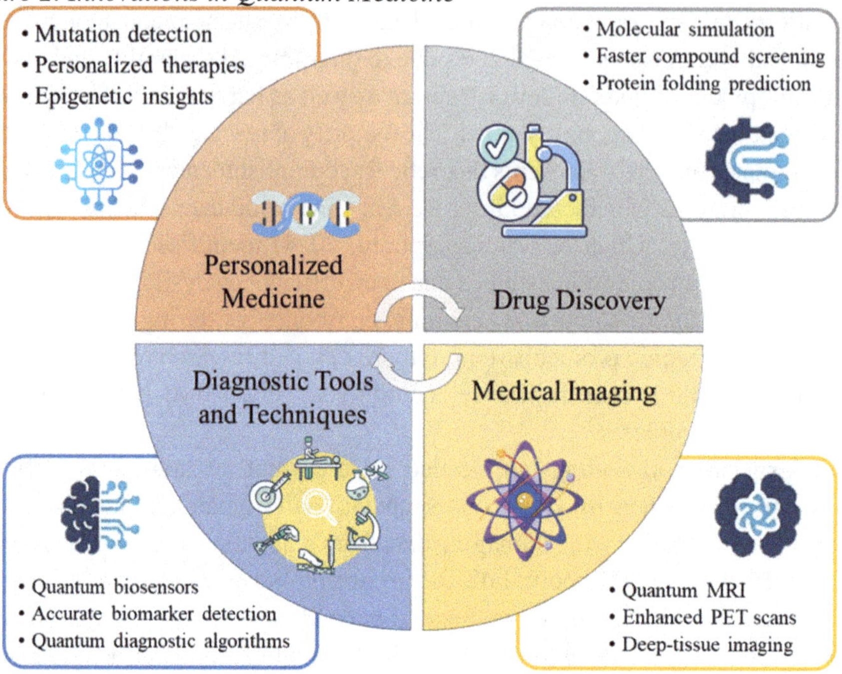

3.1 Quantum Computing in Drug Discovery

Creating new drugs takes a lot of time and money, mainly because it's hard to ensure that small drug molecules properly attach to larger targets like proteins. These tiny molecular movements are tough to simulate accurately with standard computing methods.

- **Molecular Simulation and Modeling**

Effective drug performance relies on ligand-protein pocket binding while water molecules shape both protein structures and binding outcomes in this process. The mapping process for water molecules proves both difficult and expensive particularly when the pockets are difficult to access. There was a breakthrough when PASQAL formed an alliance with Qubit Pharmaceuticals which brought together quantum computing with classical computing to pinpoint water molecules within protein structures (Ollitrault et al., 2021). The quantum principles of superposition transform their analysis technique into a faster and more specific approach for drug discovery.

- **Accelerated Compound Screening**

Protein-ligand binding knowledge stands vital for all pharmaceutical drug development activities. The binding abilities of proteins depend on water molecules present in pockets because these molecules affect the strength of ligand bindings to the protein. Quantum-based modeling systems produce accurate models of biological interactions because they provide vital details about drug protein binding actions inside natural biological conditions (Kumar, et al., 2024). Drug discovery progress gets accelerated through quantum computing data simulation methods because these approaches generate data more effectively and precisely. Qubit Pharmaceuticals together with other businesses utilizes these capabilities to improve AI models which speeds up the transition from molecule screening to preclinical testing.

- **Protein Folding Prediction**

The high-dimensional problem management capabilities of quantum computing produce effective protein folding pattern predictions. The particular three-dimensional structure of proteins exists because it enables functional activity and improper protein configurations lead to medical disorders (Pal et al., 2024). Quantum algorithms explore many protein folding solutions to create essential data which helps develop drugs that either fix or alter protein folding patterns.

The implementation of quantum computers drives fundamental changes through all stages of pharmaceutical drug discovery operations. Quantum computing simulations demonstrate elevated accuracy in molecular research which causes shorter drug development periods and lowers the associated costs and accelerates the market release of pharmaceutical products. Pharmaceutical organizations together with patients benefit from speedup since it accelerates the delivery of advanced medical treatments to those in need.

3.2 Quantum Medical Imaging

Medical imaging systems serve as essential diagnostic tools which supply clinicians with vital information about human body components inside the body. The two traditional imaging techniques Magnetic Resonance Imaging (MRI) and Positron Emission Tomography (PET) have experienced major improvements during past years. The current medical imaging systems have natural operational constraints which affect their ability to provide precise measurements and their sensitivity levels together with their capacity for detecting subtle pathological developments. Medical imaging solutions fortified with quantum technologies have advanced diagnostic capabilities by offering better image resolution and speeding up acquisition times and producing superior diagnostic precision.

- **Quantum-Enhanced MRI**

MRI serves as a non-invasive imaging practice that makes detailed pictures of bodily tissues through the combination of powerful magnetic fields and radio wave transmissions. Quantum computing along with quantum sensors proves to be a powerful tool that enhances the performance capabilities of MRI systems. The potential benefits of quantum algorithms for MRI data evaluation include optimized analysis that leads to quickening diagnostic procedures and treatment planning specifically important for urgent cases including strokes or traumatic brain injuries.

Quantum sensors which incorporate nitrogen-vacancy centers in diamonds provide an exceptional capability to detect magnetic fields at a high level of sensitivity (Balasubramani et al., 2025). Quantum sensors serve as tools to boost MRI scan spatial resolution which allows doctors to see molecular and atomic structures. These technological developments would enable medical staff to make earlier disease diagnoses and improve their ability to monitor how treatment processes evolve.

- **Advancements in Positron Emission Tomography (PET) through Quantum Entanglement**

Through PET imaging healthcare professionals use radiotracer detection of gamma rays to collect functional data on tissues and organs inside the body. Quantum entanglement now serves as a subject of research to improve PET image quality. The utilization of photon entangled states enables better image contrast together with resolution improvement that enhances the detection accuracy of abnormalities.

Using quantum-enhanced PET imaging methods doctors would achieve better lesion positioning and enhanced metabolic activity assessment that serve as critical tools for cancer diagnosis and observation.

- **Quantum Sensors in Biomedical Imaging**

Using principles of superposition and entanglement allows quantum sensors to perform highly sensitive measurements. The combination of quantum sensors enables the detection of minor changes in magnetic fields as well as electric fields and temperature and pressure fluctuations thus generating precise physiological data. Optically pumped magnetometers function as integrated sensors within wearable sensor helmets for magnetoencephalography (MEG) applications that measure brain activity when the subject moves (Aslam et al., 2023).

These quantum sensors for imaging applications show promise to produce real-time high-resolution imaging approaches that reduce medical procedures invasiveness.

Advanced medical imaging benefits greatly from quantum technologies yet developers must address various substantial hurdles when exploring this path. Quantum computer and sensor practical deployment needs to solve crucial technology barriers which involve keeping qubits stable while implementing error correction. The implementation of quantum technologies into medical imaging systems requires major funding along with team-based research between different scientific fields.

Data security together with patient privacy demand attention as quantum technologies continue to develop so ethical elements can be properly managed. The significant processing capability of quantum computers affects encryption and data security so healthcare organizations need to create new security protocols for patient data protection.

3.3 Quantum-Inspired Diagnostic Tools and Techniques

Medical diagnostics receives benefits from quantum mechanics implementations to develop superior diagnostic tools combined with new patient care methods. New diagnostic instrumentation emerges because of quantum-inspired technologies which use principles of quantum measurement along with superposition and entanglement.

- **Quantum-Inspired Machine Learning in Diagnostics**

Using quantum principles in diagnosis algorithm development produces more precise and efficient results for medical diagnostic procedures. The application of quantum-inspired support vector machines produces superior medical image classification outcomes because they enhance the detection of pneumonia in chest X-rays. These algorithms apply to complex data groups to create quick accurate medical diagnoses.

- **Quantum Activation Functions in Neural Networks**

Neural networks became more advanced through integration of quantum concepts which propelled the creation of new activation functions. The Quantum ReLU (QReLU) activation function as well as the modified Quantum ReLU (m-QReLU) serve as quantum-powered examples which improve convolutional neural networks during medical imaging classification tasks. The combination of quantum-inspired activation functions produced increases in medical image-based illness detection particularly for COVID-19 and Parkinson's disease (Maronese et al., 2022).

- **Quantum-Inspired Sensors for Biomarker Detection**

Modern technology now develops quantum-powered sensors aimed at biomarker surveillance without blood draws to track hormones and metabolites in the human body. The sensors apply electrochemical and optical biosensing methods to monitor minimal physiological changes which leads to early-stage disease recognition and persistent healthcare observation.

All potential advantages from quantum-inspired diagnostic methods need to address existing obstacles to gain clinical success. The widespread deployment of quantum diagnostics depends on resolving multiple problems which include maintaining stable quantum states and integrating these devices with standard medical equipment while building specific facilities to operate them. Medical applications of quantum-inspired diagnostic models require ongoing interdisciplinary studies between researchers to develop solutions for existing obstacles for complete system adoption.

3.4 Genomics and Personalized Medicine

Scientific experts believe quantum computing will bring radical improvements to genomics and personalized medicine because of its groundbreaking computational strength. Medical diagnostic testing achieves higher precision and the creation of patient-tailored treatments results from data analysis improvements that occur because of this innovation.

- **Accelerated Genomic Data Analysis**

Scientists use extensive dataset analysis to identify the relationship between genes and particular diseases during genomic research. Such analysis methods face challenges during processing of big complex data. Quantum computing enables researchers to process extensive genomic data better than traditional methods thus allowing them to detect connections that standard methods would miss (Robinson et al., 2021). Quantum computing analytics delivers improved capabilities to researchers who detect novel genetic markers that lead to enhanced disease mechanism understanding and therapy developments.

- **Advancements in Genome Sequencing**

The medical practice of personalized medicine requires genome sequencing because this method shows all inherited genetic elements alongside future health risks in patients. The search for genetic markers becomes faster through quantum computing thus reducing the time needed for genome sequencing.

- **Quantum-Enhanced Precision Medicine**

Medical treatments under precision medicine emerge from personal features which medical experts typically access through detailed genetic comprehension. Quantum algorithms enhance complicated biological system analysis to help medical professionals produce treatment solutions focused on individual patients. Quantum-enhanced machine learning methods identify particular genetic mutation reactions to therapeutic approaches so medical professionals can find the most suitable treatments for individual patients.

Researchers are optimistic about using quantum computation in genomic applications and personal medicine despite needing to resolve various technological challenges. Two technical barriers within quantum hardware systems restrict scientists from processing sufficient data through existing machines. The two main technical obstacles affecting quantum computing are qubit stability problems coupled with high error rates. For genetic information that has a sensitive nature, security and privacy of data remains the most important ethical consideration. The implementation of quantum computing in healthcare demands strong regulations to guarantee secure and equal utilization throughout health facilities.

4. CHALLENGES IN QUANTUM HEALTHCARE

Quantum healthcare transformation requires complete solutions for specific difficulties while implementing quantum technologies in healthcare. The implementation of quantum technology encounters various obstacles because hardware system shortcomings combine with interoperability challenges between units and data privacy ethical issues. Quantum healthcare solutions need complete implementation which demands resolving crucial barriers that this section discusses. Figure 3 describes the challenges in Quantum Healthcare.

4.1 Resource Constraints and Computational Demands

The high operational and maintenance requirements of quantum computing challenge its development because the technology remains in a state of development. The main hurdles to overcome consist of:

- The establishment and maintenance of specialized quantum environments requiring vibration-free facilities operating at extreme cold temperatures are highly expensive.
- The restricted availability of operational quantum hardware presents challenges for healthcare applications at various facilities because only few institutions hold access to it.
- The creation of quantum algorithms for healthcare shows two main problems: first it needs advanced technical expertise to develop them and second they need complex computational power to function efficiently.
- Most healthcare organizations including developing region facilities face obstacles when trying to deploy quantum technologies on a large scale.

Figure 3. Challenges in Quantum Healthcare

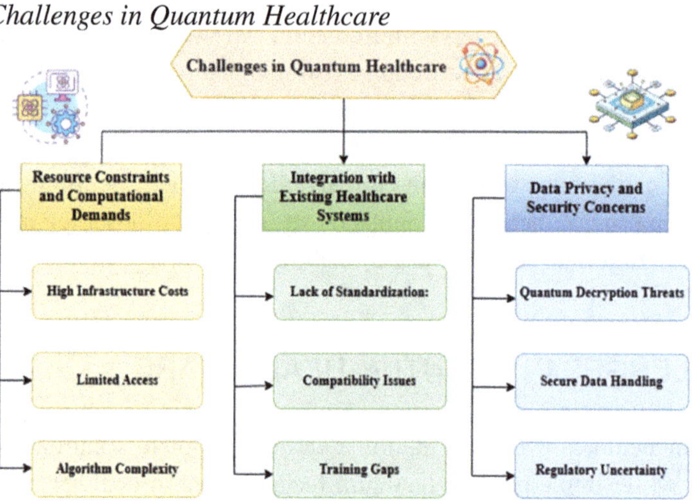

4.2 Integration with Existing Healthcare Systems

Presently it is complex to integrate quantum tools into existing healthcare systems for the following reasons:

- The health sector faces a barrier due to the absence of standard integration frameworks which detail how quantum technologies should connect to both medical imaging equipment and medical electronic health record systems.

- Compatibility problems arise between legacy systems and advanced quantum technology outputs and computational data because of their inability to handle new formats. This requires major system adaptations.
- A knowledge gap exists between developers and end-users because healthcare professionals along with IT staff lack sufficient training to comprehend and operate quantum systems.
- The technical integration problems between quantum innovations and clinical environments can prevent the successful implementation of opportunities which quantum technologies offer.The technical integration problems between quantum innovations and clinical environments can prevent the successful implementation of opportunities which quantum technologies offer.

4.3 Data Privacy and Security Concerns

The process of quantum healthcare solutions managing sensitive patient information serves as a basis for important moral and legal complications regarding:

- The key weakness of quantum computing lies in the ability to decrypt modern encryption systems which puts medical records at risk of exposure.
- Absolute security management through quantum-safe encryption and access control systems becomes essential to process the large amounts of diagnostic and genomic data through quantum systems.
- Lack of regulatory control exists for quantum healthcare applications because proper guidelines are absent regarding patient consent management of stored data and international data sharing.
- Public trust and patient rights protection depends on quantum applications which need to adhere strictly to ethical and legal standards.

5. ETHICAL ISSUES IN QUANTUM MEDICAL PRACTICES

Medical healthcare practitioners must address multiple ethical matters which occur when quantum computing systems enter healthcare operations. Quantum computing advances in medical practice require ethical analysis of the issues described in figure 4 which will affect its deployment (Malina et al., 2021).

Figure 4. Ethical Issues in Quantum Medical Practices

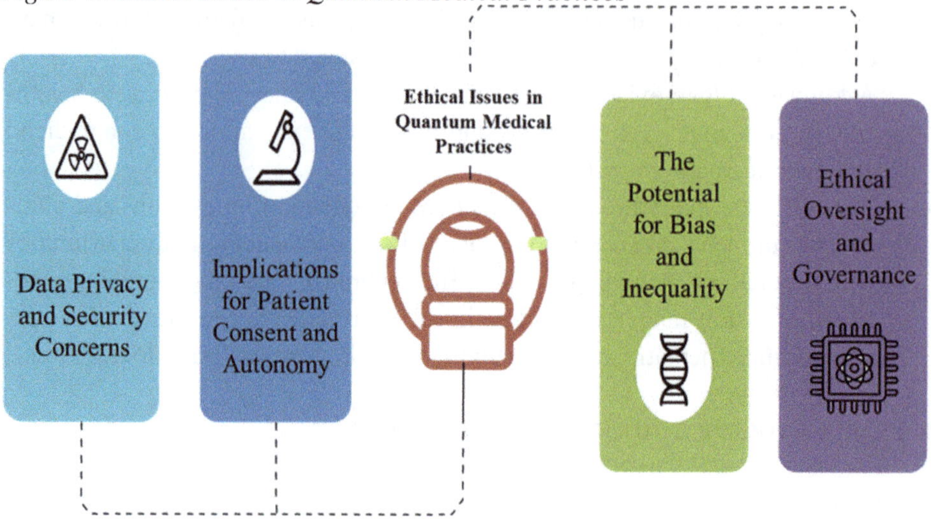

5.1 Data Privacy and Security Concerns

The strength of quantum computing enables new opportunities to protect sensitive health data because it establishes unprecedented capabilities for secure and efficient data handling. Patient information encryption enabled by quantum algorithms would produce safe data exchanges that link hospitals with their research partners and other participants. The new technology generates major privacy issues that need thorough inspection as illustrated in figure 5.

- **Encryption Vulnerability**

Quantum computers feature strong encryption vulnerabilities that severely threaten RSA (Rivest-Shamir-Adleman) in addition to ECC (Elliptic Curve Cryptography) modern encryption methods. Modern encryption shows security loopholes because quantum computers execute powerful operational patterns which surpass classical computational capabilities thereby breaking universal encryption approaches that weaken digital communication bases (Wheatley, 2024). Quantum computers will reach operational status to enable cyber criminals execute prime factorization and discrete logarithm operations that breach present encryption methods. This discovered vulnerability immediately triggered the search for quantum-safe encryption systems while these protect against quantum computer power-based attacks. The post-quantum era requires these modern encryption schemes since they provide essential protection for financial and healthcare and governmental organizations that need secure data transmission.

- **Access and Ownership**

The transition to quantum-safe encryption produces an essential issue about controlling who owns and accesses quantum-processed data. The ability of developing quantum computing systems to process vast amounts of data leads to an essential question about who currently holds ownership and control over this quantum-processed information. Data ownership boundaries become complex since quantum-capable technology enters the field but traditional data processing rules maintain their origin and location standards. The variables involved in platform-based quantum processing result in ambiguous guidelines about who controls the data and determines access rights. The control quantum computing system operators gain over data can harm information security while enabling them to monopolize owned data. Agreed regulatory standards need to be developed to decrease the risks that stem from data ownership disputes and platform access right uncertainties between quantum computing operators. Standards created by regulations provide ethical and transparent methods to handle quantum-processed data and create trust between users and stakeholders.

Figure 5. Data Privacy and Security Concerns

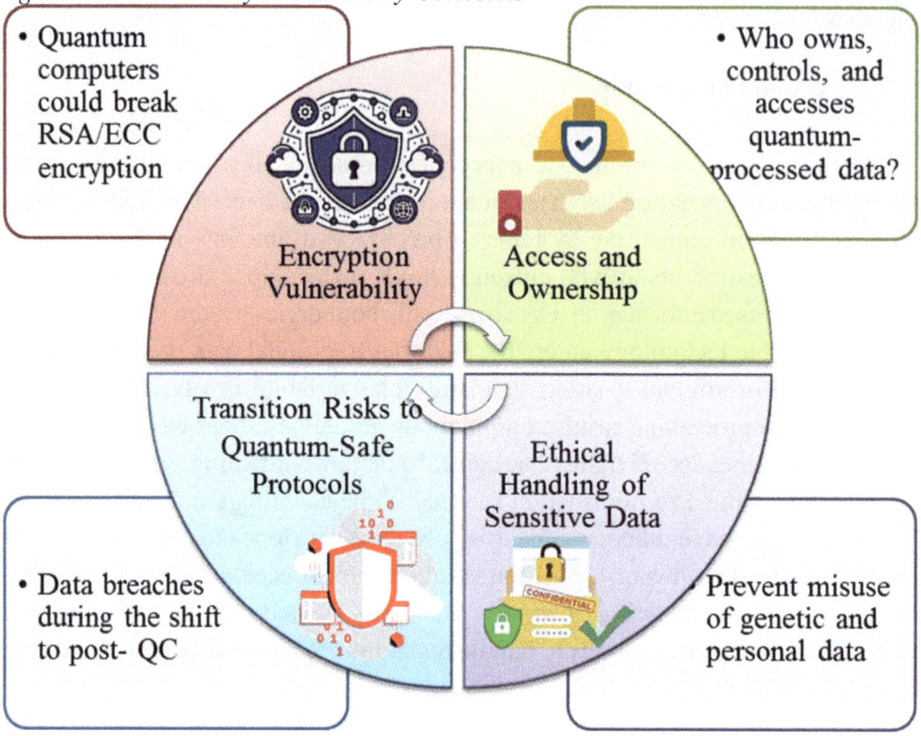

- **Ethical Data Use**

As quantum computing advances, it brings real concerns about how personal and genetic data is protected. This kind of information can reveal a lot about someone's health and background, and if misused, could lead to serious consequences. Today's encryption methods might not be strong enough in the future, so it's important to have clear rules, better safeguards, and updated laws to keep people's data private and secure.

- **Transitioning to Quantum-Safe Security**

Moving to quantum-safe encryption isn't simple. Older systems are at risk during the changeover, and that creates openings for cyber threats. Upgrading systems takes time, money, and careful planning. To make this shift safely, cybersecurity teams and experts need to work together, test thoroughly, and make sure nothing slips through the cracks.

5.2 Implications for Patient Consent and Autonomy

Healthcare quantum computing serves healthcare integration through better systems for evaluation of data and diagnostic testing along with personal treatment plans for patients (Kop et al., 2024). The advancement of quantum computing technology brings forth significant ethical concerns about patient authorization and medical independence as shown in figure 6.

- **Complexity of Quantum Processes**

The intricate operational characteristics of quantum computing systems create obstacles for patients to understand medical procedures when they need to consent to treatment. Medical providers presently explain medical procedures and their connected risks to patients who have understanding capabilities through traditional consent protocols. The intricate nature of quantum computing creates obstacles for patients to grasp the specific techniques which data goes through processing and analysis and encryption steps. The risk of uninformed consent emerges because patients accept medical procedures without comprehending their full nature. Health-care providers must present straightforward explanations about quantum system data management to patients with exact details that allow them to grasp the effects of having their data processed through quantum systems.

Figure 6. Implications for Patient Consent and Autonomy

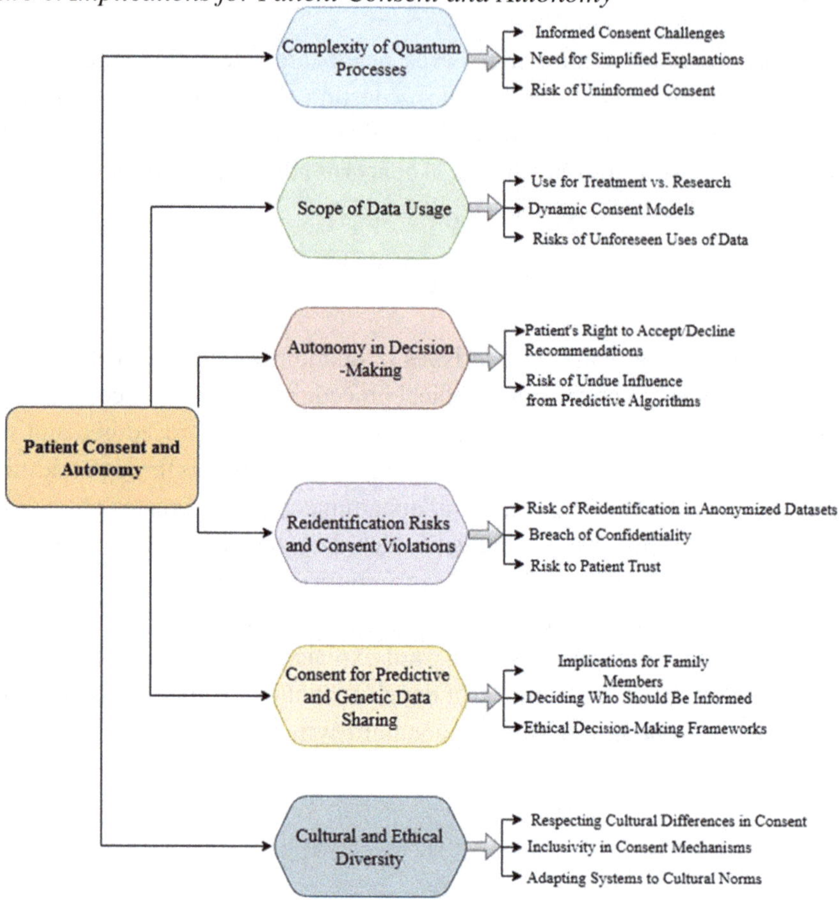

- **Scope of Data Usage**

The analyzing capabilities of quantum systems suggest they could extract complete health knowledge from genetic patterns which leads to future health prediction. Quantum systems help develop better diagnosis tools with treatment solutions but also blur the lines of patient consent authorization. Do patients who allow medical data sharing for treatment intentions simultaneously authorize researchers to use their data for extensive research activities? Quantum algorithms provide researchers the ability to detect unknown data patterns that lead to valuable new findings alongside unforeseen ways of using this information. Healthcare organizations need to create dynamic consent systems that let individuals decide about data handling for medical privacy protection.

- **Autonomy in Decision-Making**

Healthcare providers have the chance to heavily rely on quantum-derived recommendations due to the sophisticated predictive analytics and personalized medicine capabilities of quantum computing. Through probabilistic methods predictive models found in these algorithms eliminate patient choices for medical treatment decisions in healthcare. Healthcare institutions need to develop standard operating procedures which unite quantum analytic approaches with patient autonomy through their right to make healthcare choices. Patients must always keep their freedom to accept or reject expert advice regardless of what quantum systems recommend to them.

- **Reidentification Risks and Consent Violations**

The emergence of large-scale quantum computing systems increases the potential for identifying individuals from data that is supposed to be anonymous. Advanced capabilities of computing algorithms automatically link medical and genetic data points beyond patient authorization. The collapse of patient trust combined with medical ethics violations of confidentiality and patient autonomy will occur because of these data vulnerabilities. The enforcement of quantum system personal privacy regulations must protect confidentiality through standards that do not restrict individual freedom during data processing operations.

- **Approval for predictive and genetic data sharing.**

The sharing of predictive genetic data which affects relatives requires consent from every member of the involved group. Patient data that affects relatives deserves permission from the patient before being released for use. The ethical dilemma regarding how to share information about genetic predictions to family members and who holds decision-making authority over their right to know remains unresolved in quantum-based hereditary predictions. The establishment of particular ethical standards proves essential for protecting patient-family autonomy rights.

- **Cultural and Ethical Diversity**

Ethical recommendations and cultural values should determine how the consent framework develops. The public domain has more authority than personal freedom in essential decision-making choices across different communities. Quantum-powered healthcare systems require cultural sensitivity during consent design because it helps create solutions that match different healthcare contexts.

5.3 The Potential for Bias and Inequality

Quantum technology brings big promises for healthcare—faster diagnosis, better treatments, and stronger research tools. But it also raises serious ethical concerns. If these technologies are built on biased data, they risk favoring some groups over others, leaving minority populations with less accurate diagnoses and poorer care. Bias in quantum algorithms comes from the training data—if that data doesn't fairly represent all groups, the outcomes won't either.

- **Healthcare Access Gaps**

Quantum healthcare also needs expensive equipment, skilled experts, and strong infrastructure—resources often only available in well-funded institutions or developed countries. This creates a growing divide, as underserved communities miss out on these advanced tools, deepening global health inequalities and widening the digital and healthcare gap (Aggarwal, Sachdeva, & Goswami, 2023).

- **Economic Inequality in Healthcare Innovations**

Marketable healthcare solutions developed from quantum technology integration with healthcare require significant financial investments to develop. Advanced healthcare solutions maintain such high costs that only wealthy institutions and organizations can access them. The healthcare field uses quantum computing to develop personal treatment solutions but these quantum-based medical solutions are currently out of financial reach to most populations. Present conditions make it uncertain whether breakthrough lifesaving inventions will be accessible to the public.

- **Predictive Healthcare systems display biases during their operation.**

The early disease identification features of quantum-based predictive healthcare systems risk preserving current social biases throughout society. The predictive systems that analyze hereditary risk factors tend to ignore social factors which include monetary standing and educational degree and water purity and food quality. Healthcare plans use a limited analytical approach to identify biological threats yet they ignore the social elements which create health disparities between different communities.

5.4 Ethical Oversight and Governance

Healthcare operations require both ethical monitoring and governance systems to support the integration of quantum computing technology because such advanced yet complicated systems demand ethical oversight. Healthcare innovations need precise ethical standards to specifically protect privacy rights and secure equal access and enforce visible practices in quantum medical applications. The regulatory system needs to create rules for quantum system security vulnerabilities that break encryption standards and also maintain GDPR and HIPAA compliance and other international requirements. Quantum healthcare depends on independent ethical committees to evaluate projects and monitor biases and protect inclusivity from design through deployment of algorithms. Organizations need to maintain transparency by revealing their quantum system data handling and decision-making methods to users. Standard implementation development requires international cooperation as well as initiatives that remove quantum healthcare accessibility disparities. The adoption of quantum technologies requires public involvement because patients along with community members need precise information about quantum technology benefits and potential risks. Healthcare organizations that foresee and address their ethical consequences will use quantum computing ethically as they uphold social principles and respect patient rights.

6. FUTURE DIRECTIONS IN QUANTUM HEALTHCARE

Healthcare advances through quantum technologies because scientists are moving quantum discoveries into application-based healthcare practices. Research and development in quantum healthcare follows specific directions that define its modern direction:

6.1 Transition from Theory to Practice

The expected future brings experimental quantum tests into both pharmaceutical environments and hospitals as hardware advances and algorithms improve. Anticipated developments include:

- The manufacturing of quantum hardware continues to evolve toward lower prices which creates opportunities for hospitals and research centers to adopt this technology.

- Healthcare institutions will get quantum capabilities through cloud-based quantum-as-a-service platforms that eliminate the need for premise-based infrastructure.
- Real-time simulations coupled with modeling procedures through clinical decision support systems provide clinicians with data-based insights.

6.2 Personalized Quantum Medicine

Quantum computational power will transform healthcare by creating highly individualized medicines based on patient DNA information and physical health data:

- A simulation system that determines how medical therapies impact individual patient molecular structures is known as Precision Treatment Modeling.
- An integration of quantum computing and artificial intelligence trains faster diagnostic models using enhanced quantum machine learning technology.
- Patients benefit from early disease detection services because specific risk models create predictive health interventions.

6.3 Ethical and Regulatory Frameworks

A comprehensive implementation of quantum healthcare equipment depends on comprehensive legal structures and ethical frameworks. The development of global medical quantum technology usage guidelines requires international policy coordination. The development of quantum-resistant security standards must get established to create robust data protection methods which defend medical data from forthcoming quantum attacks. Medical organizations should develop transparent systems which protect patient rights while obtaining informed consent from patients throughout quantum-enhanced healthcare delivery.

6.4 Interdisciplinary Collaboration

Quantum healthcare success demands silo elimination and discipline cooperation for its achievement. The creation of research centers will unite quantum physicists with healthcare experts and engineers and ethicists into one collaborative unit.

- Public-Private Partnerships: Encouraging government, academia, and industry to co-invest in scalable quantum health solutions.
- The implementation gap requires healthcare workers to receive quantum literacy training through basic quantum tool education.

CONCLUSION

Quantum science creates new medical possibilities which lead to the development of quantum healthcare. Quantum science equips the healthcare sector with superior approaches to disease understanding and diagnostic and therapeutic procedures. The existing drug discovery process and diagnostic accuracy benefit from quantum computers which results in custom-made treatment plans for patients. Quantum cryptography acts as an additional security measure for protecting important medical data maintained through digital systems. Quantum healthcare must address three main obstacles that include its high resource requirements and integration difficulties with traditional health IT as well as patient privacy concerns and worries about fair data access. Quantum healthcare success in the future requires multi-specialty teamwork combined with rigorous rules coupled with strategies that harmonize new solutions with healthcare service needs. Perpetual research coupled with ethical practices will turn quantum technology into an essential element of healthcare systems of the future.

REFERENCES

Aggarwal, L., Sachdeva, S., & Goswami, P. (2023). Quantum healthcare computing using precision based granular approach. *Applied Soft Computing*, *144*, 110458. DOI: 10.1016/j.asoc.2023.110458

Anuradha, R., Vandana, C. P., Singh, S. V., Singh, N., Emad, R., & Nitin, V. (2024, May). Integrating Quantum Computing for Enhanced Image Reconstruction in Medical Diagnostics. In *2024 International Conference on Communication, Computer Sciences and Engineering (IC3SE)* (pp. 1294-1298). IEEE. DOI: 10.1109/IC3SE62002.2024.10593044

Arshad, M. W., Murtza, I., & Arshad, M. A. (2023). Applications of quantum computing in health sector. *Journal of Data Science and Intelligent Systems*, *1*(1), 19–24. DOI: 10.47852/bonviewJDSIS3202656

Arute, F., Arya, K., Babbush, R., Bacon, D., Bardin, J. C., Barends, R., & Burkett, B. (2019). Quantum supremacy using a programmable superconducting processor. *Nature*, *574*(7779), 505–510. DOI: 10.1038/s41586-019-1666-5 PMID: 31645734

Arya, R., & Verma, A. (2024). Quantum Computing and Healthcare. *International Journal of Advanced Research in Science. Tongxin Jishu*, *4*(2).

Aslam, N., Zhou, H., Urbach, E. K., Turner, M. J., Walsworth, R. L., Lukin, M. D., & Park, H. (2023). Quantum sensors for biomedical applications. *Nature Reviews. Physics*, *5*(3), 157–169. DOI: 10.1038/s42254-023-00558-3 PMID: 36776813

Balasubramani, S., Renjith, P. N., Kavisankar, L., Rajavel, R., Malarvel, M., & Shankar, A. (2025). A Quantum-enhanced Artificial Neural Network Model for Efficient Medical Image Compression. *IEEE Access : Practical Innovations, Open Solutions*.

Biamonte, J., Wittek, P., Pancotti, N., Rebentrost, P., Wiebe, N., & Lloyd, S. (2017). Quantum machine learning. *Nature*, *549*(7671), 195–202. DOI: 10.1038/nature23474 PMID: 28905917

Cao, Y., Romero, J., & Aspuru-Guzik, A. (2018). Potential of quantum computing for drug discovery. *IBM Journal of Research and Development*, *62*(6), 6–1. DOI: 10.1147/JRD.2018.2888987

Chandrasekaran, S., Agrawal, R., Dutt, V., & Vyas, N. (2023, January). Improved healthcare system with quantum computing. In *2023 International Conference on Artificial Intelligence and Smart Communication (AISC)* (pp. 99–103). IEEE.

Davids, J., Lidströmer, N., & Ashrafian, H. (2022). Artificial intelligence in medicine using quantum computing in the future of healthcare. In *Artificial intelligence in medicine* (pp. 423–446). Springer. DOI: 10.1007/978-3-030-64573-1_338

Dunjko, V., & Briegel, H. J. (2018). Machine learning & artificial intelligence in the quantum domain: A review of recent progress. *Reports on Progress in Physics, 81*(7), 074001. DOI: 10.1088/1361-6633/aab406 PMID: 29504942

Durant, T. J., Knight, E., Nelson, B., Dudgeon, S., Lee, S. J., Walliman, D., Young, H. P., Ohno-Machado, L., & Schulz, W. L. (2024). A primer for quantum computing and its applications to healthcare and biomedical research. *Journal of the American Medical Informatics Association : JAMIA, 31*(8), 1774–1784. DOI: 10.1093/jamia/ocae149 PMID: 38934288

Ekert, A., & Jozsa, R. (1996). Quantum computation and Shor's factoring algorithm. *Reviews of Modern Physics, 68*(3), 733–753. DOI: 10.1103/RevModPhys.68.733

Gill, S. S., Kumar, A., Singh, H., Singh, M., Kaur, K., Usman, M., & Buyya, R. (2022). Quantum computing: A taxonomy, systematic review and future directions. *Software, Practice & Experience, 52*(1), 66–114. DOI: 10.1002/spe.3039

Goswami, S., & Sharma, S. (2024, March). Artificial intelligence, quantum computing and cloud computing enabled personalized medicine in next generation sequencing bioinformatics. In *2024 IEEE International Conference on Interdisciplinary Approaches in Technology and Management for Social Innovation (IATMSI)* (Vol. 2, pp. 1–5). IEEE. DOI: 10.1109/IATMSI60426.2024.10502533

Gruska, J. (1999). *Quantum computing* (Vol. 2005). McGraw-Hill.

Gupta, S., Modgil, S., Bhatt, P. C., Jabbour, C. J. C., & Kamble, S. (2023). Quantum computing led innovation for achieving a more sustainable Covid-19 healthcare industry. *Technovation, 120*, 102544. DOI: 10.1016/j.technovation.2022.102544

Horowitz, M., & Grumbling, E. (Eds.). (2019). *Quantum computing: progress and prospects.*

Jayanthi, P., Rai, B. K., & Muralikrishna, I. (2022). The potential of quantum computing in healthcare. In *Technology road mapping for quantum computing and engineering* (pp. 81–101). IGI Global. DOI: 10.4018/978-1-7998-9183-3.ch006

Jeyaraman, N., Jeyaraman, M., Yadav, S., Ramasubramanian, S., & Balaji, S. (2024). Revolutionizing healthcare: The emerging role of quantum computing in enhancing medical technology and treatment. *Cureus, 16*(8). Advance online publication. DOI: 10.7759/cureus.67486 PMID: 39310567

Kop, M., Slijpen, S., Liu, K., Lee, J.H., Albrecht, C., & Cohen, I.G. (2024). How Quantum Technologies May Be Integrated Into Healthcare, What Regulators Should Consider. *What Regulators Should Consider (December 05, 2024).*

Kumar, G., Yadav, S., Mukherjee, A., Hassija, V., & Guizani, M. (2024). Recent advances in quantum computing for drug discovery and development. *IEEE Access : Practical Innovations, Open Solutions, 12*, 64491–64509. DOI: 10.1109/ACCESS.2024.3376408

Malina, L., Dzurenda, P., Ricci, S., Hajny, J., Srivastava, G., Matulevičius, R., Affia, A.-A. O., Laurent, M., Sultan, N. H., & Tang, Q. (2021). Post-quantum era privacy protection for intelligent infrastructures. *IEEE Access : Practical Innovations, Open Solutions, 9*, 36038–36077. DOI: 10.1109/ACCESS.2021.3062201

Maronese, M., Destri, C., & Prati, E. (2022). Quantum activation functions for quantum neural networks. *Quantum Information Processing, 21*(4), 128. DOI: 10.1007/s11128-022-03466-0

Mysore, N. R. (2022). Healthcare System 4.0 Driven by Quantum Computing and Its Use Cases: A COVID-19 Perspective. In *Artificial Intelligence, Machine Learning and Blockchain in Quantum Satellite, Drone and Network* (pp. 107–126). CRC Press.

Ollitrault, P. J., Miessen, A., & Tavernelli, I. (2021). Molecular quantum dynamics: A quantum computing perspective. *Accounts of Chemical Research, 54*(23), 4229–4238. DOI: 10.1021/acs.accounts.1c00514 PMID: 34787398

Pakela, J. M., Tseng, H. H., Matuszak, M. M., Ten Haken, R. K., McShan, D. L., & El Naqa, I. (2020). Quantum-inspired algorithm for radiotherapy planning optimization. *Medical Physics, 47*(1), 5–18. DOI: 10.1002/mp.13840 PMID: 31574176

Pal, S., Bhattacharya, M., Lee, S. S., & Chakraborty, C. (2024). Quantum computing in the next-generation computational biology landscape: From protein folding to molecular dynamics. *Molecular Biotechnology, 66*(2), 163–178. DOI: 10.1007/s12033-023-00765-4 PMID: 37244882

Pulipeti, S., & Kumar, A. (2023). Secure quantum computing for healthcare sector: A short analysis. *Security and Privacy, 6*(5), e293. DOI: 10.1002/spy2.293

Qayyum, A. (2023). Quantum computing for healthcare: A review. *Authorea Preprints.*

Rieffel, E., & Polak, W. (2000). An introduction to quantum computing for non-physicists. *ACM Computing Surveys, 32*(3), 300–335. DOI: 10.1145/367701.367709

Robinson, T., Harkin, J., & Shukla, P. (2021). Hardware acceleration of genomics data analysis: Challenges and opportunities. *Bioinformatics (Oxford, England)*, *37*(13), 1785–1795. DOI: 10.1093/bioinformatics/btab017 PMID: 34037688

Ur Rasool, R., Ahmad, H. F., Rafique, W., Qayyum, A., Qadir, J., & Anwar, Z. (2023). Quantum computing for healthcare: A review. *Future Internet*, *15*(3), 94. DOI: 10.3390/fi15030094

Wheatley, M. C. (2024). Quantum Shifts: The Societal Implications of Quantum Computing on Security, Privacy, and the Economy. *Journal of Computational Science*, *1*, 100002.

Chapter 7
Cloud Security for Healthcare:
Threat Intelligence and Risk Management

Omowunmi F. Makinde
https://orcid.org/0009-0004-9372-7539
University of the Cumberlands, USA

ABSTRACT

This chapter examines the critical role of cloud security in the healthcare sector, focusing on the integration of threat intelligence and risk management strategies. It examines the unique security challenges faced by healthcare organizations as they adopt cloud technologies, including data privacy, regulatory compliance, and the evolving threat landscape. The chapter discusses best practices for implementing robust security frameworks, leveraging threat intelligence to anticipate and mitigate cyber risks, and aligning risk management processes with industry standards. Through practical insights and case studies, it provides healthcare professionals and IT leaders with actionable guidance to safeguard sensitive health data and ensure resilient, secure cloud environments.

1. INTRODUCTION

The healthcare industry stands at a critical juncture in its digital transformation journey, with cloud computing emerging as a fundamental enabler of modern healthcare delivery. As healthcare organizations increasingly migrate their operations, data, and applications to cloud environments, the imperative for robust security measures has never been more pronounced (Zlatolas et al., 2024). This comprehensive analy-

DOI: 10.4018/979-8-3373-4918-3.ch007

sis explores the intricate landscape of cloud security for healthcare, with particular emphasis on threat intelligence and risk management frameworks that are essential for protecting sensitive patient data and maintaining operational continuity.

The convergence of healthcare and cloud computing presents both unprecedented opportunities and significant challenges. While cloud technologies offer scalability, cost-effectiveness, and enhanced collaboration capabilities, they also introduce new attack vectors and security considerations that healthcare organizations must navigate carefully. The stakes are particularly high in healthcare, where data breaches can compromise patient privacy, disrupt critical care services, and result in severe regulatory penalties (Mehrtak et al., 2021).

This paper examines the current state of healthcare cloud adoption, analyzes the evolving threat landscape specific to healthcare cloud environments, and provides a comprehensive framework for implementing effective threat intelligence and risk management strategies. Through detailed exploration of regulatory compliance requirements, emerging technologies, and best practices, this analysis aims to equip healthcare organizations with the knowledge and tools necessary to secure their cloud infrastructure while maintaining the agility and innovation that cloud computing enables. As we explore the various dimensions of healthcare cloud security, we will examine how threat intelligence can be leveraged to anticipate and mitigate emerging risks, how risk management frameworks can be tailored to healthcare-specific requirements, and how emerging technologies such as zero trust architecture and artificial intelligence can enhance security postures. The ultimate goal is to enable healthcare organizations to harness the full potential of cloud computing while maintaining the highest standards of security, privacy, and compliance.

2. HEALTHCARE CLOUD SECURITY LANDSCAPE

2.1 Current State of Healthcare Cloud Adoption

The healthcare industry's adoption of cloud computing has accelerated dramatically over the past decade, driven by the need for digital transformation, cost optimization, and improved patient outcomes. According to recent industry analyses, majority of healthcare organizations have adopted some form of cloud computing, with hybrid and multi-cloud strategies becoming increasingly prevalent. This rapid adoption has been further accelerated by the COVID-19 pandemic, which highlighted the critical importance of scalable, accessible, and resilient IT infrastructure (Sachdeva et al., 2024).

Healthcare organizations are leveraging cloud services across various domains, including electronic health records (EHR) systems, medical imaging and storage, telemedicine platforms, and clinical decision support systems. The shift from on-premises infrastructure to cloud-based solutions has enabled healthcare providers to reduce capital expenditures, improve system reliability, and enhance collaboration among care teams. However, this transition has also introduced new security challenges that require careful consideration and specialized expertise (Shojaei et al., 2024).

The current landscape is characterized by a diverse ecosystem of cloud service providers, each offering specialized healthcare solutions. Major cloud providers such as Amazon Web Services (AWS), Microsoft Azure, and Google Cloud Platform have developed healthcare-specific offerings that address regulatory compliance requirements and provide enhanced security features (Al-Issa et al., 2019). These platforms offer HIPAA-compliant services, advanced encryption capabilities, and comprehensive audit trails that are essential for healthcare operations (Yimam & Fernandez, 2016).

Despite the benefits, healthcare organizations face significant challenges in cloud adoption, including concerns about data security, regulatory compliance, and vendor lock-in (Mehrtak et al., 2021). Additionally, the shortage of skilled cybersecurity professionals in healthcare has created gaps in cloud security expertise, making organizations vulnerable to emerging threats (He et al., 2021). The current state of healthcare cloud adoption also reflects varying levels of maturity across different types of healthcare organizations. Large health systems and academic medical centers typically have more advanced cloud strategies and dedicated security teams, while smaller practices and rural hospitals may lack the resources and expertise necessary for comprehensive cloud security implementation. This disparity creates a fragmented security landscape that requires tailored approaches based on organizational size, resources, and risk tolerance (Pattanaik et al., 2024).

2.2 Regulatory Compliance in Cloud Environments

Regulatory compliance represents one of the most complex and critical aspects of healthcare cloud security. Healthcare organizations must navigate an intricate web of regulations, including the Health Insurance Portability and Accountability Act (HIPAA), the Health Information Technology for Economic and Clinical Health (HITECH) Act, and various state and international privacy laws. These regulations impose strict requirements for data protection, access controls, audit trails, and breach notification that must be maintained in cloud environments (Theodos & Sittig, 2020).

HIPAA compliance in cloud environments requires careful attention to business associate agreements (BAAs), which establish the legal framework for cloud service providers to handle protected health information (PHI). Healthcare organizations must ensure that their cloud providers are willing and able to sign comprehensive

BAAs that address all aspects of PHI handling, including data encryption, access controls, and incident response procedures (Al-Issa et al., 2019).

The HITECH Act's breach notification requirements present additional challenges in cloud environments, where data may be distributed across multiple geographic locations and managed by various third-party services. Healthcare organizations must implement robust monitoring and logging capabilities to detect potential breaches and ensure timely notification to affected individuals and regulatory authorities (Bohn & Schiereck, 2022). International regulations such as the General Data Protection Regulation (GDPR) add another layer of complexity for healthcare organizations that operate globally or serve international patients. GDPR's strict requirements for data sovereignty, consent management, and the right to be forgotten must be carefully considered when designing cloud architectures and selecting service providers (Issaoui et al., 2023). The regulation's emphasis on privacy by design aligns well with modern cloud security practices but requires proactive implementation of privacy controls throughout the data lifecycle (Shin et al., 2024).

State-level regulations further complicate the compliance landscape, with various states implementing their own privacy laws and data protection requirements. Healthcare organizations must ensure that their cloud implementations can accommodate varying regulatory requirements across different jurisdictions while maintaining operational efficiency and cost-effectiveness. This often requires sophisticated data governance frameworks and flexible cloud architectures that can adapt to changing regulatory requirements (Theodos & Sittig, 2020). The emergence of new regulations and evolving interpretations of existing laws requires healthcare organizations to maintain continuous compliance monitoring and adaptation capabilities. Cloud environments must be designed with compliance automation in mind, incorporating tools and processes that can automatically enforce regulatory requirements and generate necessary documentation for audits and assessments (Dunbar et al., 2023).

2.3 Challenges in Securing Healthcare Cloud Infrastructure

Securing healthcare cloud infrastructure presents unique challenges that stem from the intersection of complex technology environments, stringent regulatory requirements, and the critical nature of healthcare services (Mehrtak et al., 2021). One of the primary challenges is the shared responsibility model inherent in cloud computing, which requires healthcare organizations to clearly understand and manage their portion of security responsibilities while relying on cloud service providers for infrastructure-level protections (Cresswell et al., 2022). The distributed nature of cloud environments creates challenges in maintaining visibility and control over data and applications. Healthcare organizations must implement comprehensive monitoring and logging capabilities across multiple cloud services and regions while ensuring that security controls remain effective as workloads scale dynamically. This complexity is compounded by the need to integrate cloud security with existing on-premises security infrastructure in hybrid environments (He et al., 2021).

Identity and access management (IAM) represents another significant challenge in healthcare cloud environments. Healthcare organizations must manage access for diverse user populations, including clinicians, administrative staff, patients, and third-party partners, each with different access requirements and risk profiles (Glockler et al., 2023). The implementation of least-privilege access principles becomes complex when dealing with emergency access scenarios common in healthcare, where immediate access to patient information may be required to save lives (Singh et al., 2023). Data classification and protection present ongoing challenges as healthcare organizations generate and process vast amounts of sensitive information across multiple cloud services (Abouelmehdi et al., 2018). Ensuring consistent application of encryption, access controls, and data loss prevention measures across diverse cloud environments requires sophisticated data governance frameworks and automated policy enforcement mechanisms. The challenge is further complicated by the need to maintain data availability for clinical decision-making while implementing strong security controls (Morita et al., 2024).

The integration of legacy healthcare systems with modern cloud infrastructure creates additional security challenges. Many healthcare organizations rely on older systems that were not designed with cloud integration in mind, requiring complex integration approaches that may introduce security vulnerabilities. The need to maintain interoperability with various healthcare standards and protocols while implementing modern security controls adds another layer of complexity (Ewoh & Vartiainen, 2024). Incident response and forensics in cloud environments present unique challenges due to the ephemeral nature of cloud resources and the distributed architecture of cloud services. Healthcare organizations must develop specialized incident response capabilities that can effectively investigate and respond to security incidents across multiple cloud providers and services while maintaining the chain of custody required for potential legal proceedings (Alenezi et al., 2019).

The shortage of skilled cybersecurity professionals with healthcare and cloud expertise creates significant challenges for many organizations. The specialized knowledge required to effectively secure healthcare cloud environments is in high demand, and many organizations struggle to attract and retain qualified personnel. This skill gap often results in inadequate security implementations and increased vulnerability to cyber threats (He et al., 2021).

2.4 Data Protection and Privacy in Healthcare Cloud

Data protection and privacy in healthcare cloud environments require comprehensive strategies that address the entire data lifecycle, from creation and processing to storage and eventual disposal (Xiang & Cai, 2021). Healthcare data encompasses not only traditional protected health information (PHI) but also emerging data types such as genomic information, wearable device data, and artificial intelligence-generated insights, each presenting unique protection challenges (Scheibner et al., 2021). Encryption serves as a fundamental component of healthcare cloud data protection, requiring implementation at multiple levels including data at rest, data in transit, and increasingly, data in use through advanced techniques such as homomorphic encryption and secure multi-party computation (Munjal & Bhatia, 2022). Healthcare organizations must implement robust key management practices that ensure encryption keys are properly protected while remaining accessible for legitimate healthcare operations. The challenge lies in balancing strong encryption with the performance requirements of clinical applications and the need for emergency access to patient information (Abouelmehdi et al., 2018).

Data sovereignty and residency requirements add complexity to healthcare cloud data protection strategies. Many healthcare organizations must ensure that patient data remains within specific geographic boundaries to comply with local regulations or organizational policies. This requirement influences cloud provider selection and architecture design, often necessitating the use of specific cloud regions or specialized compliance offerings that guarantee data residency (Hummel et al., 2021).

Privacy-preserving technologies are becoming increasingly important in healthcare cloud environments, particularly as organizations seek to leverage data for research and analytics while protecting individual privacy (Gu et al., 2023). Techniques such as differential privacy, synthetic data generation, and federated learning enable healthcare organizations to derive insights from sensitive data without exposing individual patient information. These technologies require careful implementation to ensure that privacy protections remain effective while maintaining the utility of the data for legitimate healthcare purposes (Xu et al., 2020).

Data minimization principles require healthcare organizations to carefully consider what data is collected, processed, and stored in cloud environments. This involves implementing data classification schemes that identify the sensitivity and regulatory requirements of different data types, enabling appropriate protection measures to be applied (Mukta et al., 2022). Automated data lifecycle management becomes crucial for ensuring that data is retained only as long as necessary and is securely disposed of when no longer needed (Abouelmehdi et al., 2018).

Patient consent management in cloud environments presents unique challenges, particularly as data may be processed by multiple cloud services and third-party applications (Kassam et al., 2023). Healthcare organizations must implement comprehensive consent management frameworks that track patient preferences and ensure that data processing activities align with granted permissions. This becomes particularly complex in scenarios involving data sharing for research or public health purposes (Pietrzykowski & Smilowska, 2021).

The implementation of privacy by design principles in healthcare cloud architectures requires proactive consideration of privacy implications throughout the system design and development process. This includes implementing privacy controls at the architectural level, conducting privacy impact assessments for new cloud services, and ensuring that privacy considerations are integrated into change management processes (Semantha et al., 2020). Cross-border data transfers in global healthcare organizations require careful attention to international privacy laws and data transfer mechanisms. Organizations must implement appropriate safeguards such as standard contractual clauses or adequacy decisions to ensure that patient data receives adequate protection when transferred between different jurisdictions. The complexity of managing these requirements across multiple cloud providers and services requires sophisticated data governance frameworks and legal expertise (Xia et al., 2024).

3. THREAT INTELLIGENCE FOR HEALTHCARE CLOUD SECURITY

3.1 Healthcare-Specific Threat Landscape

The healthcare industry faces a unique and evolving threat landscape that combines traditional cybersecurity risks with sector-specific vulnerabilities and attack vectors. Healthcare organizations are particularly attractive targets for cybercriminals due to the high value of medical data, the critical nature of healthcare services, and historically weaker cybersecurity postures compared to other industries. The migration to cloud environments has introduced new dimensions to this threat landscape while also providing opportunities for enhanced security capabilities (Ewoh & Vartiainen, 2024).

Ransomware attacks represent one of the most significant threats to healthcare cloud environments, with attackers increasingly targeting cloud-based systems and data repositories. These attacks can have devastating consequences for healthcare organizations, potentially disrupting patient care, compromising sensitive data, and resulting in significant financial losses (Xu, 2024). The distributed nature of cloud environments can complicate ransomware response efforts while also providing opportunities for improved backup and recovery capabilities that can mitigate the impact of successful attacks (Seth et al., 2024).

Advanced persistent threats (APTs) targeting healthcare organizations often focus on long-term access to valuable medical data and research information. These sophisticated attacks may target cloud environments through various vectors, including compromised credentials, supply chain attacks, and exploitation of cloud service vulnerabilities (Salim et al., 2023). APT groups may establish persistent access to cloud environments and remain undetected for extended periods while exfiltrating sensitive information or preparing for more disruptive attacks (Buchta et al., 2024).

Insider threats present unique challenges in healthcare cloud environments, where authorized users may have legitimate access to sensitive patient information but may misuse this access for personal gain or malicious purposes. The shared responsibility model of cloud computing can complicate insider threat detection and response, requiring healthcare organizations to implement comprehensive user activity monitoring and behavioral analytics across cloud services (He et al., 2021). Supply chain attacks targeting cloud service providers and third-party healthcare applications pose increasing risks to healthcare organizations. These attacks may compromise cloud services used by multiple healthcare organizations, potentially affecting thousands of patients and providers simultaneously. The interconnected nature of cloud ecosystems means that a compromise of one service or provider can have cascading effects across multiple organizations and systems (Angle, 2022).

Data breaches in healthcare cloud environments may result from various factors, including misconfigured cloud services, inadequate access controls, and exploitation of application vulnerabilities. The public nature of cloud environments means that misconfigurations can expose sensitive data to unauthorized access, while the complexity of cloud security configurations increases the likelihood of human error (Seh et al., 2020). Healthcare organizations must implement comprehensive security monitoring and configuration management to prevent and detect potential data exposures (Al-Issa et al., 2019).

Nation-state actors increasingly target healthcare organizations for various purposes, including espionage, disruption of critical services, and theft of valuable research data. These sophisticated adversaries may target cloud environments as part of broader campaigns aimed at compromising healthcare infrastructure or stealing sensitive information related to medical research, patient data, or healthcare technologies (Mehrtak et al., 2021). The COVID-19 pandemic has highlighted new threat vectors specific to healthcare cloud environments, including attacks targeting telemedicine platforms, remote access systems, and cloud-based collaboration tools. The rapid adoption of new cloud services during the pandemic created security gaps that attackers have exploited, emphasizing the need for comprehensive threat intelligence and risk assessment capabilities (He et al., 2021). Emerging threats related to artificial intelligence and machine learning in healthcare cloud environments include adversarial attacks on AI models, data poisoning attempts, and exploitation of AI system vulnerabilities. As healthcare organizations increasingly rely on cloud-based AI services for clinical decision support and diagnostic assistance, these threats pose significant risks to patient safety and data integrity (Das et al., 2024).

3.2 Threat Intelligence Sources and Collection

Effective threat intelligence for healthcare cloud security requires diverse and comprehensive information sources that provide timely, relevant, and actionable insights about emerging threats and attack techniques. Healthcare organizations must develop sophisticated threat intelligence collection and analysis capabilities that combine internal security data with external threat feeds and industry-specific intelligence sources (Saeed et al., 2023). Government and regulatory sources provide critical threat intelligence for healthcare organizations, including alerts and advisories from agencies such as the Cybersecurity and Infrastructure Security Agency (CISA), the Department of Health and Human Services (HHS), and the Food and Drug Administration (FDA) (Argaw et al., 2019). These sources often provide sector-specific threat information and guidance on protecting healthcare infrastructure and medical devices. International government sources also contribute valuable intelligence about global threat trends and nation-state activities targeting healthcare organizations (Coventry & Branley, 2018).

Industry-specific threat intelligence sharing organizations, such as the Health Information Sharing and Analysis Center (H-ISAC), provide valuable platforms for healthcare organizations to share threat information and collaborate on security initiatives (Argaw et al., 2019). These organizations facilitate the exchange of indicators of compromise (IOCs), attack techniques, and mitigation strategies specific to the healthcare sector. Participation in these sharing communities enables healthcare organizations to benefit from collective intelligence and early warning capabilities (Lieneck et al., 2023).

Commercial threat intelligence providers offer specialized feeds and analysis services that can enhance healthcare organizations' threat awareness capabilities. These providers often offer healthcare-specific intelligence products that focus on threats targeting medical devices, healthcare applications, and cloud services commonly used in healthcare environments. The integration of commercial threat intelligence with internal security data can provide comprehensive visibility into the threat landscape (Botha et al., 2024).

Cloud service provider threat intelligence represents a crucial source of information for healthcare organizations operating in cloud environments. Major cloud providers offer threat intelligence services that provide insights into attacks targeting their platforms and customers. These services often include automated threat detection capabilities, security recommendations, and incident response support that can significantly enhance healthcare organizations' security postures (Wasserman & Wasserman, 2022).

Open source intelligence (OSINT) collection from various public sources, including security research publications, vulnerability databases, and social media platforms, can provide valuable insights into emerging threats and attack techniques. Healthcare organizations must develop capabilities to collect, analyze, and correlate OSINT with other intelligence sources to identify relevant threats and trends (Yadav et al., 2023). Internal threat intelligence collection from security monitoring systems, incident response activities, and vulnerability assessments provides crucial insights into organization-specific threats and attack patterns. Healthcare organizations must implement comprehensive logging and monitoring capabilities across their cloud environments to generate internal threat intelligence that can inform security decision-making and incident response activities (Saeed et al., 2023).

Threat intelligence from security vendors and technology partners can provide valuable insights into threats targeting specific technologies and platforms used by healthcare organizations. This includes intelligence from endpoint protection vendors, network security providers, and cloud security specialists who have visibility into attack trends and techniques across their customer bases (Sills et al., 2020). Academic and research institutions contribute valuable threat intelligence through security research, vulnerability discovery, and analysis of emerging attack techniques. Healthcare organizations should monitor relevant academic publications and research findings to stay informed about new threats and security technologies that may impact their cloud environments (Saeed et al., 2023).

The integration and correlation of threat intelligence from multiple sources requires sophisticated analysis capabilities and tools that can process large volumes of data and identify relevant threats and trends. Healthcare organizations must invest in threat intelligence platforms and analytical capabilities that can effectively synthesize information from diverse sources and provide actionable insights for security teams (Santos et al., 2025). Threat intelligence sharing with law enforcement and regulatory agencies can provide additional context and support for incident response activities while contributing to broader efforts to combat cybercrime targeting healthcare organizations. Healthcare organizations should establish appropriate relationships and communication channels with relevant law enforcement and regulatory agencies to facilitate effective information sharing (Ainslie et al., 2023).

3.3 Integration of Threat Intelligence in Security Operations

The effective integration of threat intelligence into healthcare cloud security operations requires sophisticated processes, technologies, and organizational structures that can transform raw intelligence data into actionable security insights and defensive measures. This integration must be seamlessly woven into existing security operations while addressing the unique requirements and constraints of healthcare environments (Abinesh Kamal & Divya, 2024). Security Information and Event Management (SIEM) systems serve as central platforms for integrating threat intelligence with security monitoring and incident response activities. Healthcare organizations must configure their SIEM systems to automatically ingest threat intelligence feeds and correlate this information with security events and alerts generated by cloud security monitoring tools. This integration enables automated threat detection and response capabilities that can identify known attack patterns and indicators of compromise in real-time (González-Granadillo et al., 2021).

Threat intelligence platforms (TIPs) provide specialized capabilities for collecting, analyzing, and disseminating threat intelligence across healthcare organizations. These platforms can aggregate intelligence from multiple sources, perform automated analysis and correlation, and distribute relevant intelligence to security teams and automated security tools. The implementation of TIPs in healthcare environments requires careful consideration of data sensitivity and sharing restrictions while ensuring that intelligence reaches the appropriate stakeholders (Mohamed, 2025).

Security orchestration, automation, and response (SOAR) platforms enable healthcare organizations to automate threat intelligence-driven security processes and responses. These platforms can automatically execute predefined response actions based on threat intelligence indicators, such as blocking malicious IP addresses, quarantining suspicious files, or initiating incident response procedures. The automation capabilities provided by SOAR platforms are particularly valuable in healthcare environments where security teams may be resource-constrained and need to focus on high-priority threats (Subudhi, 2024).

Threat hunting activities in healthcare cloud environments benefit significantly from threat intelligence integration, enabling security analysts to proactively search for signs of compromise based on known attack techniques and indicators. Threat intelligence provides the foundation for developing hunting hypotheses and guides analysts toward areas of highest risk and concern. The integration of threat intelligence with cloud security monitoring tools enables more effective and targeted threat hunting activities (Saeed et al., 2023).

Vulnerability management programs in healthcare organizations must integrate threat intelligence to prioritize remediation efforts based on active threats and attack trends. Threat intelligence can provide context about which vulnerabilities are being actively exploited in the wild, enabling healthcare organizations to focus their limited resources on addressing the most critical security gaps. This integration is particularly important in cloud environments where the attack surface may be large and constantly changing (Ewoh & Vartiainen, 2024).

Incident response procedures must incorporate threat intelligence to enhance the speed and effectiveness of response activities. Threat intelligence can provide valuable context about attack techniques, attribution, and potential impact, enabling incident response teams to make more informed decisions about containment and remediation strategies. The integration of threat intelligence with incident response tools and procedures can significantly improve the quality and speed of response activities (Kotsias et al., 2022).

Risk assessment processes in healthcare organizations benefit from threat intelligence integration by providing current and relevant information about threats targeting similar organizations and technologies. Threat intelligence can inform risk calculations and help healthcare organizations understand the likelihood and potential impact of various threat scenarios. This integration enables more accurate and dynamic risk assessments that reflect the current threat landscape (He et al., 2021).

Security awareness and training programs should incorporate relevant threat intelligence to educate healthcare staff about current threats and attack techniques. Regular communication of threat intelligence findings can help healthcare workers recognize and report suspicious activities while reinforcing the importance of security best practices. The integration of threat intelligence with training programs ensures that security awareness efforts remain current and relevant (Kruse et al., 2017). Compliance and regulatory reporting activities can benefit from threat intelligence integration by providing evidence of proactive threat monitoring and response capabilities. Threat intelligence documentation can support compliance audits and regulatory assessments while demonstrating the organization's commitment to maintaining current awareness of relevant threats and risks (Saeed et al., 2023). The measurement and evaluation of threat intelligence integration effectiveness requires the development of appropriate metrics and key performance indicators (KPIs) that assess the impact of threat intelligence on security operations. Healthcare organizations should track metrics such as threat detection rates, incident response times, and the accuracy of threat intelligence-driven alerts to continuously improve their integration processes and capabilities (Abinesh Kamal & Divya, 2024).

3.4 Proactive Threat Detection and Response

Proactive threat detection and response capabilities are essential for healthcare organizations to identify and mitigate threats before they can impact patient care or compromise sensitive health information. These capabilities must be specifically tailored to address the unique characteristics of healthcare environments and the threats they face (Mahboubi et al., 2024). Behavioral analytics and user behavior monitoring enable healthcare organizations to identify anomalous activities that may indicate insider threats or compromised accounts. These solutions must be carefully tuned to account for the legitimate variations in healthcare worker behavior, including shift patterns, emergency situations, and varying patient care responsibilities. Machine learning algorithms can help identify subtle patterns that may indicate malicious activity while minimizing false positives that could disrupt healthcare operations (Tabassum et al., 2024).

Network traffic analysis provides visibility into potential threats traversing healthcare networks, including cloud connections and inter-system communications. Healthcare organizations should implement network monitoring solutions that can identify suspicious traffic patterns, command and control communications, and data exfiltration attempts. This is particularly important in cloud environments where traditional perimeter-based security controls may be less effective (He et al., 2021). Deception technologies can provide early warning of attack activities by creating decoy systems and data that attract attackers. In healthcare environments, deception technologies must be carefully implemented to avoid interfering with legitimate healthcare operations while providing valuable intelligence about attack techniques and objectives (Morić et al., 2025).

Automated threat response capabilities enable healthcare organizations to respond rapidly to identified threats, potentially containing attacks before they can spread or cause significant damage. These capabilities must be carefully designed to account for the critical nature of healthcare systems and the potential impact of automated response actions on patient care (He et al., 2021). Threat intelligence fusion involves combining multiple sources of threat information to provide a comprehensive view of the threat landscape and enable more effective threat detection and response. Healthcare organizations should develop fusion capabilities that can correlate internal security data with external threat intelligence to identify sophisticated attacks and provide context for security incidents (Saeed et al., 2023). Continuous monitoring and assessment capabilities ensure that threat detection and response capabilities remain effective as the threat landscape evolves. Healthcare organizations should implement processes for regularly evaluating and updating their threat detection capabilities based on new threats, attack techniques, and changes in their environment (Elendu et al., 2024).

4. RISK MANAGEMENT FRAMEWORKS FOR HEALTHCARE CLOUD

4.1 Risk Assessment Methodologies

Healthcare organizations require robust risk assessment methodologies specifically designed to address the unique challenges and requirements of cloud computing in healthcare environments. These methodologies must account for regulatory compliance requirements, patient safety considerations, and the complex interdependencies inherent in healthcare systems (Ali et al., 2024). The NIST Risk Management Framework (RMF) provides a comprehensive foundation for healthcare cloud risk assessment. This framework emphasizes a continuous, organization-wide approach to risk management that aligns well with the dynamic nature of cloud computing. Healthcare organizations can adapt the RMF to address healthcare-specific requirements by incorporating HIPAA security requirements, FDA medical device guidance, and other relevant regulatory frameworks into their risk assessment processes (Veeraballi, 2025).

Healthcare-specific risk assessment methodologies must address the unique characteristics of health information and healthcare operations. The HITRUST Common Security Framework (CSF) provides a comprehensive approach to healthcare information security risk assessment that incorporates multiple regulatory and industry standards. This framework is particularly valuable for healthcare organizations because it provides a unified approach to addressing various compliance requirements while maintaining focus on healthcare-specific risks (He et al., 2021). Cloud-specific risk assessment considerations include evaluating the shared responsibility model, assessing cloud service provider security controls, and analyzing the risks associated with data migration and integration. Healthcare organizations must develop risk assessment processes that can evaluate cloud services against healthcare-specific requirements and identify potential gaps in security coverage (Fathullah et al., 2023).

Quantitative risk assessment methods enable healthcare organizations to assign monetary values to potential risks, facilitating more informed decision-making about risk mitigation investments (Pascarella et al., 2021). These methods are particularly valuable for healthcare organizations that must balance security investments with patient care priorities and budget constraints. However, quantitative methods must account for the difficulty of assigning monetary values to patient safety risks and regulatory compliance failures (Rigaud et al., 2024). Qualitative risk assessment approaches focus on categorizing risks based on likelihood and impact without assigning specific monetary values (Pascarella et al., 2021). These approaches may be more practical for healthcare organizations that lack the data or resources necessary for quantitative analysis. Qualitative methods can effectively communicate risk levels to healthcare leadership and support risk-based decision-making (Ferdosi et al., 2020). Dynamic risk assessment capabilities are essential in cloud environments where configurations, threats, and business requirements change frequently. Healthcare organizations should implement continuous risk assessment processes that can adapt to changes in their cloud environment and provide real-time visibility into risk levels (Cheimonidis & Rantos, 2023).

4.2 Risk Mitigation Strategies

Effective risk mitigation strategies for healthcare cloud environments must address identified risks through a combination of technical controls, administrative procedures, and risk transfer mechanisms. These strategies must be tailored to the specific risk profile of each healthcare organization while maintaining compliance with applicable regulations and standards (He et al., 2021). Technical risk mitigation controls form the foundation of healthcare cloud security. Encryption strategies must address both data at rest and data in transit, with key management practices that ensure healthcare organizations maintain control over their encryption keys. Multi-factor authentication and privileged access management solutions help mitigate risks associated with unauthorized access to healthcare systems and data (Wani et al., 2020).

Network security controls, including network segmentation, intrusion detection and prevention systems, and secure network architectures, help contain potential security incidents and prevent lateral movement within healthcare cloud environments. These controls must be designed to accommodate the complex communication patterns inherent in healthcare operations while maintaining security effectiveness (Chinnasamy & Deepalakshmi, 2021). Administrative risk mitigation strategies include developing comprehensive security policies and procedures, implementing security awareness training programs, and establishing incident response capabilities. Healthcare organizations must ensure that their administrative controls address the unique requirements of cloud computing while maintaining alignment with healthcare operational requirements (Angle, 2022).

Risk transfer mechanisms, including cyber insurance and contractual risk allocation, enable healthcare organizations to transfer certain risks to third parties. Cyber insurance policies specifically designed for healthcare organizations can provide financial protection against data breach costs, business interruption, and regulatory fines. However, healthcare organizations must carefully evaluate insurance coverage to ensure it addresses their specific risk profile and cloud computing arrangements (Amah et al., 2023).

Vendor risk management strategies are critical for healthcare organizations that rely on cloud service providers and other third-party vendors. These strategies should include comprehensive vendor assessment processes, ongoing monitoring of vendor security postures, and contractual provisions that address security requirements and incident response procedures (Angle, 2022). Business continuity and disaster recovery planning represent essential risk mitigation strategies for healthcare organizations. Cloud computing can enhance business continuity capabilities by providing geographically distributed infrastructure and automated backup and recovery capabilities. However, healthcare organizations must ensure their continuity plans address cloud-specific risks and dependencies (Amah et al., 2023).

5. TRUST MODELS AND CLOUD SERVICE PROVIDER EVALUATION

5.1 Cloud Trust Frameworks for Healthcare

Trust frameworks for healthcare cloud computing establish the foundation for evaluating and managing relationships with cloud service providers. These frameworks must address the unique requirements of healthcare organizations, including regulatory compliance, patient safety, and data protection requirements (Chiregi & Navimipour, 2018). The concept of zero trust architecture has gained significant traction in healthcare cloud security, emphasizing the principle of "never trust, always verify." This approach assumes that no user, device, or network should be trusted by default, requiring continuous verification and validation of access requests. In healthcare cloud environments, zero trust principles help address the challenges of securing distributed systems and protecting sensitive health information across multiple cloud services and locations (Vukotich, 2023).

Healthcare-specific trust frameworks must incorporate regulatory requirements and industry standards into their evaluation criteria. The HITRUST CSF provides a comprehensive trust framework that addresses multiple regulatory requirements while providing a standardized approach to evaluating cloud service providers. This framework enables healthcare organizations to assess cloud providers against consistent criteria and compare different service offerings (Udroiu et al., 2022).

Cloud security certification programs, such as SOC 2 Type II, ISO 27001, and FedRAMP, provide independent validation of cloud service provider security controls. Healthcare organizations should require appropriate certifications from their cloud service providers and understand the scope and limitations of these certifications. However, certifications alone are not sufficient; healthcare organizations must conduct their own due diligence to ensure cloud services meet their specific requirements (Kabra et al., 2022).

Shared responsibility models define the division of security responsibilities between healthcare organizations and their cloud service providers. Trust frameworks must clearly articulate these responsibilities and ensure that healthcare organizations understand their obligations for securing data, applications, and user access in cloud environments. This clarity is essential for maintaining regulatory compliance and ensuring comprehensive security coverage (Mehrtak et al., 2021).

Transparency and auditability requirements in healthcare trust frameworks ensure that cloud service providers can demonstrate their security controls and provide necessary documentation for regulatory compliance. Healthcare organizations should require cloud providers to provide detailed security documentation, audit reports, and incident notification procedures that meet healthcare regulatory requirements (Kiseleva et al., 2022).

5.2 Cloud Service Provider Assessment

Comprehensive cloud service provider assessment is critical for healthcare organizations to ensure their chosen providers can meet the stringent security and compliance requirements of the healthcare industry. This assessment process must evaluate multiple dimensions of cloud service provider capabilities and align with healthcare-specific requirements (Al-Issa et al., 2019). Security control assessment forms the core of cloud service provider evaluation for healthcare organizations. This assessment should evaluate the provider's implementation of administrative, physical, and technical safeguards required by HIPAA and other applicable regulations. Healthcare organizations should conduct detailed reviews of provider security policies, procedures, and technical implementations to ensure they meet healthcare requirements (Mehrtak et al., 2021).

Compliance and certification evaluation involves reviewing the cloud service provider's compliance with relevant standards and regulations. Healthcare organizations should verify that providers maintain appropriate certifications and can demonstrate ongoing compliance with healthcare-specific requirements. This evaluation should also assess the provider's ability to support the healthcare organization's own compliance obligations (Dunbar et al., 2023). Data protection and privacy capabilities must be thoroughly evaluated to ensure cloud service providers can adequately protect health information. This includes assessing encryption capabilities, key management practices, data loss prevention controls, and privacy-preserving technologies. Healthcare organizations should also evaluate the provider's data handling practices, including data retention, deletion, and cross-border transfer capabilities (Hassan et al., 2022).

Incident response and business continuity capabilities are critical evaluation criteria for healthcare organizations that cannot tolerate extended service disruptions. Healthcare organizations should assess the provider's incident response procedures, communication protocols, and recovery time objectives to ensure they align with healthcare operational requirements (Sachdeva et al., 2024). Financial stability and business continuity of cloud service providers represent important considerations for healthcare organizations that may depend on cloud services for critical operations. Healthcare organizations should evaluate provider financial health, business continuity plans, and succession planning to ensure service continuity over the long term (Alshammari et al., 2016). Geographic and jurisdictional considerations may impact cloud service provider selection for healthcare organizations subject to data residency requirements or operating in multiple regulatory jurisdictions. Healthcare organizations should evaluate provider data center locations, data handling practices, and ability to meet jurisdictional requirements (Gao et al., 2018).

5.3 Patient Trust and Transparency

Patient trust represents a fundamental requirement for healthcare organizations adopting cloud computing, as patients must have confidence that their health information is being protected appropriately. Building and maintaining patient trust requires transparency about cloud computing practices and clear communication about data protection measures (Kerasidou & Kerasidou, 2023). Transparency requirements for healthcare cloud computing include providing clear information to patients about how their health information is stored, processed, and protected in cloud environments. Healthcare organizations should develop patient-facing communications that explain cloud computing benefits and security measures in understandable terms while addressing common patient concerns about data security and privacy (Rockwern et al., 2021).

Consent management in cloud environments must address patient rights and preferences regarding the use of their health information. Healthcare organizations should implement consent management systems that can accommodate patient preferences about cloud-based data processing while maintaining operational efficiency and regulatory compliance (Kassam et al., 2023). Patient rights and access requirements must be maintained in cloud environments, including the right to access, correct, and request deletion of health information. Healthcare organizations should ensure their cloud implementations support patient rights while maintaining appropriate security controls and audit trails (Sachdeva et al., 2024). Data portability and interoperability considerations impact patient trust by ensuring that patients can access and transfer their health information as needed. Healthcare organizations should evaluate cloud service providers' support for data portability standards and interoperability requirements that enable patient access and care coordination (Li et al., 2022).

Breach notification and communication procedures must be designed to maintain patient trust while meeting regulatory requirements. Healthcare organizations should develop clear procedures for communicating with patients about security incidents involving cloud services, providing appropriate information about the incident and steps being taken to address it (Seh et al., 2020). Patient education and engagement initiatives can help build trust in healthcare cloud computing by providing patients with information about cloud security measures and their benefits. Healthcare organizations should develop educational materials and programs that help patients understand how cloud computing can improve their care while maintaining appropriate security and privacy protections (Asan et al., 2021).

6. EMERGING TECHNOLOGIES AND FUTURE DIRECTIONS

6.1 Zero Trust Architecture in Healthcare Cloud

Zero Trust Architecture (ZTA) represents a paradigm shift in healthcare cloud security, moving away from traditional perimeter-based security models toward a comprehensive approach that assumes no implicit trust within the network. This architectural approach is particularly relevant for healthcare organizations operating in cloud environments where traditional network boundaries are blurred or non-existent (Vukotich, 2023). The implementation of Zero Trust in healthcare cloud environments requires a fundamental rethinking of security architecture design. Rather than relying on network location as a primary security control, Zero Trust architectures continuously verify and validate every access request based on multiple factors, including user identity, device posture, location, and behavioral patterns. This approach is particularly valuable in healthcare environments where users may access systems from various locations and devices while maintaining the need for secure access to sensitive patient information (Azad et al., 2024).

Identity and access management forms the cornerstone of Zero Trust implementation in healthcare cloud environments. Healthcare organizations must implement comprehensive identity governance programs that can manage complex user hierarchies, role-based access controls, and dynamic access requirements (Vukotich, 2023). This includes implementing strong authentication mechanisms, such as multi-factor authentication and risk-based authentication, that can adapt to changing threat conditions while maintaining user experience (Suleski et al., 2023). Device trust and endpoint security become critical components of Zero Trust architectures in healthcare environments. Healthcare organizations must implement comprehensive device management and security solutions that can assess device posture, enforce security policies, and prevent unauthorized devices from accessing healthcare systems and data. This is particularly challenging in healthcare environments where personal devices, medical devices, and traditional IT equipment must coexist securely (Wang et al., 2023).

Network micro-segmentation enables healthcare organizations to implement granular access controls that limit lateral movement and contain potential security incidents. In cloud environments, micro-segmentation can be implemented through software-defined networking, cloud-native security groups, and application-level access controls that provide fine-grained control over network communications (Sheikh et al., 2021). Data-centric security approaches within Zero Trust architectures focus on protecting data regardless of its location or the network it traverses. Healthcare organizations must implement comprehensive data classification, encryption, and access control mechanisms that can protect health information throughout its lifecycle. This includes implementing data loss prevention solutions, rights management systems, and privacy-preserving technologies that maintain data protection in distributed cloud environments (Sarkar et al., 2022). Continuous monitoring and analytics capabilities are essential for Zero Trust implementation, providing the visibility and intelligence necessary to make real-time access decisions. Healthcare organizations must implement comprehensive monitoring solutions that can collect and analyze data from multiple sources, including network traffic, user behavior, and system logs, to identify potential threats and anomalous activities (Weinberg & Cohen, 2024).

6.2 AI and Machine Learning for Cloud Security

Artificial Intelligence (AI) and Machine Learning (ML) technologies are transforming healthcare cloud security by enabling more sophisticated threat detection, automated response capabilities, and predictive security analytics. These technologies are particularly valuable in healthcare environments where the volume and complexity of security data exceed human analytical capabilities (Mohamed, 2025). Anomaly detection using machine learning algorithms enables healthcare organizations to identify subtle patterns and behaviors that may indicate security threats. These algorithms can analyze user behavior, network traffic, and system activities to identify deviations from normal patterns that may indicate insider threats, compromised accounts, or advanced persistent threats. In healthcare environments, ML-based anomaly detection must be carefully tuned to account for the legitimate variations in healthcare workflows and emergency situations (Khan & Alkhathami, 2024).

Automated threat response capabilities powered by AI enable healthcare organizations to respond rapidly to identified threats, potentially containing attacks before they can impact patient care or compromise sensitive data. These capabilities must be carefully designed to account for the critical nature of healthcare systems and the potential impact of automated actions on patient care operations (Arefin, 2024). Predictive security analytics leverage machine learning algorithms to identify potential security risks before they materialize into actual threats. These capabilities can analyze historical security data, threat intelligence, and environmental factors to predict likely attack vectors and recommend proactive security measures. In healthcare environments, predictive analytics can help organizations prioritize security investments and prepare for emerging threats (Salem et al., 2024).

Natural Language Processing (NLP) technologies enable healthcare organizations to analyze unstructured security data, including incident reports, threat intelligence feeds, and security logs. NLP can help identify patterns and relationships in textual data that may not be apparent through traditional analysis methods, providing valuable insights for threat detection and response (Islam et al., 2022). AI-powered vulnerability management solutions can help healthcare organizations prioritize vulnerability remediation based on threat intelligence, exploit availability, and potential impact on healthcare operations. These solutions can analyze vulnerability data in the context of the organization's specific environment and threat landscape to provide risk-based prioritization recommendations (Yazdi et al., 2024). Machine learning-enhanced identity and access management solutions can adapt access controls based on user behavior patterns, risk assessments, and contextual factors. These solutions can provide more granular and dynamic access controls while maintaining user experience and operational efficiency in healthcare environments (Aboukadri et al., 2024).

6.3 Quantum-Resistant Security Measures

The emergence of quantum computing technologies poses significant long-term challenges to current cryptographic systems, requiring healthcare organizations to begin preparing for the post-quantum cryptography era. While practical quantum computers capable of breaking current encryption algorithms may still be years away, the sensitive nature of health information and long data retention requirements make quantum-resistant security measures a critical consideration for healthcare cloud security (SaberiKamarposhti et al., 2024). Post-quantum cryptography (PQC) algorithms are being developed to resist attacks from both classical and quantum computers. Healthcare organizations should begin evaluating these algorithms and planning for their eventual implementation in cloud environments. This planning must account for the performance implications of PQC algorithms, which may require more computational resources than current cryptographic methods (Liu & Moody, 2024).

Cryptographic agility represents a critical capability for healthcare organizations to adapt to changing cryptographic requirements, including the transition to quantum-resistant algorithms. Healthcare organizations should implement cryptographic frameworks that can support multiple algorithms and enable rapid transitions between different cryptographic methods as needed (Marengo & Santamato, 2025). Key management systems must evolve to support quantum-resistant cryptography while maintaining the security and operational requirements of healthcare environments. This includes implementing quantum key distribution (QKD) technologies where appropriate and developing key management practices that can support the larger key sizes and different operational characteristics of post-quantum algorithms (Gitonga, 2025).

Risk assessment for quantum threats requires healthcare organizations to evaluate their current cryptographic implementations and identify systems and data that may be vulnerable to quantum attacks. This assessment should consider the timeline for quantum computer development, the sensitivity and retention periods of protected data, and the feasibility of implementing quantum-resistant measures (Baseri et al., 2025). Hybrid security approaches may be necessary during the transition to quantum-resistant cryptography, combining current cryptographic methods with quantum-resistant algorithms to provide defense against both classical and quantum attacks. Healthcare organizations should develop transition strategies that maintain security throughout the migration process (Radanliev, 2024). Standards and compliance considerations for quantum-resistant security measures are still evolving, with organizations like NIST working to standardize post-quantum cryptographic algorithms. Healthcare organizations should monitor these standardization efforts and plan for compliance with emerging requirements while maintaining alignment with existing healthcare regulations (Chen, 2022).

7. IMPLEMENTATION AND BEST PRACTICES

7.1 Security Architecture Design

Effective security architecture design for healthcare cloud environments requires a comprehensive approach that integrates security controls throughout the technology stack while maintaining alignment with healthcare operational requirements and regulatory compliance obligations. The architecture must be designed to scale with organizational growth and adapt to evolving threats and technologies (Mehrtak et al., 2021). Layered security architecture principles provide the foundation for robust healthcare cloud security implementations. This approach implements multiple layers of security controls that provide defense in depth, ensuring that the failure of any single control does not compromise the entire security posture. In healthcare cloud environments, layered security includes network security controls, endpoint protection, application security, data protection, and identity management controls that work together to provide comprehensive protection (Al-Issa et al., 2019).

Cloud-native security architecture leverages the inherent capabilities of cloud platforms to implement security controls that are integrated with cloud services and infrastructure. This approach takes advantage of cloud provider security services, such as identity and access management, network security, and data protection services, while supplementing them with healthcare-specific controls and third-party solutions as needed (Theodoropoulos et al., 2023). Secure by design principles ensure that security considerations are integrated into system design from the beginning rather than added as an afterthought. Healthcare organizations should adopt secure development practices that incorporate security requirements into system design, implement security testing throughout the development lifecycle, and maintain security considerations throughout system operations and maintenance (Del-Real et al., 2025).

Integration architecture for healthcare cloud environments must address the complex interconnections between cloud services, on-premises systems, and third-party applications. This includes implementing secure API gateways, message queuing systems, and data integration platforms that can maintain security while enabling the interoperability required for healthcare operations (Seth et al., 2025). Scalability and performance considerations in security architecture design ensure that security controls can adapt to changing workloads and performance requirements without compromising security effectiveness. Healthcare organizations must design security architectures that can handle peak loads, emergency situations, and growth in data volumes and user populations (Haque et al., 2023). Disaster recovery and business continuity architecture must be integrated with security architecture to ensure that security controls remain effective during disaster recovery operations and business continuity scenarios. This includes implementing secure backup and recovery procedures, maintaining security controls in alternate processing sites, and ensuring that security monitoring and incident response capabilities remain operational during disruptions (Drinkwater & Saeed, 2022).

7.2 Incident Response and Business Continuity

Healthcare organizations require specialized incident response and business continuity capabilities that account for the critical nature of healthcare operations and the potential impact of security incidents on patient care. These capabilities must be designed to operate effectively in cloud environments while maintaining coordination with on-premises systems and third-party partners (Sachdeva et al., 2024). Incident response planning for healthcare cloud environments must address the unique characteristics of cloud computing, including the shared responsibility model, distributed infrastructure, and potential for rapid scaling and configuration changes. Healthcare organizations should develop incident response procedures that can effectively coordinate with cloud service providers while maintaining control over incident response activities and patient care operations (He et al., 2022).

Healthcare-specific incident classification and prioritization procedures must account for the potential impact of security incidents on patient safety and care delivery. Incidents that may impact life-supporting systems or emergency care capabilities require immediate response, while incidents affecting administrative systems may be handled with lower priority. This classification system must be clearly communicated to incident response teams and integrated into response procedures (Cooper et al., 2018). Communication and notification procedures for healthcare security incidents must address multiple stakeholder groups, including clinical staff, administrative personnel, patients, regulatory authorities, and business partners. Healthcare organizations should develop communication templates and procedures that can provide appropriate information to each stakeholder group while maintaining operational security and regulatory compliance (He et al., 2022).

Evidence collection and forensic analysis capabilities in cloud environments require specialized tools and procedures that can effectively gather and analyze evidence from cloud services and infrastructure. Healthcare organizations should develop forensic capabilities that can work with cloud service providers to collect necessary evidence while maintaining chain of custody requirements and regulatory compliance (Mishra et al., 2022). Business continuity planning for healthcare cloud environments must ensure that critical healthcare operations can continue during security incidents and system disruptions. This includes implementing alternate processing capabilities, maintaining access to critical patient information, and ensuring that clinical decision support systems remain available during incidents (Mehrtak et al., 2021). Recovery and restoration procedures must be designed to restore normal operations while ensuring that security vulnerabilities are addressed and systems are properly secured before returning to production use. Healthcare organizations should implement comprehensive testing procedures that validate both functional and security aspects of recovered systems (Cremer et al., 2022).

7.3 Continuous Monitoring and Compliance

Continuous monitoring and compliance capabilities are essential for healthcare organizations to maintain security effectiveness and regulatory compliance in dynamic cloud environments. These capabilities must provide real-time visibility into security posture while supporting ongoing compliance assessment and reporting requirements (Vashishth et al., 2025). Security monitoring architecture for healthcare cloud environments must provide comprehensive visibility across cloud services, on-premises systems, and hybrid infrastructure. This includes implementing centralized logging and monitoring solutions that can collect and analyze security data from multiple sources while maintaining appropriate data protection and privacy controls (Krotsiani et al., 2015).

Compliance monitoring and reporting capabilities must address the multiple regulatory frameworks that apply to healthcare organizations, including HIPAA, HITECH, state privacy laws, and industry standards. Healthcare organizations should implement automated compliance monitoring solutions that can continuously assess compliance posture and generate reports for regulatory authorities and internal stakeholders (Theodos & Sittig, 2020). Key performance indicators (KPIs) and metrics for healthcare cloud security should provide meaningful insights into security effectiveness and compliance posture. These metrics should include both technical indicators, such as incident response times and vulnerability remediation rates, and business-focused indicators, such as compliance assessment results and patient trust measures (Brenner et al., 2023).

Automated compliance assessment capabilities can help healthcare organizations maintain ongoing compliance with regulatory requirements while reducing the manual effort required for compliance activities. These capabilities should be able to assess cloud configurations, security controls, and operational procedures against regulatory requirements and provide recommendations for addressing identified gaps (Dunbar et al., 2023). Audit and assessment procedures for healthcare cloud environments must address the distributed nature of cloud computing while maintaining the rigor required for healthcare regulatory compliance. Healthcare organizations should develop audit procedures that can effectively evaluate cloud service providers, internal controls, and integrated systems while providing necessary documentation for regulatory authorities (Kedi et al., 2024). Continuous improvement processes ensure that monitoring and compliance capabilities evolve to address changing threats, regulatory requirements, and business needs. Healthcare organizations should implement regular reviews of monitoring effectiveness, compliance procedures, and security controls to identify opportunities for improvement and ensure ongoing effectiveness (Endalamaw et al., 2024).

8. CONCLUSION

The intersection of healthcare and cloud computing represents both tremendous opportunity and significant challenge for healthcare organizations worldwide. As this comprehensive analysis has demonstrated, the successful implementation of cloud security in healthcare environments requires a multifaceted approach that addresses regulatory compliance, threat intelligence integration, risk management, and emerging technologies while maintaining focus on patient care and safety. The healthcare cloud security landscape continues to evolve rapidly, driven by technological advancement, regulatory changes, and an increasingly sophisticated threat environment. Healthcare organizations that successfully navigate this landscape will be those that adopt comprehensive security frameworks, implement robust threat intelligence capabilities, and maintain a proactive approach to risk management and security architecture design.

The integration of threat intelligence into healthcare cloud security operations represents a critical capability for modern healthcare organizations. By leveraging comprehensive threat intelligence sources and implementing proactive threat detection and response capabilities, healthcare organizations can identify and mitigate threats before they impact patient care or compromise sensitive health information. Risk management frameworks specifically tailored for healthcare cloud environments provide the foundation for making informed decisions about cloud adoption, security investments, and risk mitigation strategies. These frameworks must account for the unique characteristics of healthcare operations while providing practical guidance for managing the complex risks associated with cloud computing.

Trust models and cloud service provider evaluation processes ensure that healthcare organizations can confidently select and manage relationships with cloud service providers while maintaining appropriate security and compliance standards. These processes must evolve to address emerging technologies and changing regulatory requirements while maintaining focus on patient trust and transparency. Emerging technologies, including Zero Trust Architecture, AI and machine learning, and quantum-resistant security measures, will continue to shape the future of healthcare cloud security. Healthcare organizations must begin preparing for these technologies while maintaining focus on current security requirements and operational needs.

The implementation of comprehensive security architectures, incident response capabilities, and continuous monitoring programs provides the operational foundation for effective healthcare cloud security. These capabilities must be designed to scale with organizational growth and adapt to changing threats while maintaining the reliability and availability required for healthcare operations. As healthcare organizations continue their digital transformation journeys, the principles and practices outlined in this analysis will serve as essential guidance for building secure, compliant, and resilient cloud environments that protect patient information while enabling improved healthcare delivery. The future of healthcare depends on the successful integration of cloud computing technologies with robust security practices that maintain patient trust and ensure the confidentiality, integrity, and availability of health information. The path forward requires continued collaboration between healthcare organizations, cloud service providers, technology vendors, and regulatory authorities to address emerging challenges and opportunities in healthcare cloud security. By maintaining focus on patient care and safety while embracing the transformative potential of cloud computing, healthcare organizations can build the secure, scalable, and innovative technology foundations necessary for the future of healthcare delivery.

REFERENCES

Abinesh Kamal, K. U., & Divya, S. V. (2024). Integrated Threat Intelligence Platform for security operations in organizations. *Automatika (Zagreb), 65*(2), 401–409. DOI: 10.1080/00051144.2023.2295146

Abouelmehdi, K., Beni-Hessane, A., & Khaloufi, H. (2018). Big Healthcare data: Preserving Security and Privacy. *Journal of Big Data, 5*(1), 1. Advance online publication. DOI: 10.1186/s40537-017-0110-7

Aboukadri, S., Ouaddah, A., & Mezrioui, A. (2024). Machine learning in identity and Access Management Systems: Survey and Deep Dive. *Computers &amp. Computers & Security, 139*, 103729. DOI: 10.1016/j.cose.2024.103729

Ainslie, S., Thompson, D., Maynard, S., & Ahmad, A. (2023). Cyber-threat Intelligence for Security Decision-making: A review and research agenda for practice. *Computers &amp. Computers & Security, 132*, 103352. DOI: 10.1016/j.cose.2023.103352

Al-Issa, Y., Ottom, M. A., & Tamrawi, A. (2019). EHealth Cloud Security Challenges: A survey. *Journal of Healthcare Engineering, 2019*, 1–15. DOI: 10.1155/2019/7516035

Alenezi, A., Atlam, H. F., & Wills, G. B. (2019). Experts reviews of a cloud forensic readiness framework for organizations. *Journal of Cloud Computing (Heidelberg, Germany), 8*(1), 11. Advance online publication. DOI: 10.1186/s13677-019-0133-z

Ali, T., Al-Khalidi, M., & Al-Zaidi, R. (2024). Information security risk assessment methods in cloud computing: Comprehensive review. *Journal of Computer Information Systems*, •••, 1–28. DOI: 10.1080/08874417.2024.2329985

Alshammari, M. M., Alwan, A. A., & Aishaikhli, I. (2016, December). *Data Recovery and Business continuity in Cloud computing: A review of the research literature.* International Journal of Advancements in Computing Technology. https://www.researchgate.net/publication/312166397_Data_recovery_and_business_continuity_in_Cloud_computing_A_Review_of_the_Research_Literature

Amah, U., Mart, J., & Oyetoro, A. (2023). *Cloud Security Governance Guidelines.* DOI: 10.14293/PR2199.000062.v1

Angle, J. (2022, May). *Healthcare Supply Chain Cybersecurity Risk Management 2*. Cloud Security Alliance. https://www.researchgate.net/publication/360550527_Healthcare_Supply_Chain_Cybersecurity_Risk_Management_2

Arefin, S. (2024). Strengthening Healthcare data security with AI-powered threat detection. [IJSRM]. *International Journal of Scientific Research and Management, 12*(10), 1477–1483. DOI: 10.18535/ijsrm/v12i10.ec02

Argaw, S. T., Bempong, N.-E., Eshaya-Chauvin, B., & Flahault, A. (2019). The state of research on cyberattacks against hospitals and available best practice recommendations: A scoping review. *BMC Medical Informatics and Decision Making, 19*(1), 10. Advance online publication. DOI: 10.1186/s12911-018-0724-5

Asan, O., Yu, Z., & Crotty, B. H. (2021). How clinician-patient communication affects trust in health information sources: Temporal Trends from a national cross-sectional survey. *PLoS One, 16*(2), e0247583. Advance online publication. DOI: 10.1371/journal.pone.0247583

Azad, M. A., Abdullah, S., Arshad, J., Lallie, H., & Ahmed, Y. H. (2024). Verify and trust: A multidimensional survey of Zero-trust security in the age of IOT. *Internet of Things : Engineering Cyber Physical Human Systems, 27*, 101227. DOI: 10.1016/j.iot.2024.101227

Baseri, Y., Chouhan, V., Ghorbani, A., & Chow, A. (2025). Evaluation framework for Quantum Security Risk Assessment: A Comprehensive Strategy for Quantum-Safe Transition. *Computers &amp. Computers & Security, 150*, 104272. DOI: 10.1016/j.cose.2024.104272

Bohn, L., & Schiereck, D. (2022). Regulation of data breach publication: The case of US healthcare and the hitech act. *Journal of Economics and Finance, 47*(2), 386–399. DOI: 10.1007/s12197-022-09607-6

Botha, N. N., Segbedzi, C. E., Dumahasi, V. K., Maneen, S., Kodom, R. V., Tsedze, I. S., Akoto, L. A., Atsu, F. S., Lasim, O. U., & Ansah, E. W. (2024). Artificial Intelligence in Healthcare: A scoping review of perceived threats to patient rights and safety. *Archives of Public Health = Archives Belges de Santé Publique, 82*(1), 188. Advance online publication. DOI: 10.1186/s13690-024-01414-1

Brenner, M., Weir, A., McCann, M., Doyle, C., Hughes, M., Moen, A., Ingvar, M., Nauwelaerts, K., Turk, E., & McCabe, C. (2023). Development of the key performance indicators for Digital Health Interventions: A scoping review. *Digital Health, 9*, 20552076231152160. Advance online publication. DOI: 10.1177/20552076231152160

Buchta, R., Gkoktsis, G., Heine, F., & Kleiner, C. (2024). Advanced persistent threat attack detection systems: A review of approaches, challenges, and Trends. *Digital Threats : Research and Practice, 5*(4), 1–37. DOI: 10.1145/3696014

Cheimonidis, P., & Rantos, K. (2023). Dynamic Risk Assessment in cybersecurity: A systematic literature review. *Future Internet, 15*(10), 324. DOI: 10.3390/fi15100324

Chen, L. (2022, February 1). *Paving the runway for standardization of Post-Quantum Cryptography*. CSRC. https://csrc.nist.gov/pubs/journal/2022/02/paving-the-runway-for-standardization-of-pqc/final

Chinnasamy, P., & Deepalakshmi, P. (2021). HCAC-EHR: Hybrid cryptographic access control for secure EHR retrieval in Healthcare Cloud. *Journal of Ambient Intelligence and Humanized Computing, 13*(2), 1001–1019. DOI: 10.1007/s12652-021-02942-2

Chiregi, M., & Navimipour, N. J. (2018). Cloud computing and trust evaluation: A systematic literature review of the state-of-the-art mechanisms. *Journal of Electrical Systems and Information Technology, 5*(3), 608–622. DOI: 10.1016/j.jesit.2017.09.001

Cooper, J., Williams, H., Hibbert, P., Edwards, A., Butt, A., Wood, F., Parry, G., Smith, P., Sheikh, A., Donaldson, L., & Carson-Stevens, A. (2018). Classification of patient-safety incidents in primary care. *Bulletin of the World Health Organization, 96*(7), 498–505. DOI: 10.2471/BLT.17.199802

Coventry, L., & Branley, D. (2018). Cybersecurity in healthcare: A narrative review of trends, threats and Ways Forward. *Maturitas, 113*, 48–52. DOI: 10.1016/j.maturitas.2018.04.008

Cremer, F., Sheehan, B., Fortmann, M., Kia, A. N., Mullins, M., Murphy, F., & Materne, S. (2022). Cyber risk and cybersecurity: A systematic review of data availability. *The Geneva Papers on Risk and Insurance. Issues and Practice, 47*(3), 698–736. DOI: 10.1057/s41288-022-00266-6

Cresswell, K., Hernández, A. D., Williams, R., & Sheikh, A. (2022). Key challenges and opportunities for Cloud Technology in health care: Semistructured interview study. *JMIR Human Factors, 9*(1), e31246. Advance online publication. DOI: 10.2196/31246

Das, A., Tariq, A., Batalini, F., Dhara, B., & Banerjee, I. (2024). Exposing vulnerabilities in clinical llms through data poisoning attacks: Case study in breast cancer. *The National Library of Medicine*. DOI: 10.1101/2024.03.20.24304627

Del-Real, C., De Busser, E., & van den Berg, B. (2025). A systematic literature review of security and privacy by design principles, norms, and strategies for Digital Technologies. *International Review of Law, Computers &amp. International Review of Law Computers & Technology*, 1–32. DOI: 10.1080/13600869.2025.2457227

Drinkwater, K., & Saeed, S. (2022, April). *Integrating Cybersecurity and Disaster Recovery: A Unified Approach to Business Continuity*. ResearchGate. https://www.researchgate.net/publication/383268245_Integrating_Cybersecurity_and_Disaster_Recovery_A_Unified_Approach_to_Business_Continuity

Dunbar, P., Keyes, L. M., & Browne, J. P. (2023). Determinants of regulatory compliance in health and Social Care Services: A systematic review using the Consolidated Framework for Implementation Research. *PLoS One*, *18*(4), e0278007. Advance online publication. DOI: 10.1371/journal.pone.0278007

Elendu, C., Omeludike, E. K., Oloyede, P. O., Obidigbo, B. T., & Omeludike, J. C. (2024). Legal implications for clinicians in cybersecurity incidents. *Medicine*, *103*(39), e39887. Advance online publication. DOI: 10.1097/MD.0000000000039887

Endalamaw, A., Khatri, R. B., Mengistu, T. S., Erku, D., Wolka, E., Zewdie, A., & Assefa, Y. (2024). A scoping review of continuous quality improvement in healthcare system: Conceptualization, models and tools, barriers and facilitators, and impact. *BMC Health Services Research*, *24*(1), 487. Advance online publication. DOI: 10.1186/s12913-024-10828-0

Ewoh, P., & Vartiainen, T. (2024). Vulnerability to cyberattacks and sociotechnical solutions for Health Care Systems: Systematic review. *Journal of Medical Internet Research*, *26*, e46904. Advance online publication. DOI: 10.2196/46904

Fathullah, M. A., Subbarao, A., & Muthaiyah, S. (2023). A systematic review: Risk Management of cloud computing projects in Healthcare. *International Journal of Management. Finance and Accounting*, *4*(2), 83–115. DOI: 10.33093/ijomfa.2023.4.2.5

Ferdosi, M., Rezayatmand, R., & Molavi Taleghani, Y. (2020). Risk management in executive levels of healthcare organizations: Insights from a scoping review (2018). *Risk Management and Healthcare Policy*, *13*, 215–243. DOI: 10.2147/RMHP.S231712

Gao, F., Thiebes, S., & Sunyaev, A. (2018). Rethinking the meaning of cloud computing for Health Care: A taxonomic perspective and future research directions. *Journal of Medical Internet Research*, *20*(7), e10041. Advance online publication. DOI: 10.2196/10041

Gitonga, C. K. (2025). The impact of quantum computing on cryptographic systems: Urgency of quantum-resistant algorithms and practical applications in cryptography. *European Journal of Information Technologies and Computer Science*, *5*(1), 1–10. DOI: 10.24018/compute.2025.5.1.146

Glockler, J., Sedlmeir, J., Frank, M., & Fridgen, G. (2023). A systematic review of identity and Access Management Requirements in enterprises and potential contributions of self-sovereign identity. *Business &amp. Business & Information Systems Engineering*, *66*(4), 421–440. DOI: 10.1007/s12599-023-00830-x

González-Granadillo, G., González-Zarzosa, S., & Diaz, R. (2021). Security Information and Event Management (SIEM): Analysis, trends, and usage in critical infrastructures. *Sensors (Basel)*, *21*(14), 4759. DOI: 10.3390/s21144759

Gu, X., Sabrina, F., Fan, Z., & Sohail, S. (2023). A review of Privacy Enhancement Methods for Federated Learning in healthcare systems. *International Journal of Environmental Research and Public Health*, *20*(15), 6539. DOI: 10.3390/ijerph20156539

Haque, R. U., Hasan, A. S. M. T., Daria, A., Rasool, A., Chen, H., Jiang, Q., & Zhang, Y. (2023). A novel secure and distributed architecture for privacy-preserving healthcare system. *Journal of Network and Computer Applications*, *217*, 103696. DOI: 10.1016/j.jnca.2023.103696

Hassan, J., Shehzad, D., Habib, U., Aftab, M. U., Ahmad, M., Kuleev, R., & Mazzara, M. (2022). The Rise Of Cloud Computing: Data Protection, Privacy, and open research challenges—a systematic literature review (SLR). *Computational Intelligence and Neuroscience*, *2022*, 1–26. DOI: 10.1155/2022/8303504

He, Y., Aliyu, A., Evans, M., & Luo, C. (2021). Health Care Cybersecurity challenges and solutions under the climate of covid-19: Scoping review. *Journal of Medical Internet Research*, *23*(4), e21747. Advance online publication. DOI: 10.2196/21747

He, Y., Maglaras, L., Aliyu, A., & Luo, C. (2022). Healthcare Security Incident Response Strategy - A Proactive Incident Response (IR) procedure. *Security and Communication Networks*, *2022*, 1–10. DOI: 10.1155/2022/2775249

He, Y., Zamani, E. D., Lloyd, S., & Luo, C. (2022). Agile incident response (air): Improving the incident response process in healthcare. *International Journal of Information Management*, *62*, 102435. DOI: 10.1016/j.ijinfomgt.2021.102435

Hummel, P., Braun, M., Tretter, M., & Dabrock, P. (2021). Data sovereignty: A Review. *Big Data &amp. Big Data & Society*, *8*(1), 2053951720982012. Advance online publication. DOI: 10.1177/2053951720982012

Islam, S., Papastergiou, S., & Silvestri, S. (2022). Cyber threat analysis using natural language processing for a secure healthcare system. *2022 IEEE Symposium on Computers and Communications (ISCC)*, 1–7. DOI: 10.1109/ISCC55528.2022.9912768

Issaoui, A., Örtensjö, J., & Islam, M. S. (2023). Exploring the General Data Protection Regulation (GDPR) compliance in cloud services: Insights from Swedish public organizations on privacy compliance. *Future Business Journal*, *9*(1), 107. Advance online publication. DOI: 10.1186/s43093-023-00285-2

Kabra, M., C, P. H., & Rao, M. (2022). Design and evaluation of performance-efficient SOC-on-FPGA for cloud-based healthcare applications. *2022 IEEE Nordic Circuits and Systems Conference (NorCAS)*, 1–6. DOI: 10.1109/NorCAS57515.2022.9934217

Kassam, I., Ilkina, D., Kemp, J., Roble, H., Carter-Langford, A., & Shen, N. (2023a). Patient perspectives and preferences for consent in the digital health context: State-of-the-art literature review. *Journal of Medical Internet Research*, *25*, e42507. Advance online publication. DOI: 10.2196/42507

Kassam, I., Ilkina, D., Kemp, J., Roble, H., Carter-Langford, A., & Shen, N. (2023b). Patient perspectives and preferences for consent in the digital health context: State-of-the-art literature review. *Journal of Medical Internet Research*, *25*, e42507. Advance online publication. DOI: 10.2196/42507

Kedi, W. E., Ejimuda, C., & Ajegbile, M. D. (2024). Cloud computing in healthcare: A comprehensive review of data storage and Analysis Solutions. *World Journal of Advanced Engineering Technology and Sciences*, *12*(2), 290–298. DOI: 10.30574/wjaets.2024.12.2.0291

Kerasidou, A., & Kerasidou, C. (2023). Data-driven research and Healthcare: Public Trust, data governance and the NHS. *BMC Medical Ethics*, *24*(1), 51. Advance online publication. DOI: 10.1186/s12910-023-00922-z

Khan, M. M., & Alkhathami, M. (2024). Anomaly detection in IOT-based healthcare: Machine Learning for Enhanced Security. *Scientific Reports*, *14*(1), 5872. Advance online publication. DOI: 10.1038/s41598-024-56126-x

Kiseleva, A., Kotzinos, D., & De Hert, P. (2022). Transparency of AI in healthcare as a multilayered system of accountabilities: Between legal requirements and technical limitations. *Frontiers in Artificial Intelligence*, *5*, 879603. Advance online publication. DOI: 10.3389/frai.2022.879603

Kotsias, J., Ahmad, A., & Scheepers, R. (2022). Adopting and integrating cyber-threat Intelligence in a commercial organisation. *European Journal of Information Systems*, *32*(1), 35–51. DOI: 10.1080/0960085X.2022.2088414

Krotsiani, M., Spanoudakis, G., & Kloukinas, C. (2015). Monitoring-based certification of Cloud Service Security. *Lecture Notes in Computer Science*, *9415*, 644–659. DOI: 10.1007/978-3-319-26148-5_44

Kruse, C. S., Frederick, B., Jacobson, T., & Monticone, D. K. (2017). Cybersecurity in Healthcare: A systematic review of modern threats and Trends. *Technology and Health Care*, *25*(1), 1–10. DOI: 10.3233/THC-161263

Li, E., Clarke, J., Ashrafian, H., Darzi, A., & Neves, A. L. (2022). The impact of electronic health record interoperability on safety and quality of care in high-income countries: Systematic Review. *Journal of Medical Internet Research*, *24*(9), e38144. Advance online publication. DOI: 10.2196/38144

Lieneck, C., McLauchlan, M., & Phillips, S. (2023). Healthcare cybersecurity ethical concerns during the COVID-19 Global Pandemic: A Rapid Review. *Healthcare (Basel)*, *11*(22), 2983. DOI: 10.3390/healthcare11222983

Liu, Y.-K., & Moody, D. (2024). Post-quantum cryptography and the Quantum Future of Cybersecurity. *Physical Review Applied*, *21*(4), 040501. Advance online publication. DOI: 10.1103/PhysRevApplied.21.040501

Mahboubi, A., Luong, K., Aboutorab, H., Bui, H. T., Jarrad, G., Bahutair, M., Camtepe, S., Pogrebna, G., Ahmed, E., Barry, B., & Gately, H. (2024). Evolving techniques in cyber threat hunting: A systematic review. *Journal of Network and Computer Applications*, *232*, 104004. DOI: 10.1016/j.jnca.2024.104004

Marengo, A., & Santamato, V. (2025). Quantum algorithms and complexity in healthcare applications: A systematic review with machine learning-optimized analysis. *Frontiers of Computer Science*, *7*, 1584114. Advance online publication. DOI: 10.3389/fcomp.2025.1584114

Mehrtak, M., SeyedAlinaghi, S. A., MohsseniPour, M., Noori, T., Karimi, A., Shamsabadi, A., Heydari, M., Barzegary, A., Mirzapour, P., Soleymanzadeh, M., Vahedi, F., Mehraeen, E., & Dadras, O. (2021). Security challenges and solutions using healthcare cloud computing. *Journal of Medicine and Life*, *14*(4), 448–461. DOI: 10.25122/jml-2021-0100

Mishra, A. K., Govil, M. C., Pilli, E. S., & Bijalwan, A. (2022). Digital Forensic Investigation of healthcare data in cloud computing environment. *Journal of Healthcare Engineering*, *2022*, 1–11. DOI: 10.1155/2022/9709101

Mohamed, N. (2025). Artificial Intelligence and machine learning in cybersecurity: A deep dive into state-of-the-art techniques and future paradigms. *Knowledge and Information Systems*, *67*(8), 6969–7055. Advance online publication. DOI: 10.1007/s10115-025-02429-y

Morić, Z., Dakić, V., & Regvart, D. (2025). Advancing Cybersecurity with honeypots and deception strategies. *Informatics (MDPI), 12*(1), 14. DOI: 10.3390/informatics12010014

Morita, P. P., Kaur, J., & Miranda, P. A. (2024a). Enhancing public health research: A viewpoint report on the transition to secure, cloud-based systems. *Frontiers in Public Health, 11*, 1270450. Advance online publication. DOI: 10.3389/fpubh.2023.1270450

Morita, P. P., Kaur, J., & Miranda, P. A. (2024b). Enhancing public health research: A viewpoint report on the transition to secure, cloud-based systems. *Frontiers in Public Health, 11*, 1270450. Advance online publication. DOI: 10.3389/fpubh.2023.1270450

Mukta, R., Paik, H., Lu, Q., & Kanhere, S. S. (2022). A survey of data minimisation techniques in blockchain-based healthcare. *Computer Networks, 205*, 108766. DOI: 10.1016/j.comnet.2022.108766

Munjal, K., & Bhatia, R. (2022). A systematic review of homomorphic encryption and its contributions in healthcare industry. *Complex &amp. Complex & Intelligent Systems*, *9*(4), 3759–3786. DOI: 10.1007/s40747-022-00756-z

Pascarella, G., Rossi, M., Montella, E., Capasso, A., De Feo, G., Botti, G., Nardone, A., Montuori, P., Triassi, M., D'Auria, S., & Morabito, A. (2021). Risk analysis in healthcare organizations: Methodological Framework and critical variables. *Risk Management and Healthcare Policy, 14*, 2897–2911. DOI: 10.2147/RMHP.S309098

Pattanaik, P. K., Gupta, S., Pani, A. K., Himanshu, U., & Pappas, I. O. (2024). Impact of inter and intra organizational factors in healthcare digitalization: A Conditional Mediation Analysis. *Information Systems Frontiers*. Advance online publication. DOI: 10.1007/s10796-024-10522-w

Pietrzykowski, T., & Smilowska, K. (2021). The reality of informed consent: Empirical studies on patient comprehension—systematic review. *Trials*, *22*(1), 57. Advance online publication. DOI: 10.1186/s13063-020-04969-w

Radanliev, P. (2024). Artificial Intelligence and Quantum Cryptography. *Journal of Analytical Science and Technology*, *15*(1), 4. Advance online publication. DOI: 10.1186/s40543-024-00416-6

Rigaud, M., Buekers, J., Bessems, J., Basagaña, X., Mathy, S., Nieuwenhuijsen, M., & Slama, R. (2024). The methodology of Quantitative Risk Assessment Studies. *Environmental Health : A Global Access Science Source*, *23*(1), 13. Advance online publication. DOI: 10.1186/s12940-023-01039-x

Rockwern, B., Johnson, D., & Snyder Sulmasy, L. (2021). Health Information Privacy, protection, and use in the expanding digital health ecosystem: A position paper of the American College of Physicians. *Annals of Internal Medicine*, *174*(7), 994–998. DOI: 10.7326/M20-7639

SaberiKamarposhti, M., Ng, K.-W., Chua, F.-F., Abdullah, J., Yadollahi, M., Moradi, M., & Ahmadpour, S.SaberiKamarposhti. (2024). Post-quantum Healthcare: A roadmap for cybersecurity resilience in medical data. *Heliyon*, *10*(10), e31406. Advance online publication. DOI: 10.1016/j.heliyon.2024.e31406

Sachdeva, S., Bhatia, S., Al Harrasi, A., Shah, Y. A., Anwer, M., Philip, A. K., Shah, S. F. A., Khan, A., & Ahsan Halim, S. (2024). Unraveling the role of Cloud Computing in health care system and biomedical sciences. *Heliyon*, *10*(7), e29044. Advance online publication. DOI: 10.1016/j.heliyon.2024.e29044

Saeed, S., Suayyid, S. A., Al-Ghamdi, M. S., Al-Muhaisen, H., & Almuhaideb, A. M. (2023). A systematic literature review on Cyber Threat Intelligence for Organizational Cybersecurity Resilience. *Sensors (Basel)*, *23*(16), 7273. DOI: 10.3390/s23167273

Salem, A. H., Azzam, S. M., Emam, O. E., & Abohany, A. A. (2024). Advancing cybersecurity: A comprehensive review of AI-Driven Detection Techniques. *Journal of Big Data*, *11*(1), 105. Advance online publication. DOI: 10.1186/s40537-024-00957-y

Salim, D. T., Singh, M. M., & Keikhosrokiani, P. (2023). A systematic literature review for APT detection and Effective Cyber Situational Awareness (ECSA) conceptual model. *Heliyon*, *9*(7), e17156. Advance online publication. DOI: 10.1016/j.heliyon.2023.e17156

Santos, P., Abreu, R., Reis, M. J., Serôdio, C., & Branco, F. (2025). A systematic review of Cyber Threat Intelligence: The effectiveness of technologies, strategies, and collaborations in Combating modern threats. *Sensors (Basel)*, *25*(14), 4272. DOI: 10.3390/s25144272

Sarkar, S., Choudhary, G., Shandilya, S. K., Hussain, A., & Kim, H. (2022). Security of zero trust networks in cloud computing: A comparative review. *Sustainability (Basel)*, *14*(18), 11213. DOI: 10.3390/su141811213

Scheibner, J., Raisaro, J. L., Troncoso-Pastoriza, J. R., Ienca, M., Fellay, J., Vayena, E., & Hubaux, J.-P. (2021). Revolutionizing medical data sharing using advanced privacy-enhancing technologies: Technical, legal, and ethical synthesis. *Journal of Medical Internet Research*, *23*(2), e25120. Advance online publication. DOI: 10.2196/25120

Seh, A. H., Zarour, M., Alenezi, M., Sarkar, A. K., Agrawal, A., Kumar, R., & Ahmad Khan, R. (2020). Healthcare data breaches: Insights and implications. *Healthcare (Basel)*, *8*(2), 133. DOI: 10.3390/healthcare8020133

Semantha, F. H., Azam, S., Yeo, K. C., & Shanmugam, B. (2020). A systematic literature review on privacy by design in the healthcare sector. *Electronics (Basel)*, *9*(3), 452. DOI: 10.3390/electronics9030452

Seth, D., Najana, M., & Ranjan, P. (2024). Compliance and regulatory challenges in cloud computing: A sector-wise analysis. *International Journal of Global Innovations and Solutions (IJGIS)*. DOI: 10.21428/e90189c8.68b5dea5

Seth, M., Jalo, H., Högstedt, Å., Medin, O., Sjöqvist, B. A., & Candefjord, S. (2025). Technologies for interoperable internet of medical things platforms to manage medical emergencies in home and Prehospital Care: Scoping Review. *Journal of Medical Internet Research*, *27*, e54470. Advance online publication. DOI: 10.2196/54470

Sheikh, N., Pawar, M., & Lawrence, V. (2021). Zero Trust Using Network Micro Segmentation. *IEEE INFOCOM 2021 - IEEE Conference on Computer Communications Workshops (INFOCOM WKSHPS)*, 1–6. DOI: 10.1109/INFOCOMWKSHPS51825.2021.9484645

Shin, H., Ryu, K., Kim, J.-Y., & Lee, S. (2024). Application of privacy protection technology to Healthcare Big Data. *Digital Health*, *10*, 20552076241282242. Advance online publication. DOI: 10.1177/20552076241282242

Shojaei, P., Vlahu-Gjorgievska, E., & Chow, Y.-W. (2024). Security and privacy of technologies in Health Information Systems: A systematic literature review. *Computers*, *13*(2), 41. DOI: 10.3390/computers13020041

Sills, M., Ranade, P., & Mittal, S. (2020). Cybersecurity threat intelligence augmentation and embedding improvement - A healthcare USECASE. *2020 IEEE International Conference on Intelligence and Security Informatics (ISI)*, 1–6. DOI: 10.1109/ISI49825.2020.9280482

Singh, C., Thakkar, R., & Warraich, J. (2023). IAM identity access management—Importance in maintaining security systems within organizations. *European Journal of Engineering and Technology Research*, *8*(4), 30–38. DOI: 10.24018/ejeng.2023.8.4.3074

Subudhi, S. (2024). Effectiveness of AI/ML in SOAR (security automation and orchestration) platforms. [IJSR]. *International Journal of Science and Research (Raipur, India)*, *13*(8), 201–206. DOI: 10.21275/MR24802085215

Suleski, T., Ahmed, M., Yang, W., & Wang, E. (2023). A review of multi-factor authentication in the internet of healthcare things. *Digital Health*, *9*, 20552076231177144. Advance online publication. DOI: 10.1177/20552076231177144

Tabassum, M., Mahmood, S., Bukhari, A., Alshemaimri, B., Daud, A., & Khalique, F. (2024). Anomaly-based threat detection in Smart Health Using Machine Learning. *BMC Medical Informatics and Decision Making*, *24*(1), 347. Advance online publication. DOI: 10.1186/s12911-024-02760-4

Theodoropoulos, T., Rosa, L., Benzaid, C., Gray, P., Marin, E., Makris, A., Cordeiro, L., Diego, F., Sorokin, P., Girolamo, M. D., Barone, P., Taleb, T., & Tserpes, K. (2023). Security in cloud-native services: A survey. *Journal of Cybersecurity and Privacy*, *3*(4), 758–793. DOI: 10.3390/jcp3040034

Theodos, K., & Sittig, S. (2020, December 7). *Health Information Privacy Laws in the digital age: HIPAA doesn't apply*. Perspectives in health information management. https://pmc.ncbi.nlm.nih.gov/articles/PMC7883355/

Udroiu, A.-M., Dumitrache, M., & Sandu, I. (2022). Improving the cybersecurity of medical systems by applying the NIST framework. *2022 14th International Conference on Electronics, Computers and Artificial Intelligence (ECAI)*, 1–7. DOI: 10.1109/ECAI54874.2022.9847498

Vashishth, T. K., Sharma, V., Sharma, K. K., Kumar, B., Chaudhary, S., & Panwar, R. (2025). Securing the cloud: Strategies for protecting sensitive patient data in cloud-based Healthcare Recommender Systems. *Healthcare Recommender Systems*, 185–220. DOI: 10.1007/978-3-031-80056-6_9

Veeraballi, V. R. (2025). Implementing the NIST risk management framework in cloud environments: A comprehensive approach. *INTERNATIONAL JOURNAL OF COMPUTER ENGINEERING AND TECHNOLOGY*, *16*(1), 3655–3670. DOI: 10.34218/IJCET_16_01_252

Vukotich, G. (2023). Healthcare and cybersecurity: Taking a Zero trust approach. *Health Services Insights*, *16*, 11786329231187826. Advance online publication. DOI: 10.1177/11786329231187826

Wang, Z., Yu, X., Xue, P., Qu, Y., & Ju, L. (2023). Research on medical security system based on Zero trust. *Sensors (Basel)*, *23*(7), 3774. DOI: 10.3390/s23073774

Wani, T. A., Mendoza, A., & Gray, K. (2020). Hospital bring-your-own-device security challenges and solutions: Systematic review of Gray Literature. *JMIR mHealth and uHealth*, *8*(6), e18175. Advance online publication. DOI: 10.2196/18175

Wasserman, L., & Wasserman, Y. (2022). Hospital cybersecurity risks and gaps: Review (for the non-cyber professional). *Frontiers in Digital Health*, *4*, 862221. Advance online publication. DOI: 10.3389/fdgth.2022.862221

Weinberg, A. I., & Cohen, K. (2024). Zero trust implementation in the emerging technologies era: A survey. *Complex Engineering Systems*, *4*(3). Advance online publication. DOI: 10.20517/ces.2024.41

Xia, L., Cao, Z., & Zhao, Y. (2024). Paradigm transformation of global health data regulation: Challenges in governance and human rights protection of cross-border data flows. *Risk Management and Healthcare Policy*, *17*, 3291–3304. DOI: 10.2147/RMHP.S450082

Xiang, D., & Cai, W. (2021). Privacy protection and secondary use of health data: Strategies and methods. *BioMed Research International, 2021*(1). DOI: 10.1155/2021/6967166

Xu, J. (2024). The current status and promotional strategies for Cloud Migration of Hospital Information Systems in China: Strengths, weaknesses, opportunities, and threats analysis. *JMIR Medical Informatics*, *12*, e52080. Advance online publication. DOI: 10.2196/52080

Xu, J., Glicksberg, B. S., Su, C., Walker, P., Bian, J., & Wang, F. (2020). Federated Learning for Healthcare Informatics. *Journal of Healthcare Informatics Research*, *5*(1), 1–19. DOI: 10.1007/s41666-020-00082-4

Yadav, A., Kumar, A., & Singh, V. (2023). Open-source intelligence: A comprehensive review of the current state, applications and future perspectives in Cyber Security. *Artificial Intelligence Review*, *56*(11), 12407–12438. DOI: 10.1007/s10462-023-10454-y

Yazdi, M., Zarei, E., Adumene, S., & Beheshti, A. (2024). Navigating the power of Artificial Intelligence in Risk Management: A comparative analysis. *Safety (Basel, Switzerland)*, *10*(2), 42. DOI: 10.3390/safety10020042

Yimam, D., & Fernandez, E. B. (2016). A survey of compliance issues in cloud computing. *Journal of Internet Services and Applications*, *7*(1), 5. Advance online publication. DOI: 10.1186/s13174-016-0046-8

Zlatolas, L. N., Welzer, T., & Lhotska, L. (2024). Data breaches in Healthcare: Security Mechanisms for attack mitigation. *Cluster Computing*, *27*(7), 8639–8654. DOI: 10.1007/s10586-024-04507-2

Chapter 8
Blockchain-Based Trust and Data Integrity Models for Healthcare Security

Shalini Jaiswal
https://orcid.org/0000-0003-0137-7734
Amity University, Greater Noida, India

Yaduvir Singh
https://orcid.org/0000-0002-2552-4797
NIET, Greater Noida, India

ABSTRACT

Blockchain technology offers a decentralized framework to enhance trust and data integrity in healthcare security. By leveraging blockchain, sensitive electronic health records (EHRs) can be securely stored, shared, and accessed with tamper-proof mechanisms. Smart contracts automate access control, ensuring that only authorized entities can retrieve data. The consensus mechanism upholds the validity of transactions across the network, eliminating single points of failure. With privacy preservation and interoperability, blockchain enhances secure communication among diverse systems. These models promote data integrity, reduce fraud, and increase trust in healthcare systems by ensuring transparency, accountability, and resistance to cyberattacks.

1. INTRODUCTION

Effective interchange of health information has been hampered by information security issues brought by, among other things, data sharing laws and "fear of financial

DOI: 10.4018/979-8-3373-4918-3.ch008

consequences associated with data sharing (Zhang et al., 2018). With the increasing use of wearable health technology, telemedicine, electronic health records (EHRs), and AI-driven diagnostic tools, the healthcare sector is rapidly getting digital. Unauthorized access, data manipulation, and the opaqueness of data management and sharing procedures are some of the urgent issues (Lau, 2018).

One promising way to deal with these issues is through blockchain technology (Anderson, 2018). Fundamentally, blockchain is a distributed and decentralized ledger technology that uses consensus processes, cryptographic hashing, and data integrity. This database consists of several geographically unrestricted networked devices, such as computers, phones, and embedded systems. Because of its built-in trust mechanism, which is cryptographically enabled, network participants do not need to trust one another. This ledger's entries are referred to as blocks, which are made up of messages and transactions that are connected, time-stamped using cryptographic hashes, and verified by other members of the network.

Blockchain has the potential to improve trust and accountability in healthcare systems by eliminating the need for centralized middlemen and facilitating transparent peer-to-peer interactions. Furthermore, blockchain is especially well-suited for applications where data integrity and trust are crucial due to its intrinsic qualities, which include immutability, transparency, and traceability. Blockchain can facilitate clinical trials, pharmaceutical supply chains, consent management, audit trails, safe patient record sharing, and real-time health data monitoring via IoT devices in the healthcare industry (Agbo et al., 2019). Fast and dependable services are guaranteed by blockchain technology (Prashanth Joshi et al., 2018). The blockchain systems are regarded as a secure platform where users' actions are tracked and any modifications to the block are computationally difficult to detect due to the chain's constant accumulation (Zhu et al., 2019).

This chapter will provide a comprehensive exploration frameworks and architectures that integrate blockchain with healthcare IT systems, covering data provenance, audit trails, smart contracts, and secure identity management, like my previous work related to Technology in different fields (Jaiswal et al., 2023a; Jaiswal et al., 2023b; Jaiswal et al., 2024; Jaiswal et al., 2025)

2. FUNDAMENTAL TECHNOLOGY OF BLOCKCHAIN

The protection of this data has become important. In this context, security and privacy are regarded as prominent concerns. To address these concerns, emerging technologies such as blockchain are being recognized for their significant role in enhancing data security and ensuring privacy (Kshetri, 2025). Figure 1 illustrates the structure and operation of a blockchain using a Merkle tree, and the transactions are hashed pairwise and progressively combined to form a Merkle Root. This ensures integrity, as any modifications in a transaction alter the root hash, maintaining data immutability and block linkage.

Figure 1. Blockchain structure and operation.

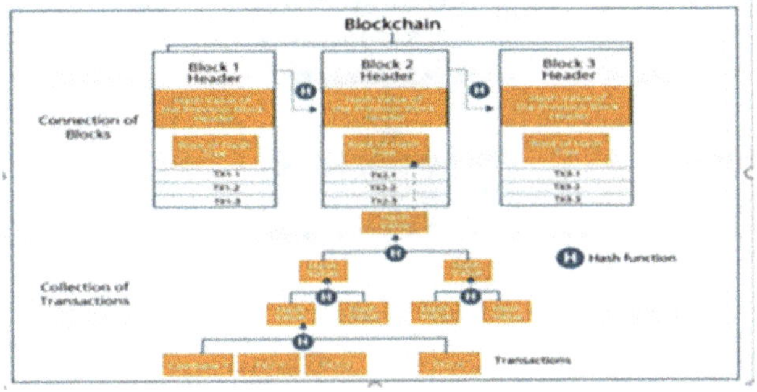

2.1 Distributed Ledger Technology

In a blockchain network, nodes comprise computers or devices that are utilized to store and maintain copies of the blockchain. Transactions are grouped into blocks, which are subsequently linked in a linear sequence, with each block containing a timestamp and a reference to a preceding block (R. Islam et al., 2025). Figure 2 illustrates the structure of the blockchain chain, highlighting how the individual blocks are interconnected. Each block consists of a block header and the block. The block header contains a hash of the previous block header, establishing a cryptographic link between the consecutive blocks, and a Merkle Root, which is a hash representing all transactions in that block. The block body stores all the transactions. this chained arrangement ensures data integrity and immutability, as an alteration in one block would require all subsequent blocks due to the dependency on the previous hashes. This structure facilitates the formation of a secure and decentralized database that is resistant to tampering and unauthorized modifications. Instead, the network is maintained by a distributed set of nodes that collaboratively validate and record the transactions. This design focuses on the secure and tamper-evident distributed ledger.

Figure 2. Interconnection of blocks in the structure of blockchain.

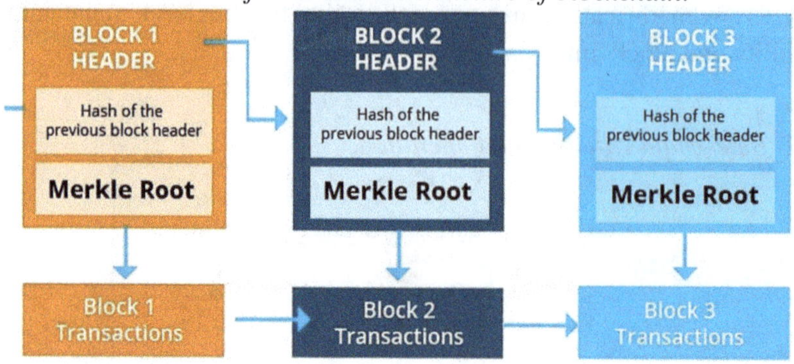

2.2 Cryptography and Network Security

In the context of blockchain, cryptography plays a fundamental role in securing the data, and this form of protection is commonly referred to as cryptographic security. Cryptographic hashing is one of the most important components that keep the blockchain technology secure and trustworthy. It plays a vital role in maintaining the integrity of the data stored on the blockchain. A cryptographic hash is a function that takes an input (like a message or transaction) and converts it into a fixed-length string of characters, often it is known as "hash". What makes it powerful is that even a small change in the input, such as changing a single character, completely changes the hash output. This makes it incredibly difficult for anyone to alter or fake data without it being detected. Hashing functions used in blockchain, like SHA-256,are one-way functions (Jasim et al., 2023). This means it is nearly impossible to figure out the original input just by looking at the hash. That's why hashes are perfect for verifying the data, like any transactions and any secure information as passwords. For example, if you want the hash message of "Blockchain" using a SHA-256, you will receive a specific one-time hash value which cannot be regenerated and this ensures the sensitivity an any tampering with the original data becomes almost impossible (Guo & Yu, 2022) .Cryptographic hash functions offer several critical benefits when employed within blockchain systems. The Advantages of the Cryptographic Hash functions are mentioned in Table 1, and Table 2 shows the comparison of Cryptographic Hash Functions.

Table 1. Advantages of Cryptographic Hash Functions

Feature	Description
Security	Blockchain's cryptographic functions are designed to resist tampering and unauthorized modifications. They ensure collision resistance, making it computationally infeasible to find two distinct inputs that produce the same hash.
Preimage Resistance	Prevents attackers from reversing a hash to discover the original input. It ensures that it is highly unlikely to find another input that yields the same hash, enhancing data confidentiality.
Integrity	Integrity is ensured by including the hash of the previous block in each new block, forming a tamper-evident chain of transactions. Any unauthorized change would break the hash linkages, making such manipulations easily detectable and thereby preventing fraud.
Efficiency	Cryptographic hashes enable compact data representation, reducing storage needs and speeding up verification. This results in faster transmission and improved scalability of the blockchain. *(Sevin & Osman Mohammed, 2024)*

Table 2. Comparison of the Cryptographic Hash Functions

Hash Functions	Output Length (Bits)	Speed	Resistance to the attacks	Applications
MD5	128	Low	Weak	Integrity of the Files
SHA -1	160	Fast	Weak	Legal systems, Git for the Version Control
SHA-256	256	Moderate	Strong	Bitcoin and Digital Certificates
SHA-3	Variable (up to 512)	Moderate	Very Strong	Cryptographic applications
Blake2	Variable (up to 512)	Very Fast	Very Strong	Cryptography
Blake 3	Variable (up to 256)	Fast	Strong	File Hashing
Scrypt	Variable (up to 256)	Fast	Strong	Dodge Coin
Ethash	Variable (up to 256)	Fast	Strong	Ethereum

The comparison of the cryptographic functions highlights key factors such as the speed, output size, security features, and resistance to hardware attacks. The output size represents the fixed length of the hash produced, while speed varies depending on the algorithm's complexity and hardware implementation. Security features are assessed based on the algorithm's complexity and hardware implementation. (Singh et al., 2024) Additionally, some algorithms are designed to be memory hard, intentionally requiring significant memory resources to resist specialized hardware attacks, thus allowing the fairness and decentralization of blockchain-based systems. A consensus algorithm is employed to ensure that all participating nodes possess a consistent view of the blockchain and concur on the sequence of the transactions. This mechanism is essential for enabling the maintenance of a unified, consistent, and tamper–evident ledger of the transactions across the network, eliminating the necessity for a centralized authority.

2.3 Consensus Mechanism

When the concept of the blockchain is applied, all participating nodes must agree on the consensus so that the transparency of the information is maintained during the completion of any transaction. Consensus algorithms are essential for maintaining data consistency across the nodes in the blockchain network. Each type of algorithm offers different mechanisms for ensuring non-biased accounting rights to all the participants. A well-designed consensus algorithm not only sustains the network activity but also delivers a consistent flow of effective computational power across all the systems. In comparison, a badly designed consensus algorithm can lead to a vulnerable network that can be attacked. (Hussein et al., 2023). The Characteristics of the Consensus Algorithms are mentioned in Table 3.

Table 3. Characteristics of the Consensus Algorithms

Feature	Description
Agreement	Ensures all network participants reach consensus on transaction validity and order, maintaining a consistent and reliable distributed ledger.
Security	Protects the network from tampering, double-spending, and attacks by assuming most participants act honestly.
Fault Tolerance	Maintains functionality even with faulty or malicious nodes, preserving system integrity and availability.
Decentralization	Distributes decision-making across the network to prevent central control, enhancing transparency and resilience.
Scalability	Supports increasing transactions and participants without sacrificing performance or security.
Fairness	Ensures equal opportunity for participants to validate transactions and earn rewards, promoting inclusivity and decentralization.
Speed	Aims for fast block confirmations and low transaction delays to enhance user experience and enable real-time applications.
Energy	Promotes energy-efficient algorithms to reduce environmental impact while maintaining network security.
Rewards	Provides incentives to participants for maintaining network operation and security, aligning individual efforts with system goals.

2.3.1 Different Categories of the Consensus Algorithm

The consensus mechanism can be applied with the different categories of the consensus algorithm, which are as follows:

a) **Proof of Work (PoW)**

Mining is the process of adding new blocks to a blockchain using the Proof of Work (PoW) consensus algorithm, where miners compete to solve complex mathematical puzzles. The first miner to solve the puzzle adds a new block and is rewarded with cryptocurrency, getting the rewards for the participation and securing the network. Each block links to the previous one via a cryptographic hash, making the tampering extremely difficult. Pow uses significant computational power and in Bitcoin, relies on the SHA-256 hash function with difficulty adjusted every 2016 blocks. Forking can occur when two miners add blocks simultaneously, resolved by choosing the longest chain. Pow is used in networks like Bitcoin and Ethereum. Figure 3 shows the relation of the header block and an input block connected with SHA256 Hash Function, and in PoW, the hash value is mined, and the person who can get the rewards.

Figure 3. The relation of the header block and an input block.

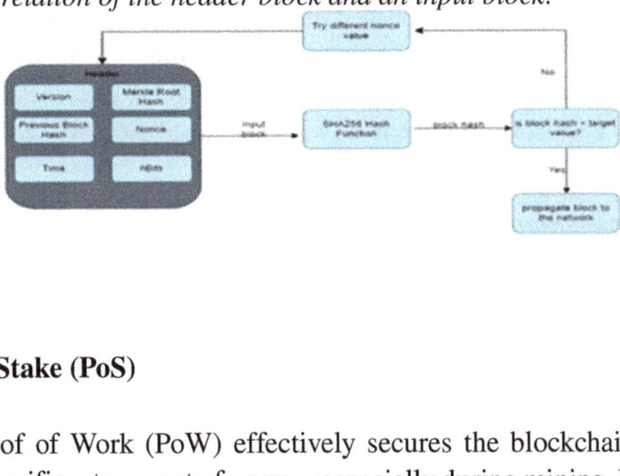

b) **Proof of Stake (PoS)**

While Proof of Work (PoW) effectively secures the blockchain networks, it consumes a significant amount of energy, especially during mining. Pow also gives an advantage to entities with greater computational power, increasing their chances of adding new blocks. In addition to high energy consumption, Pow has several drawbacks. A more energy-efficient alternative is the Proof of Stake (Pos)consensus algorithm. In PoS, validators are chosen based on the amount of the cryptocurrency they stake, rather than their computing power. Nodes stake their coins to become eligible, and an algorithm selects a validator using factors such as stake size, coin age, and randomization to ensure fairness. In some cases, the node with the best combination of the highest stake and lowest hash is selected to validate the next block. (Hussein et al., 2023) Figure 4 shows the PoS algorithm workflow.

Figure 4. PoS algorithm workflow.

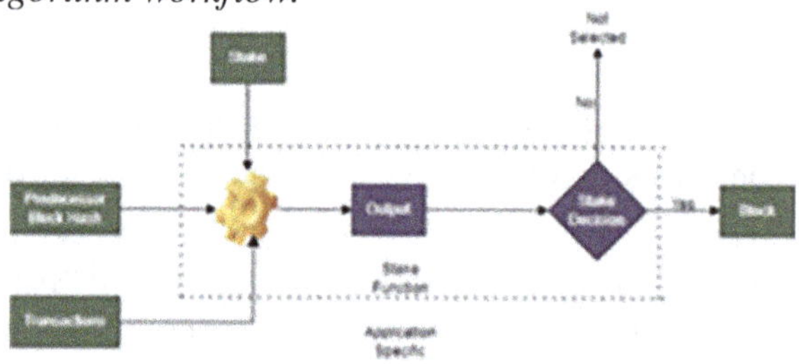

c) **Proof of Activity (PoA)**

PoA is a hybrid consensus mechanism that combines aspects of Proof of Work (PoW) and Proof of Stake (PoS). It begins with miners solving a PoW puzzle to create an almost empty block containing only header data and the reward address. Once a miner successfully mines this block, the process shifts to the PoS phase. A group of validators is selected based on their staked cryptocurrency to sign the block. After receiving the required number of signatures, the block is completed by adding transactions from the pool and is then appended to the blockchain. Figure 5 shows how this Proof of activity can be represented.

Figure 5. Representation of the Proof of activity.

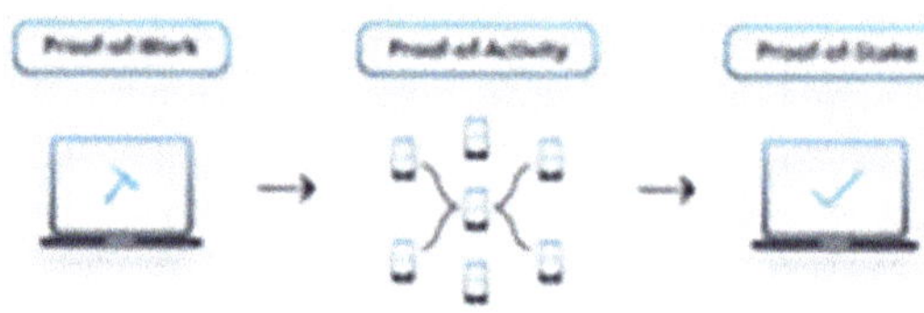

d) **Proof of Burn (PoB)**

Proof of Burn is a consensus mechanism where participants permanently destroy a portion of their cryptocurrency by sending it to an unrecoverable address (Figure 6). This act signals the long-term commitment as validators give up the immediate value for a chance to earn future rewards. The more coins a validator burns, the higher their chances of being selected to create the next block and receive the rewards. To prevent the early dominance, PoB often requires ongoing coin burning, encouraging continuous participation. While PoB often requires ongoing chain burning, it encourages continuous participation. While PoB is more energy efficient than PoW, it can still lead to centralization and raises concerns for the long-term sustainability due to the continual loss of coins.

Figure 6. Proof of burn.

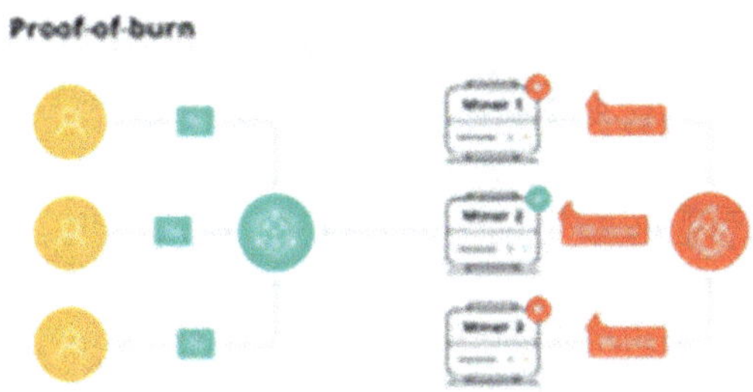

e) **Delegated Proof of Stake (DPoS)**

Delegated Proof of Stake (DPoS) is a consensus mechanism that secures blockchain networks through user voting and delegation (Figure 7). Users can vote directly or delegate their voting power to elect "witnesses" responsible for validating transactions and creating blocks. Witnesses earn rewards for successfully verifying blocks, which are often shared with their voters. If a witness fails to validate in time, the block is missed and picked by the next witness, termed as a "stolen block". Witnesses must stake tokens, risking penalties for the malicious behavior. Reputation and performance are key to maintaining a top position. Users also elect "delegates" to manage the network governance, such as proposing protocol changes. Delegates do not validate transactions but influence network policies. Full node validators verify that the witness created blocks follow consensus rules, though they do not benefit in the form of rewards (Regueiro et al., 2021).

Figure 7. DPoS.

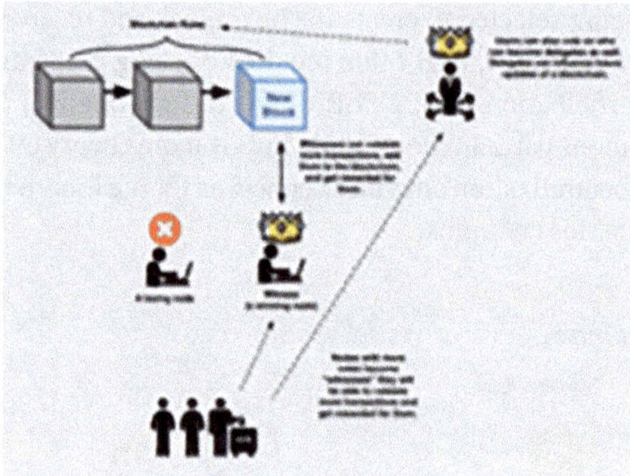

f) **Paxos Algorithm**

The Paxos algorithm is a fault-tolerant consensus mechanism that allows distributed network nodes to agree on a single proposed value without relying on a central authority (Figure 8). It operates through message exchanges among the three types of nodes: proposers, acceptors, and learners. The basic process involves a proposer sending a value to acceptors. if a majority accepts it, the proposer notifies he learners who then update their local data. If conflicting values are received, the process restarts to reach an agreement. Paxos is widely used in distributed systems due to its resilience to node failures and malicious behavior. The algorithm is designed to ensure safety and consistency, even in asynchronous environments. It tolerates message delays, duplication, and reordering without compromising correctness. Multiple rounds of the proposals can occur, but only one value is ultimately chosen. Variants like Multi-Paxos and Fast Paxos improve efficiency for practical deployment. Paxos remains a foundational protocol for achieving consensus in distributed databases, file systems, and cloud infrastructures (Hussein et al., 2023).

Figure 8. PAXOS Algorithm

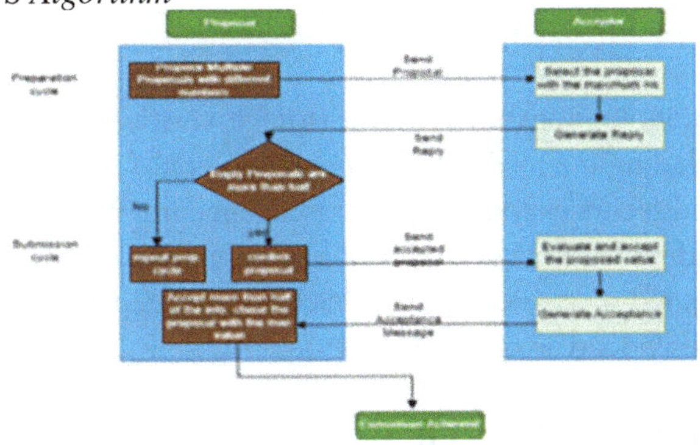

g) **Raft Algorithm**

RAFT is a distributed consensus-based algorithm designed to help a group of nodes agree on a single system state or value (Figure 9). Created as a more understandable and implementable alternative to algorithms like Paxos, RAFT divided nodes into leaders and followers. The leader proposes new values and replicates them to followers, who accept or reject proposals based on predefined rules. Once a majority accepts, the value is committed and logged. If the leader fails, followers hold an election to select the node with the most up–to–date log as the new leader. RAFT ensures strong consistency, guaranteeing all nodes eventually agree and fault tolerance, allowing the system to operate despite node failures. Its simplicity and reliability have made it popular in distributed databases, key-value stores, configuration management, and file systems. Paxos and RAFT are both non-Byzantine-based algorithms.

Figure 9. RAFT algorithm.

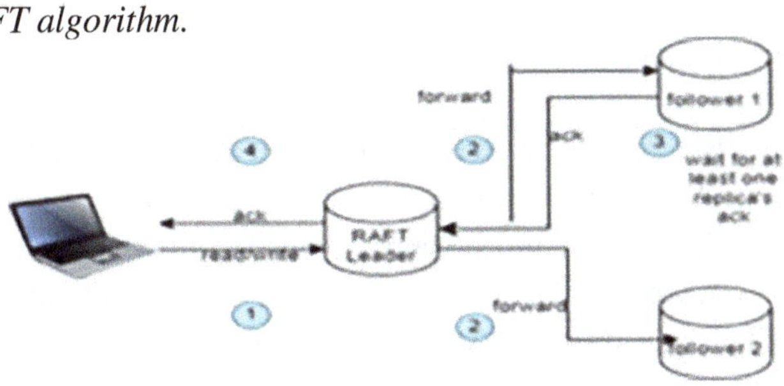

3. ARCHITECTURAL MODELS AND FRAMEWORKS OF BLOCKCHAIN

Blockchain technology encompasses the storage, verification, and sharing of data in industries, including the medical field (Esposito et al., 2018). Its decentralized, unchangeable, and secure characteristics present encouraging answers to persistent problems in the administration of health data. The degree to which blockchain technology can be applied successfully in various industries depends on its architectural models and frameworks (Casino et al., 2019).

3.1 Classification of Blockchain for Healthcare Systems

Blockchain networks are classified into three main types: public, private, and consortium (Figure 10). Each type varies in terms of access permissions, decentralization, scalability, and use cases.

Figure 10. Types of blockchain networks.

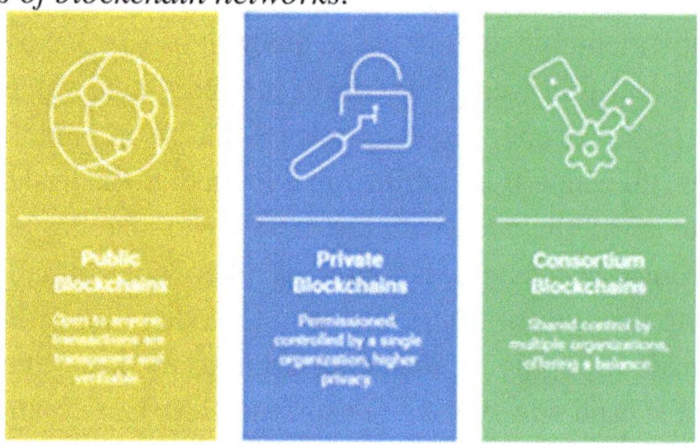

a) **Public Blockchains**

Anyone who wishes to participate can do so on public blockchains, which are completely decentralized. Ethereum and Bitcoin are notable examples. Anyone can read, write, and audit a public blockchain. To verify transactions, these networks use consensus techniques like Proof of Work (PoW) or Proof of Stake (PoS). Public blockchains can be applied to patient-centric data models in the healthcare industry, where patients have control over who can access their medical records. These solutions improve privacy and autonomy by giving patients the ability to allow or revoke access to their data. Public blockchains have privacy and scalability issues despite these benefits. Healthcare laws like HIPAA and GDPR, which mandate stringent data confidentiality, may clash with their open nature. Additionally, real-time healthcare applications may be constrained by transaction throughput and latency (Agbo et al., 2019).

b) **Private Blockchains**

Private blockchains limit participation to a certain group of people or to a single business. In terms of speed and resource usage, they are more effective and more centralized. Private blockchains can be used in healthcare for internal hospital operations like supply chain logistics, billing, and patient record administration. These blockchains provide greater control over access privileges, high efficiency, and regulatory compliance.

Enforcing fine-grained data access and guaranteeing low latency are two important advantages of private blockchains. For example, a hospital can facilitate compliance with privacy rules by controlling who has access to sensitive information. However, when several institutions are involved, this centralization may reduce transparency and create problems with trust. Private blockchains are suitable for internal hospital systems where only authorized personnel need access to medical records.

c) **Consortium Blockchains**

Semi-decentralized, consortium blockchains are run by multiple organizations as opposed to one. Selected participants are given access credentials. They are perfect for cooperative healthcare networks since they are run by a collection of institutions rather than a single organization. To securely and effectively share patient data, for instance, a consortium of several hospitals, insurance providers, and government agencies can be established.

This architecture preserves data privacy and governance control while fostering interoperability and trust. Applications include clinical research collaboration, insurance claim processing. Electronic health record (EHR) sharing is ideal for consortium blockchains. Consortium blockchains decrease redundancies, optimize workflows, and enhance patient care coordination by granting many stakeholders access to and verification of data (Zhang et al., 2018). One prominent example is the MIT MedRec project, which uses a blockchain-based system to manage EHRs and allows physicians and patients to share access safely and transparently. Consortium blockchain's advantages include improved privacy through shared governance, balanced control and decentralization, and adaptability for multi-institutional cooperation. Their drawback is that they necessitate multi-party consensus and more intricate governance structures. For healthcare networks that include hospitals, insurance companies, and regulatory agencies, consortium blockchains are perfect.

3.2 Layered Architectures for Healthcare Applications

Each block that makes up the blockchain contains digital data. A chain is formed by tying each block together. There are three components in each block. Information on the transactions, the parties to the transactions, and the cryptographic algorithms that set each block apart are all stored in the block. Four steps can be used to summarize how blockchain operates. Indeed, they are.

1. The transaction is carried out.
2. After verification, the transaction is validated.
3. The block contains the transaction.
4. After hashing, the block is appended to the blockchain.

The fingerprints of each block are connected. Consensus will assist in confirming and connecting blockchains. A layered method is used to comprehend how blockchain technology operates. To accommodate the variety of any application, the architectural layers are more widely applicable. Businesses that need great scalability and reliability might use the blockchain to enhance their services and draw in more clients. The application layer, execution engine layer, data model layer, consensus layer, and network layer are the layers that make up the architecture. The blockchain's layer hierarchy is depicted in Figure 11. Table 4 lists the various blockchain development platforms available based on these layers (Brakeville and Perepa, 2018).

Figure 11. Blockchain's layer hierarchy.

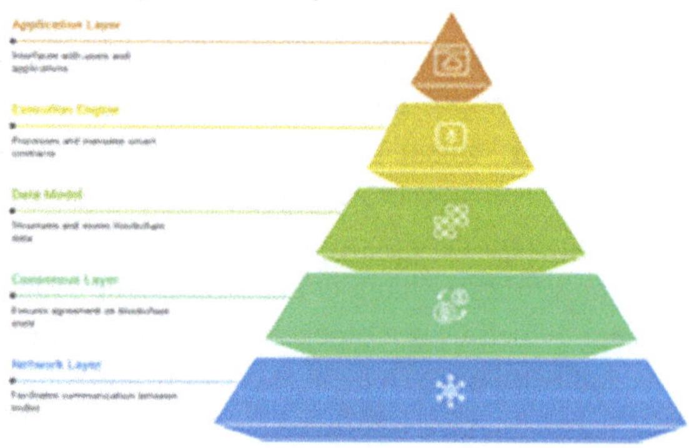

Table 4. Comparison of Blockchain Platforms

Layers	Ethereum	Ripple	Hyperledger	Parity	Sawtooth Lake
Application	Cryptocurrency	Cryptocurrency	Smart Contract	Smart Contract	Smart Contract
Execution Engine	EVM	–	Dockers	EVM	TEE
Data Model	Account-based	UTXO based	Account-based	Account-based	Account-based
Consensus	PoW	Ripple Consensus Ledger	PBFT	PoA	PoET
Network	P2P	P2P	P2P	P2P	P2P

a) **Application layer**

In the blockchain architecture, it is the highest layer. For consumers to engage with the system, it offers a graphical user interface. Ethereum, Solidity, Parity, and other tools are among them. Blockchain data is visible, unchangeable, and unalterable. It is resistant to fraudulent activity and unauthorized access. The application layer and the execution layer are the two sub-layers that make up the application layer. The application layer is how end users communicate with the blockchain network. Frameworks, user interfaces, APIs, and other components make up the application layer. The execution layer contains the chain code, underlying rules, and smart contracts. This sublayer contains the rules and executes the actual code. Instructions are transmitted from the application layer to the execution layer. The centralized nodes that are involved in Bitcoin transactions are the source of this layer's security challenges. A few of the difficulties include denial-of-service attacks, illegal access to the server, password cracking, host security, etc. App developers must thus ensure that their software is thoroughly tested and free of known vulnerabilities (Wang et al., 2019).

b) **Execution engine**

The execution engine, a crucial feature of the blockchain's architectural concept, oversees processing and carrying out transactions. It is the central processing unit that applies business logic to the data on the blockchain and is positioned between the consensus layer and the application layer. The execution engines used by different blockchain systems are implemented differently. For example, Ethereum executes smart contracts written in languages like Solidity using the Ethereum Virtual Machine (EVM). Docker containers are used with Hyperledger Fabric to isolate and execute chain code.

When several contracts are being executed in a single transaction block, the execution time should be deterministic and quick. Deterministic execution is used to prevent transaction inconsistencies. One blockchain execution engine that offers functions like process model deployment, instance generation for the deployed model, and control and record execution is the Caterpillar engine. Smart card implementation reduces third-party expenses while increasing security and dependability (Chen et al., 2018). The hazards and dangers of smart contracts are the difficulties of this layer.

The attack aims to take over the control flow and interfere with the atomicity of the transaction. An attacker can access or change a function or variable that shouldn't be available in most of these assaults because proper permission checks or explicit function visibility were not carried out. Therefore, it is crucial to safeguard against current vulnerabilities before building smart contracts to prevent data manipulation and build trust. Before its deployment, it should undergo several security inspections. Professionals must perform regular code audits, timely code optimizations, and anomalous behavior monitoring of deployed contracts to prevent losses.

c) **Data model.**

For cryptocurrency, the data model guarantees simplicity. Each application has a different data model. It stands for physical storage, the blockchain data structure, and the shared database. On a P2P network, the transactions on a blockchain are organized into blocks. Data cannot be changed in the absence of a consensus. Pointers and linked lists are the two primary parts of blockchain data structures. There are numerous hashes in a Merkel tree. Each block contains the Merkel root, which includes the version number, timestamp, nonce, and details from the preceding block. The hash power of the participants determines the blockchain's security. To encourage node participation, the blockchain typically compensates members in virtual currency. However, if the members don't cooperate with this, a centralization issue occurs.

d) **Consensus layer**

One of the most crucial blockchain layers is the consensus layer. The conclusion algorithm is the name given to the consensus algorithm. A blockchain cannot exist without a consensus algorithm. A consensus algorithm is used to validate blocks. Of all the layers in the blockchain, this one is referred to as the most important. The consensus layer's job is to get everyone on board with a single transaction rule. Information verification is assigned to globally recognized groups of transactions. Blockchain consensus algorithms come in two varieties: permissionless and permissioned. A probabilistic model, which encompasses networks like Ethereum, Bitcoin, and others, is another name for a permissionless blockchain. The other kind, called Permitted, uses a deterministic algorithm like Hyperledger Fabric. Some nodes on these blockchains verify the ordering nodes and determine if they are false. Numerous attack methods, including bribery, long-range, and Sybil attacks, pose a danger to the consensus layer. Therefore, it's critical to investigate a consensus process that is both faster and more secure while also making current attacks more challenging.

e) **Network layer**

The network layer is also known as the peer-to-peer (P2P) layer. In a P2P computer network, the computer nodes are dispersed and share to accomplish the purpose. The nodes on the blockchain carry out the transaction. The nodes can be classified as either whole or half. To guarantee the validity, transaction, and verification of the mining rules, a complete node is utilized. By interacting, spreading, and learning through every node, the P2P layer keeps the blockchain network's present state legitimate. Propagating or broadcasting transactions among peers is its duty. Making the most of the underlying network bandwidth for transmission is one of the main concerns.

4. APPLICATION OF BLOCKCHAIN IN HEALTHCARE SECURITY AND CASE STUDIES

Maintaining and managing an e-health record is challenging for the healthcare industry (Zhang et al., 2018a). Blockchain offers numerous applications in the healthcare industry, including enhancing mobile health apps, tracking devices, exchanging and storing electronic medical records, and managing data from clinical trials, as well as storing insurance information, among other uses (Omar et al., 2021). The different uses of the blockchain in the healthcare sector are depicted in Figure 12. Blockchain technology can be used to guarantee that private data, including patient records, disease records, lab results, treatment received, ambulance services, and compilation of episodes, is securely transferred, verified by each user's digital signature, and entered the ledger in the shortest amount of time possible (Zhang et al.,2022a). Hyperledger Fabric is a solution for electronic health records that uses blockchain as a distributed ledger among networks to transmit information across enterprises (Wutthikarn & Hui, 2018). Numerous Blockchain platforms have been introduced by firms such as Ripple, Ethereum, Quorum, Corda, NEO, NEM, and a few more. One use of telemedicine is telesurgery, which enables a physician to perform actual procedures with the aid of robots and wireless communication equipment. It reduces costs and time, and it can help address the physician shortage. One blockchain-based application that aims to improve the medical and other disciplines through decentralization is called Medblocks (Enescu et al., 2018).

Figure 12. Uses of blockchain in the healthcare sector.

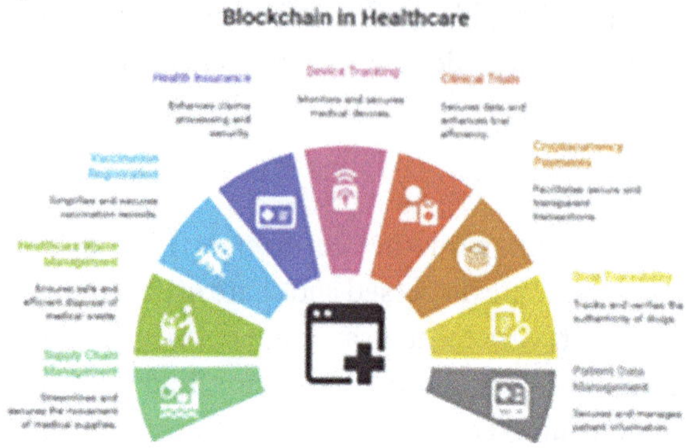

4.1 Management of patient data

Blockchain has been widely utilized to manage patient data, primarily to increase cost-effectiveness and security. Lab tests are conducted, patient appointments are scheduled, billing and accounts are handled, and medical data is maintained electronically (Shahnaz et al., 2019). Many of the EHR systems used in the healthcare sector have them installed. Delivering safe, tamper-proof, and multi-platform medical records is the primary objective. Blockchain keeps track of a patient's whole medical history, providing a secure means of recording and preserving all their health information. This allows for a wide range of management granularities by the patient, doctors, regulators, hospitals, insurers, and others.

4.2 Drug traceability

Drug counterfeiting causes pharmaceutical businesses to lose a lot of money and damage their brand. By avoiding fraud and counterfeit goods, blockchain-based medicine traceability allows for increased supply chain efficiency without the need for a traditional supply chain management system. The authors designed a drug traceability system that allows stakeholders to engage with the smart contract and the medicine monitoring system (Musamih et al., 2021a). It is anticipated that stakeholders would be able to access the smart contract, decentralized storage system, and on-chain resources using software devices with a front-end layer represented by a dApp that is linked to the smart contract, on-chain services, and decentralized storage system by an API. Tseng et al. (2018) created a G-coin blockchain to safeguard public health data and facilitate transparent medicine sales.

4.3 Cryptocurrency payments

Cryptocurrency payments in healthcare provide many advantages. Blockchain technology records every transaction in a ledger. All the coin owners' information is contained in the saved data. This ensures that the transactions occurring are authentic. Since digital currency is decentralized, neither the government nor the bank has control over it. The digital currency is still owned by the person who generated it. Blockchain makes it possible for patients to trade. The lack of intermediaries, such as banks, merchants, and representatives, does not require the support of a central office to carry out the transactions. It simplifies the charging process. The framework efficiently identifies the patients who attempt clinical activities (Kombe et al., 2018). It checks the legitimacy of the subtleties presented by them and the qualification of the exchanges.

4.4 Clinical trials and data security

Accurate and genuine data collection is essential for clinical research. Correlation, measurement, and analysis are all crucial. Additionally, from the perspective of the patient, it provides an additional degree of protection and security to the sensitive and personally identifiable data that the patient would be worried about if it were compromised in areas where identity theft may take place. The significance of blockchain for clinical trials has been examined in several studies (Jahankhani et al., 2019; Omar et al., 2020). Blockchain technology is making clinical trials more open and transparent from the start, with registration and informed consent, to the results release and medication administration.

4.5 Device tracking

Monitoring medical devices from production to decommissioning is another crucial step in transforming healthcare. Managing a pool of medical equipment used by multiple departments and patients is a challenge for all hospitals. Finding the right materials in a medical emergency requires time. To provide quick equipment recovery and prevent needless repurchasing and fraud analytics from the supply chain to decommissioning, medical device monitoring and tracking are therefore essential (Jafri and Singh, 2022). Compared to traditional location monitoring techniques, a blockchain-based strategy offers several benefits. The immutability and tamper-proof nature of blockchain are its most obvious characteristics. The location of the item, its history, its creator, reseller, and serial number can all be revealed in an immutable log created using blockchain technology to aid with regulatory compliance. A bad individual cannot alter or delete a device's location history from the database using this blockchain-based method. Blockchain allows us to verify that the medical equipment is in approved locations, ensure that clients use it, and obtain important information about how the loaned-out equipment is used. Among the advantages are the ability to quickly locate equipment in an emergency, keep an inventory process log, and automate the usage process.

4.6 Secure healthcare setups

In terms of effectively providing and prescribing medical care to patients while protecting the privacy of their data, as well as the process of providing medical professionals with up-to-date, reliable, and accurate data in real-time, smart healthcare has reached a high level of sophistication (Chakraborty et al., 2019). IoT has also done a great job in the healthcare industry, making patient monitoring and diagnosis easier.

4.7 Health insurance: claims processing

Health insurance has become essential in people's life due to the increase in health problems. People who cannot afford significant medical expenses may find it challenging to deal with medical emergencies. Health insurance provides financial security from the worry of debt and assists consumers in paying for medical treatments in the event of an emergency. Concerns about fraud, security, and privacy may surface concerning health insurance and its many benefits. Fraud has been a touchy subject in the health insurance sector in recent years because of the enormous losses it causes to people, companies, and governments. Therefore, both commercial businesses and governmental authorities need to build systems that can detect fraudulent payments and incidents. One of the most annoying procedures is filing an insurance claim, which requires the insurance processors to search for false claims, fragmented data sources, and cancelled policies that the clients have mentioned. The procedure is also rather extensive. This technology enables the insurers to acquire ownership of the assets to be protected and offers risk-free management and transparency (Raikwar et al., 2018). These days, transactions play a major role in the insurance sector. Many Fintech systems use an immutable ledger, developed by Blockchain technology, to detect cryptocurrency double-spending to meet productivity and security criteria (Raikwar et al., 2018). Two insurance service models are offered by blockchain-based insurance systems: one for end users' web identity security and another for the data security of commercial websites, which is suggested for web identity security. The claim's supporting documentation is automatically uploaded for authentication. Contracts are implemented automatically to strengthen the confidence between the policyholder and the insurer (Guo et al., 2018).

4.8 Vaccination registration and monitoring

Governments all over the world-imposed lockdowns to reduce the rate of transmission. For medical professionals, managing the population's testing and vaccination program was an enormous undertaking. Streamlining processes is necessary to improve efficacy and save more lives. Smart contracts were developed to automate the process of recording and tracking events related to the distribution and delivery of COVID-19 vaccinations to guarantee data provenance. A Digital Vaccine Passport (DVP) system was designed to prioritize safe vaccinations for the people who require them and use blockchain technology to automate testing certifications to help control the severity of the pandemic crisis (Nabil et al., 2022).As blockchain offers a distributed system with increased privacy, transparency, and authenticity, the DVP system incorporated private blockchain Hyperledger Fabric to provide seamless testing and immunization. The system was able to improve cost efficiency.

4.9 Vaccine distribution

Vaccination is one of the most effective approaches to prevent the spread of infectious illnesses. The vaccine supply chain differs from conventional supply chains because of the perishability of the products and the need for strict transportation and storage rules to protect people's health and safety (Musamih et al., 2021b). Inefficiencies, including ineffective delivery strategies or a lack of interoperability, lead to a halt or delay in the immunization supply. Furthermore, governments must establish a suitable logistical network and plan a prompt and efficient vaccination distribution in the case of a pandemic due to the enormous number of doses needed for the implementation of a mass vaccination campaign. Physical limitations include inadequate storage systems, limited infrastructure, and a lack of medical personnel. To guarantee that the vaccines are preserved, specialized storage equipment is required. Ultra-freezers have limited capacity and availability, so an efficient management system is required to ensure vaccination validity time. The supply and demand for vaccines might be unpredictable due to communication problems among supply chain players, which can lead to inefficiencies and regional imbalances. Maintaining the integrity of health data is crucial when it comes to security issues like possible cyberattacks or data manipulation. Starting with the actual and current vaccine allocation criteria, a model was developed to mimic the possible blockchain-based supply chain performance improvement, which would include improved player communication as well as the automation of the procurement process through smart contracts (Rinaldi et al., 2022). The nationwide immunization campaign was thus carried out in response to demand. The established simulation model made it possible to use smart contracts to automate the vaccination acquisition process. Smart contracts were used to track each region's inventory, and suitable inventory regulations were established and implemented. According to the investigation, lowering stock levels through integrated and transparent data sharing throughout the whole supply chain increased vaccine distribution performance (Sookhak et al., 2021).

4.10 Healthcare Waste Management

The rise of COVID-19 has made managing healthcare waste a difficult issue. Hospital and vaccination waste are to blame for the rise in waste. One tactic to control COVID-19 is the widespread usage of face masks. In addition to wearing other personal protection equipment, health personnel must ensure patient and staff safety. The bulk of masks are composed of non-renewable petroleum-based materials, which has led to a sharp rise in hospital waste and increased environmental contamination. These leftovers could be classified as healthcare waste together with sharps, contaminated blood, body and tissue parts, chemicals, pharmaceuticals, and radioactive materials. For the efficient management of healthcare waste, reverse logistics (RL), which involves handling and getting rid of hazardous or non-hazardous waste from products and packaging, has become a major alternative. Indicators for healthcare waste management have shown themselves to be highly important for evaluating hospital waste and supporting environmental management. Therefore, to prioritize the criteria and weigh the many indicators, a multi-criteria analysis method called the Analytic Hierarchy Process (AHP) was employed (De Aguiar et al., 2020). The purpose of the assessment tool was to find reliable waste indicators. The overproduction and underutilization of vaccinations because of large-scale vaccine production constitute another kind of waste. Today's processes and technologies for handling waste data on COVID-19 vaccinations usually lack transparency, traceability, accountability, trust, and security components. As a result, a blockchain-based solution with five phases was suggested. Trash assessment, production and delivery, consumption, production, and commitment are all included in the blockchain-based solution. The whole life cycle of a COVID-19 vaccine is controlled by multiple smart contracts to guarantee responsibility for all actions taken by the involved parties and reduce any further waste caused by overproduction, overordering, or underconsumption. Using the REMIX IDE, an Ethereum-based smart contract was created and deployed on the Kovan Testnet (Musamih et al., 2022). By employing the PoA consensus process, the suggested approach was able to get around the problem of large-scale data storage and achieve higher throughput.A private permissioned Ethereum blockchain was used to improve data privacy. By employing a private permissioned blockchain devoid of centralized authorities, regulators were able to take use of smart contracts and modify the blockchain's configuration to meet their needs. trash was decreased by using the commitment smart contract, which made sure that each organization was accountable for any trash produced.

4.11 Supply chain management

Effective management of the Healthcare Supply Chain (HCSC) is essential for healthcare providers in both their daily operations and during pandemics like COVID-19. Despite significant improvements in new technologies and treatment options, healthcare providers still face challenges with purchasing, ordering, forecasting, and distribution processes as large amounts of cargo are delivered both domestically and internationally daily. Like manufacturing supply chains, the healthcare sector has a difficult time managing and simplifying healthcare processes. Group Purchasing Organizations (GPOs) are important participants in the HCSC and offer vendors and providers savings for large purchases. A blockchain-based solution that utilizes Ethereum smart contracts and a decentralized storage system was suggested to improve the efficiency of the contracting process in HCSC and to expedite the administration of GPO contracts (Omar et al., 2021). With a blockchain-based GPO contract solution, manufacturing, distribution, GPOs, and healthcare providers may all be integrated into a single decentralized Ethereum network. The solution includes the essential procedures for purchasing drugs and devices. The suggested architecture ensured trust and transparency and restricted access to smart contracts to registered stakeholders. By preventing price disparities with stakeholders, the approach increased cost efficiency. The presence of a functional, transparent distribution network that can be audited by all important stakeholders is essential to the success of a worldwide vaccination campaign and the prompt introduction of a vaccine. Food, commodities, and prescription medications are among the items in the vaccination supply chain that may sustain damage during transportation. This could be caused by a variety of things, such as improper storage procedures, exposure to air or sunlight, and improper storage conditions. The Internet of Things (IoT) has made basic shipment tracking better by making these transportation systems more visible and transparent. A blockchain-based smart container system called CryptoCargo was developed to track shipping conditions and spot any violations that can endanger the shipment's contents (Alkhoori et al., 2021). These infractions are recorded using smart contracts on the blockchain, which provides safe and unchangeable storage, increasing its credibility in a situation where there are several parties and minimal opportunity for trust. Smart contracts are designed to manage and monitor the proper vaccine distribution conditions in relation to the safe handling guidelines given by vaccine manufacturers, allowing all network peers to be informed of the situation. A prototype was created to provide vaccines, a transparent side effect solution that is impenetrable, and an Ethereum test network called Ropsten (Antal et al., 2021).

The results of every on-chain action were examined and validated on the Etherscan. The results for an implementation based on Ethereum show that it is feasible in terms of transaction throughput and gas consumption cost. Increased COVID-19 vaccine distribution efficiency and transparency, traceability, and a rigorous audit of storage and delivery conditions were all satisfactorily addressed by the suggested approach. Accuracy and transparency were ensured in the registration process and in the administration of the vaccination waiting list. The comparison of current businesses that have used blockchain technology for healthcare services is shown in Table 4. Some of the most recent leading businesses that use blockchain technology to offer healthcare system solutions are listed in the table.

CASE STUDIES

Numerous pilot projects, practical applications, and research prototypes have been used to investigate the potential of blockchain technology in the healthcare industry. These case studies demonstrate how blockchain technology may help with urgent healthcare security issues, especially when it comes to maintaining data integrity, privacy, and stakeholder trust. Here are a few noteworthy instances that illustrate various blockchain uses in the healthcare industry.

a) **Decentralized Record Management (MedRec)**

MedRec, one of the first blockchain-based electronic health record (EHR) management systems, was created by MIT Media Lab researchers. The platform handles access control, data exchange, and authentication via a private, permissioned Ethereum blockchain. MedRec contains metadata that connects to patient records found in pre-existing hospital databases on the blockchain rather than actual medical data. Permissions and consent are managed using smart contracts. Patients have authority over who can access their records from various providers. Transparency and auditability are also guaranteed. MedRec showed how blockchain technology may decentralize medical data management without interfering with the hospital's current infrastructure. By giving patients control over who can access their data, it improves security and trust.

b) **Estonia's National Blockchain Health Infrastructure**

Estonia has adopted blockchain technology to protect the integrity of its national healthcare system and is regarded as a global leader in digital governance. To incorporate KSI Blockchain into its eHealth system, the nation teamed up with cybersecurity company Guardtime. All access to people's medical records is recorded using blockchain technology. Data integrity and non-repudiation are ensured by tamper-evident logs. integration of government agencies, clinics, and hospitals nationwide. The Estonian approach demonstrates how blockchain technology can be implemented on a national scale. The method increases public trust in digital services, guarantees adherence to privacy laws, and enhances transparency. Similar efforts to establish safe and compatible health data systems have been sparked by it in other nations.

c) **Robomed Network: Smart Contract-Based Care Management**

Robomed Network is a blockchain-based digital health platform that uses smart contracts to optimize patient care. It was introduced in Russia and the Middle East and uses a value-based care paradigm to link patients and healthcare providers. Treatment plans and anticipated results are specified using smart contracts. Care is given to patients according to pre-established quality measures. Every medical encounter and result are documented on the blockchain. Robomed emphasizes the application of blockchain technology to clinical responsibility. It avoids treatment data manipulation, improves care delivery transparency, and matches provider incentives with patient outcomes. A new paradigm of programmable healthcare contracts is also made possible by it.

d) **Chronicled and MediLedger: Securing the Pharmaceutical Supply Chain**

Pfizer, Gilead, and Amgen are among the pharmaceutical corporations that are part of the MediLedger Project, which is headed by Chronicled. It complies with the U.S. Drug Supply Chain Security Act (DSCSA) by utilizing blockchain technology to guarantee the integrity of the pharmaceutical supply chain. traces the origin of drugs from producer to retailer. uses cryptographic verification to stop fake medications. Zero-knowledge proofs are used to protect transactional data. MediLedger provides immutable audit trails and real-time traceability, which enhance supply chain security. It tackles major security risks in international pharmaceutical logistics, such as fraud, diversion, and counterfeit medications (Mackey & Nayyar, 2017).

e) **Solve. Care: Blockchain for Care Coordination and Payments**

A blockchain technology called Solve Care focuses on healthcare payment and administrative procedures (Solve Care, 2021). It offers decentralized scheduling, claims processing, and patient journey management systems. Tokens are used in this for incentive schemes and transparent healthcare payments. uses decentralized apps (dApps) and smart contracts to manage care plans. This makes cross-border insurance and telemedicine services possible. Solve Care lowers fraud and administrative burden in medical transactions. Particularly in intricate, multi-party healthcare settings, its blockchain architecture facilitates value-based care and enhances patient-provider collaboration.

f) **BurstIQ: Secure Health Data Marketplace**

A blockchain platform located in the United States, BurstIQ facilitates safe data sharing across healthcare organizations (BurstIQ, 2021). It creates a marketplace for health data by fusing blockchain, AI, and big data. Key features include data sharing that complies with HIPAA, smart contracts that allow data licensing, monetization, and privacy enforcement, and the ability to support population health studies, research, and personalized care. BurstIQ enables safe data sharing between people and organizations while upholding ownership and consent controls. It encourages the commercial use of anonymised health data and a trust-based environment for cooperative health research. From supply chain integrity and fraud protection to patient data management and care coordination, the mentioned case studies demonstrate the blockchain's broad applicability in the healthcare industry.

5. HEALTHCARE-SPECIFIC SECURITY CHALLENGES

5.1 Electronic Health Records

As healthcare continues to evolve into an increasingly complex and multi-layered system, the need for efficient, secure, and patient-centered data management has never been so critical and take care. While blockchain technology is often associated with financial transactions, and its underlying fundamentals of immutability, decentralization, and transparency offer an effective solution to many of the problems faced in managing of electronic health records (Figure 13). The blockchain can be used efficiently for the healthcare domain for storing, accessing, and sharing purposes. The blockchain role in EHRs in the current scenario can never be neglected as it will provide the privacy and security to the user-centric health records information, and the vast number of researchers are working on it. When dealing with electronic health records, there also exist numerous challenges associated with it. The Challenges of electronic health records without blockchain are given below.

Figure 13. blockchain based HER

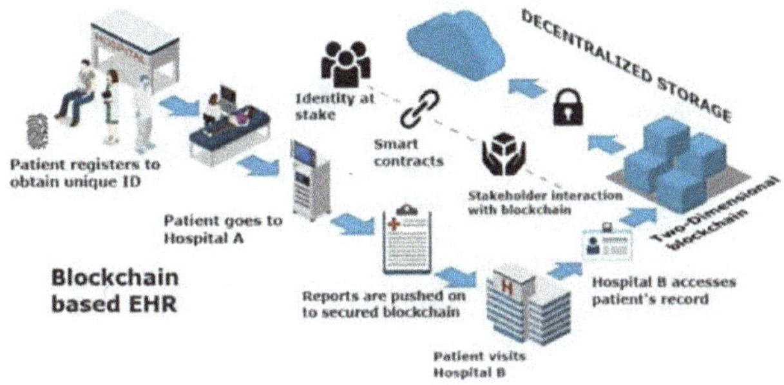

a) **Complexity in Modern Healthcare:**

The modern healthcare system is no longer limited to single-point care. Instead, it includes a wide network of general practitioners, insurance companies, specialists, consultants, and allied health professionals. Over a patient's lifetime, these varied interactions generate the fragmented trail of the medical records. The maintenance of the records of the patient as per the individual is a matter of concern.

b) **Barriers to accessibility and Interoperability:**

Current Electronic health records are typically designed for use in a single organization and have limited interoperability between different healthcare providers. This type of architecture lowers the performance for timely data sharing and disrupts the continuity of care.

Blockchain offers a decentralized framework that can unify different healthcare records into a singular, tamper-proof ledger (Figure 14). Each health-related interaction, be it a doctor's visit, lab result, or prescription, can be recorded as a time-stamped block on the chain. These blocks form a chronological, immutable patient history accessible by the authorized parties.(Pu et al., 2024)

Figure 14. Benefits of blockchain-enabled data systems.

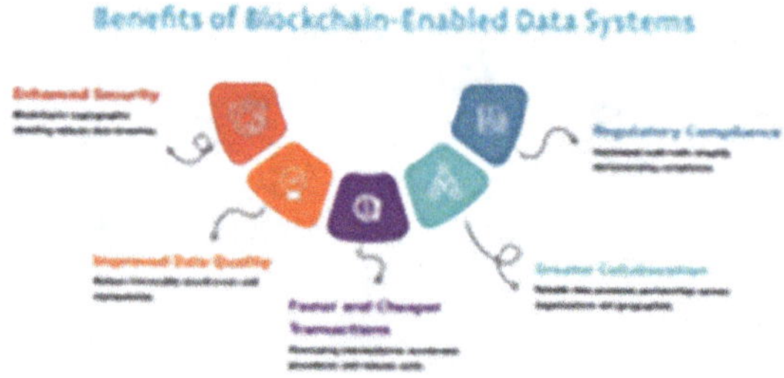

a) **Securing Access and Safeguarding Patient Privacy:**

Block Chain does not just improve accessibility, it enhances security and patient autonomy. Using encryption and smart contracts, patients can determine exactly who accesses their data and under what circumstances.

b) **Interoperability and Consent:**

Interoperability is the ability for systems to work together, is inherently supported by the blockchain's distributed architectures. Additionally, smart contracts can automate the process of managing patient consent and eliminate the need for manual approvals and paperwork,

Blockchain technology presents a unique opportunity to reshape electronic health records management. By addressing core issues of fragmentation, inaccessibility, and lack of interoperability block blockchain enables a more integrated and patient-focused approach to healthcare. The application of the blockchain in EHRs allows up-to-date information that enhances decision-making and ultimately improves patient outcomes (M. S. Islam & Rahman, 2025).

5.2 Data Privacy Laws

In today's digital world, personal data is constantly collected, shared and stored often without individuals being fully aware. As data breaches and cyber threats continue to rise, governments across the world are enforcing stronger data privacy laws to safeguard citizen's information. Two of the most significant and influential regulations in this space are the General Data Protection Regulation (GDPR) and the Health Insurance Portability and Accountability Act(HIPAA) .Both laws, while differing in scope, reflect a global commitment to privacy, accountability and trust. (Merlec et al., 2021)

a) **General Data Protection Regulation (GDPR):**

The General Data Protection Regulation (GDPR), created by the European Union in 2018, has become the global benchmark for data privacy. GDPR applies to any organization, regardless of location, that handles the personal data of EU citizens. Its core principles include transparency, accountability, and individual control over personal information. (Lee et al., 2023) Under the GDPR, individuals have the following rights:

1. Right to Erasure (right to be forgotten).
2. Right to access and correct their data.
3. Right to data portability and restriction of processing.

The different organizations must obtain the explicit information consent, ensuring the lawful data processing, appointing the Data Protection Officers (DPOs) when required, and report data breaches in 72 hours. If the organizations are not following the process can lead to higher fines, which ensures the importance of securing ethical data practices.

b) **Health Insurance Portability and Accountability Act (HIPAA):**

HIPAA focuses specifically on the privacy and security of protected health information (PHI). The act was passed in the year 1996, and it regulates how healthcare providers, insurers, and business associates handle the electronic health records of medical data. HIPAA ensures the following rules for accessing the Electronic Health Records(EHRs):

1. *Privacy Rule:* It restricts how the protected health information(PHI's) can be used and shared.
2. *The Security Rule:* This rule allows the user to have mandated safeguards (technical, physical, and administrative) to protect electronic health records information.
3. *The Breach Notification Rule:* It required the covered entities to notify individuals and regulators when data breach occurs.

HIPAA is basically designed for the healthcare industry, but both laws enforce patient trust, data accuracy, and responsible handling. Data privacy is no longer just a compliance issue it is a matter of trust and ethical responsibility. Laws like GDPR and HIPAA represent a global shift toward protecting individuals in the age of digital vulnerability.

7. CONCLUSION

Blockchain technology's use in healthcare systems offers a revolutionary chance to solve persistent problems with security, data integrity, and trust. The potential of blockchain as a fundamental infrastructure to safeguard electronic health records (EHRs), expedite data interchange, and provide patients greater control over their medical data has been examined in this chapter. Healthcare stakeholders may reduce the risks of data breaches, illegal access, and tampering with sensitive patient records by utilizing the fundamental characteristics of blockchain technology, which include immutability, decentralization, transparency, and cryptographic security. Blockchain-based trust models improve credibility and auditability within healthcare networks by promoting distributed consensus processes rather than relying on centralized authorities. Additionally, digital signatures and cryptographic hashing guarantee that data integrity is verifiable and impervious to manipulation.

Scalability, regulatory compliance, compatibility with legacy healthcare systems, and the requirement for strong off-chain data management are just a few of the significant issues that still exist. These drawbacks highlight how crucial it is to create hybrid solutions that combine blockchain's advantages with complementary technologies like edge devices, cloud computing, and safe data storage protocols.

The legal and ethical environment about patient consent and privacy is equally significant. Although blockchain can increase transparency, it also creates issues with data permanence and the right to be forgotten, particularly in areas where strict laws like GDPR and HIPAA are in effect. Therefore, a careful balance between innovation and compliance must direct the implementation of blockchain in the healthcare industry. As the healthcare sector shifts to more patient-centred, interoperable, and data-driven care models, blockchain holds promise as a tool for improving trust and data integrity. In addition to technology developments, cross-sector cooperation between patients, legislators, technologists, and healthcare practitioners will be essential to its successful implementation. Blockchain has the ability to completely rethink the digital trust architecture of healthcare, resulting in safer, more effective, and more fair systems of care as research and pilot applications develop further.

REFERENCES

Agbo, C. C., Mahmoud, Q. H., & Eklund, J. M. (2019). Blockchain technology in healthcare: A systematic review. *Health Care*, *7*(2), 56. DOI: 10.3390/healthcare7020056 PMID: 30987333

Alkhoori, O., Hassan, A., Almansoori, O., Debe, M., Salah, K., Jayaraman, R., Arshad, J., & Rehman, M. H. U. (2021). Design and implementation of CryptoCargo: A blockchainpowered smart shipping container for vaccine distribution. *IEEE Access : Practical Innovations, Open Solutions*, *9*, 9. DOI: 10.1109/ACCESS.2021.3070911

. Anderson, J. (2018). Record audit logs through permissioned blockchain technology, Tech. Report.

Antal, C., Cioara, T., Antal, M., & Anghel, I. (2021). Blockchain platform for COVID-19 vaccine supply management. *IEEE Open Journal of the Computer Society*, *2*, 164–178. DOI: 10.1109/OJCS.2021.3067450

Brakeville, S., & Perepa, B. (2018). *Blockchain basics: Introduction to distributed ledgers*. IBM Developer.

Casino, F., Dasaklis, T. K., & Patsakis, C. (2019). A systematic literature review of blockchain-based applications: Current status, classification and open issues. *Telematics and Informatics*, *36*, 55–81. DOI: 10.1016/j.tele.2018.11.006

Chakraborty, S., Aich, S., & Kim, H. C. 2019. A secure healthcare system design framework using blockchain technology. Int. Conf. Adv. Commun. Technol. ICACT 260–264., 2019-Febru.DOI: 10.23919/ICACT.2019.8701983

Chen, G., Xu, B., Lu, M., & Chen, N.-S. (2018). Exploring blockchain technology and its potential applications for education. *Smart Learn. Environ.*, *5*(1), 1. DOI: 10.1186/s40561-017-0050-x

Chronicled. (2021). *MediLedger Network*. https://www.mediledger.com

De Aguiar, E. J., Faiçal, B. S., Krishnamachari, B., & Ueyama, J. (2020). A survey of blockchain-based strategies for healthcare. *ACM Computing Surveys*, *53*(2), 1–27. Advance online publication. DOI: 10.1145/3376915

Enescu, F. M., Bizon, N., Stirbu, C., & Ionescu, V. M. 2018. Blockchain technology applied in health the study of blockchain application in the health system (II). In: Proceedings of the 10th International Conference on Electronics, Computers and Artificial Intelligence. ECAI. https://doi.org/DOI: 10.1109/ECAI.2018.8679029

Esposito, C., De Santis, A., Tortora, G., Chang, H., & Choo, K.-K. R. (2018). Blockchain: A panacea for healthcare cloud-based data security and privacy? *IEEE Cloud Computing*, *5*(1), 31–37. DOI: 10.1109/MCC.2018.011791712

Guo, H., & Yu, X. (2022). A survey on blockchain technology and its security. *Blockchain: Research and Applications*, *3*(2), 100067.

Hussein, Z., Salama, M. A., & El-Rahman, S. A. (2023). Evolution of blockchain consensus algorithms: A review on the latest milestones of blockchain consensus algorithms. *Cybersecurity*, *6*(1), 30. DOI: 10.1186/s42400-023-00163-y

Islam, M. S., & Rahman, M. S. (2025). LogStamping: A blockchain-based log auditing approach for large-scale systems. *arXiv Preprint arXiv:2505.17236*.

Islam, R., Bose, R., Roy, S., Khan, A. A., Sutradhar, S., Das, S., Ali, F., & AlZubi, A. A. (2025). Decentralized trust framework for smart cities: A blockchain-enabled cybersecurity and data integrity model. *Scientific Reports*, *15*(1), 23454. DOI: 10.1038/s41598-025-06405-y PMID: 40603417

Jafri, R., & Singh, S. (2022). Blockchain applications for the healthcare sector: Uses beyond Bitcoin. In *Elsevier eBooks* (71–92). DOI: 10.1016/B978-0-323-90615-9.00022-0

Jahankhani, H., Kendzierskyj, S., Jamal, A., & Epiphaniou, G. H. 2019. In: Al-Khateeb(Ed.), Blockchain and Clinical Trial Securing Patient Data (Advanced Sciences and Technologies for Security Applications).

Jaiswal, S., Bahadur, P. S., Singh, S., & Rajpoot, S. (2023a, September). Progressive Technology of InfraRed Spectroscopy for Characterization of Materials. In Proceedings of the 6th International Conference on Contemporary Computing and Informatics (IC3I). IEEE. DOI: 10.1109/IC3I59117.2023.10397795

Jaiswal, S., & Khanam, S. Z. (2025). Techno-Economic Analysis of Green Hydrogen Production for Industrial Use. In Mabrouki, J. (Ed.), *Obstacles Facing Hydrogen Green Systems and Green Energy* (pp. 479–506). IGI Global Scientific Publishing., DOI: 10.4018/979-8-3693-8980-5.ch028

Jaiswal, S., Machiraju, M. S., & Kaustubh, M. H. (2023b, November 24–26). Review of novel technology in cochlear implants among special needs children. In Proceedings of the 2023 10th IEEE Uttar Pradesh Section International Conference on Electrical, Electronics and Computer Engineering (UPCON) (pp. 370–374). IEEE. DOI: 10.1109/UPCON59197.2023.10434570

Jaiswal, S., Singh, P., Srivastav, S., Chaudhary, R., & Kumar, A. (2024, November 14–16). Noval technology of nano-robot for promising drug delivery system. In Proceedings of the 2024 7th International Conference on Contemporary Computing and Informatics (IC3I) (pp. 858–863). IEEE. DOI: 10.1109/IC3I61595.2024.10829002

Jasim, L. H., Mishra, A., Joshi, S. K., & Sapaev, I. B., DR, P., & Babu, A. N. (2023). Analysing blockchain-based cryptography: Enhancing security, transparency, and practical implementations. *2023 International Conference for Technological Engineering and Its Applications in Sustainable Development (ICTEASD)*, 39–44. DOI: 10.1109/ICTEASD57136.2023.10585016

Kombe, C., Ally, M., & Sam, A. (2018). A review on healthcare information systems and consensus protocols in blockchain technology. *Int. J. Adv. Technol. Eng. Explor.*, *5*(49), 473–483. DOI: 10.19101/IJATEE.2018.547023

. Lau, E. (2018). Decoding the hype: Blockchain in Healthcare - A Software Architecture for the provision of a patient summary to overcome interoperability issues.

Lee, T.-F., Chang, I.-P., & Su, G.-J. (2023). Compliance with hipaa and gdpr in certificateless-based authenticated key agreement using extended chaotic maps. *Electronics (Basel)*, *12*(5), 1108. DOI: 10.3390/electronics12051108

Mackey, T. K., & Nayyar, G. (2017). A review of existing and emerging digital technologies to combat the global trade in fake medicines. *Expert Opinion on Drug Safety*, *16*(5), 587–602. DOI: 10.1080/14740338.2017.1313227 PMID: 28349715

Merlec, M. M., Lee, Y. K., Hong, S.-P., & In, H. P. (2021). A smart contract-based dynamic consent management system for personal data usage under GDPR. *Sensors (Basel)*, *21*(23), 7994. DOI: 10.3390/s21237994 PMID: 34883997

Musamih, A., Jayaraman, R., Salah, K., Hasan, H. R., Yaqoob, I., & Al-Hammadi, Y. (2021b). Blockchain-based solution for distribution and delivery of COVID-19 vaccines. *IEEE Access : Practical Innovations, Open Solutions*, *9*, 71372–71387. DOI: 10.1109/ACCESS.2021.3079197 PMID: 34812393

Musamih, A., Salah, K., Jayaraman, R., Arshad, J., Debe, M., Al-Hammadi, Y., & Ellahham, S. (2021a). A Blockchain-Based approach for drug traceability in healthcare supply chain. *IEEE Access : Practical Innovations, Open Solutions*, *9*, 9728–9743. DOI: 10.1109/ACCESS.2021.3049920

Musamih, A., Salah, K., Jayaraman, R., Yaqoob, I., Al-Hammadi, Y., & Antony, J. (2022). Blockchain-based solution for COVID-19 vaccine waste reduction. *Journal of Cleaner Production*, *372*(August), 133619. DOI: 10.1016/j.jclepro.2022.133619 PMID: 35999948

Nabil, S. S., Alam Pran, M. S., Al Haque, A. A., Chakraborty, N. R., Chowdhury, M. J. M., & Ferdous, M. S. (2022). Blockchain-based COVID vaccination registration and monitoring. *Blockchain Res. Appl., 3*(4), 100092. Advance online publication. DOI: 10.1016/j.bcra.2022.100092

Omar, I. A., Jayaraman, R., Debe, M. S., Salah, K., Yaqoob, I., & Omar, M. (2021). Automating procurement contracts in the healthcare supply chain using blockchain smart contracts. *IEEE Access : Practical Innovations, Open Solutions, 9*, 37397–37409. DOI: 10.1109/ACCESS.2021.3062471

Prashanth Joshi, A., Han, M., & Wang, Y. (2018). A survey on security and privacy issues of blockchain technology. *Mathematical Foundations of Computing, 1*(2), 121–147. DOI: 10.3934/mfc.2018007

Pu, X., Jiang, R., Song, Z., Liang, Z., & Yang, L. (2024). A medical big data access control model based on smart contracts and risk in the blockchain environment. *Frontiers in Public Health, 12*, 1358184. DOI: 10.3389/fpubh.2024.1358184 PMID: 38605878

Raikwar, M., Mazumdar, S., Ruj, S., Sen Gupta, S., Chattopadhyay, A., & Lam, K. Y. 2018.A blockchain framework for insurance processes. In: 2018 9th IFIP International Conference On New Technologies, Mobility And Security, NTMS 2018 - Proceedings,vol. 2018, pp. 1–4. https://doi.org/DOI: 10.1109/NTMS.2018.8328731

Regueiro, C., Seco, I., Gutiérrez-Agüero, I., Urquizu, B., & Mansell, J. (2021). A blockchain-based audit trail mechanism: Design and implementation. *Algorithms, 14*(12), 341. DOI: 10.3390/a14120341

. Rinaldi, M., et al., 2022. Improving the Distribution Vaccines Using the Blockchain Technology: the Italian Case Study, 2023.

Sevin, A., & Osman Mohammed, A. A. (2024). Comparative Study of Blockchain Hashing Algorithms with a Proposal for HashLEA. *Applied Sciences (Basel, Switzerland), 14*(24), 11967. DOI: 10.3390/app142411967

Shahnaz, A., Qamar, U., & Khalid, A. (2019). Using blockchain for electronic health records. *IEEE Access : Practical Innovations, Open Solutions, 7*, 147782–147795. DOI: 10.1109/ACCESS.2019.2946373

Singh, Y., Jaiswal, S., & Kumar, V. (2024). A Comprehensive Literature Review on Privacy, Security, and Data Management in Healthcare. *2024 2nd International Conference on Disruptive Technologies (ICDT)*, 220–224.

Solve.Care. (2021). *Solve.Care Platform Overview*. https://solve.care

Sookhak, M., Jabbarpour, M. R., Safa, N. S., & Yu, F. R. (2021). Blockchain and smart contract for access control in healthcare: A survey, issues and challenges, and open issues. *Journal of Network and Computer Applications*, *178*, 102950. DOI: 10.1016/j.jnca.2020.102950

Tseng, J. H., Liao, Y. C., Chong, B., & Liao, S. W. (2018). Governance on the drug supply chain via gcoin blockchain. *International Journal of Environmental Research and Public Health*, *15*(6), 1055. Advance online publication. DOI: 10.3390/ijerph15061055 PMID: 29882861

Wang, H., Wang, Y., Cao, Z., Li, Z., & Xiong, G. (2019). *An Overview of Blockchain Security Analysis* (Vol. 970). Springer Singapore., DOI: 10.1007/978-981-13-6621-5_5

Wutthikarn, R., & Hui, Y. G. 2018. Prototype of blockchain in dental care service application based on hyperledger composer in hyperledger fabric framework, 2018. In: International Computer Science and Engineering Conference, *22nd*. ICSEC. . Jul. 2018.DOI: 10.1109/ICSEC.2018.8712639

Zhang, G., Yang, Z., & Liu, W. (2022a). Blockchain-based privacy preserving e-health system for healthcare data in cloud. *Computer Networks*, *203*, 108586. DOI: 10.1016/j.comnet.2021.108586

Zhang, P., Schmidt, D. C., White, J., & Lenz, G. (2018). Blockchain technology use cases in healthcare. In *Advances in computers*,1–41. https://doi.org/DOI: 10.1016/bs.adcom.2018.03.006

Zhang, P., Schmidt, D. C., White, J., & Lenz, G. (2018a). Blockchain technology use cases in healthcare. In *Advances in Computers* (Vol. 111, pp. 1–41). Academic Press Inc., DOI: 10.1016/bs.adcom.2018.03.006

Zhu, L., Wu, Y., Gai, K., & Choo, K. K. R. (2019). Controllable and trustworthy blockchain-based cloud data management. *Future Generation Computer Systems*, *91*, 527–535. DOI: 10.1016/j.future.2018.09.019

Compilation of References

Abbasi, I. A., Jan, S. U., Alqahtani, A. S., Khan, A. S., Algarni, F., Nyangaresi, V. O., Nyangaresi, V. O., Nyangaresi, V. O., & Nyangaresi, V. O. (2024). A lightweight and robust authentication scheme for the healthcare system using public cloud server. *PLoS One*, *19*(1), e0294429. Advance online publication. DOI: 10.1371/journal.pone.0294429 PMID: 38289970

Abbou, B., Klein, A., Dudkiewicz, M., Goldschmid, N., Dahan Shriki, D., Gabbay-Benziv, R., Ophir, A., Kessel, B., Ben Natan, M., & Roguin, A. (2024). When all computers shut down: The clinical impact of a major cyber-attack on a general hospital. *Frontiers in Digital Health*, *6*, 1321485. Advance online publication. DOI: 10.3389/fdgth.2024.1321485 PMID: 38433989

Abdulmalek, S., Nasir, A., Jabbar, W. A., Almuhaya, M. A. M., Bairagi, A. K., Khan, M. A.-M., & Kee, S.-H. (2022). IoT-Based Healthcare-Monitoring System towards Improving Quality of Life: A Review. *Healthcare (Basel)*, *10*(10), 1993. DOI: 10.3390/healthcare10101993 PMID: 36292441

Abedi, S., Arvani, A., & Jamalzadeh, R. (2015). Cyber security of plug-in electric vehicles in smart grids: Application of intrusion detection methods. In *Plug In Electric Vehicles in Smart Grids: Integration Techniques* (pp. 129–147). Springer. DOI: 10.1007/978-3-319-22204-2_6

Abinesh Kamal, K. U., & Divya, S. V. (2024). Integrated Threat Intelligence Platform for security operations in organizations. *Automatika (Zagreb)*, *65*(2), 401–409. DOI: 10.1080/00051144.2023.2295146

Abomhara, M., & Køien, G. M. (2015). Cyber security and the internet of things: Vulnerabilities, threats, intruders and attacks. *Journal of Cyber Security and Mobility*, *4*(1), 65–88. DOI: 10.13052/jcsm2245-1439.414

Abouelmehdi, K., Khaloufi, H., & Beni-Hessane, A. (2018). Big healthcare data: Preserving security and privacy. *Journal of Big Data*, *5*(1), 1. Advance online publication. DOI: 10.1186/s40537-017-0110-7

Aboukadri, S., Ouaddah, A., & Mezrioui, A. (2024). Machine learning in identity and Access Management Systems: Survey and Deep Dive. *Computers &amp. Computers & Security*, *139*, 103729. DOI: 10.1016/j.cose.2024.103729

Abujaber, A. A., & Nashwan, A. J. (2024). Ethical framework for artificial intelligence in healthcare research: A path to integrity. *World Journal of Methodology*, *14*(3). Advance online publication. DOI: 10.5662/wjm.v14.i3.94071 PMID: 39310239

Acharya, S., Dvorkin, Y., & Karri, R. (2020). Public plug-in electric vehicles + grid data: Is a new cyberattack vector viable? *IEEE Transactions on Smart Grid*, *11*(6), 5099–5113. DOI: 10.1109/TSG.2020.2994177

Adler-Milstein, J., & Jha, A. K. (2017). HITECH Act drove large gains in hospital electronic health record adoption. *Health Affairs*, *36*(8), 1416–1422. DOI: 10.1377/hlthaff.2016.1651 PMID: 28784734

Agbo, C. C., Mahmoud, Q. H., & Eklund, J. M. (2019). Blockchain technology in healthcare: A systematic review. *Health Care*, *7*(2), 56. DOI: 10.3390/healthcare7020056 PMID: 30987333

Aggarwal, L., Sachdeva, S., & Goswami, P. (2023). Quantum healthcare computing using precision based granular approach. *Applied Soft Computing*, *144*, 110458. DOI: 10.1016/j.asoc.2023.110458

Ahmad, I., Shahid, F., Islam, J., Haque, K., & Harjula, E. (2024). *Adaptive Lightweight Security for Performance Efficiency in Critical Healthcare Monitoring*. / arxiv.2406.03786DOI: 10.1109/ISMICT61996.2024.10738175

Ahmed, S. (2019). *BYOD, Personal Area Networks (PANs) and IOT: Threats to Patients Privacy*. Cornell University. https://doi.org//arxiv.1902.06462DOI: 10.48550

Ainslie, S., Thompson, D., Maynard, S., & Ahmad, A. (2023). Cyber-threat Intelligence for Security Decision-making: A review and research agenda for practice. *Computers &amp. Computers & Security*, *132*, 103352. DOI: 10.1016/j.cose.2023.103352

Ajish, D. (2024). The significance of artificial intelligence in zero trust technologies: A comprehensive review. *Journal of Electrical Systems and Information Technology*, *11*(1), 30. Advance online publication. DOI: 10.1186/s43067-024-00155-z

Akinsanya, O. O., Papadaki, M., & Sun, L. (2020). Towards a maturity model for health-care cloud security (M2HCS). *Information &amp. Information and Computer Security, 28*(3), 321–345. DOI: 10.1108/ICS-05-2019-0060

Alagic, G., Alagic, G., Apon, D., Cooper, D., Dang, Q., Dang, T., Kelsey, J., Lichtinger, J., Liu, Y.K., Miller, C. and Moody, D. (2022). Status report on the third round of the NIST post-quantum cryptography standardization process.

Alanazi, A. T. (2023). Clinicians' Perspectives on Healthcare Cybersecurity and Cyber Threats. *Cureus, 15*(10). Advance online publication. DOI: 10.7759/cureus.47026 PMID: 37965389

Alarfaj, K. A., & Rahman, M. M. H. (2024). The Risk Assessment of the Security of Electronic Health Records Using Risk Matrix. *Applied Sciences (Basel, Switzerland), 14*(13), 5785. DOI: 10.3390/app14135785

Alatawi, E., & Albalawi, U. (2025). Harnessing AI for Cyber Defense: Honeypot-Driven Intrusion Detection Systems. *Symmetry, 17*(5), 628. DOI: 10.3390/sym17050628

Alenezi, A., Atlam, H. F., & Wills, G. B. (2019). Experts reviews of a cloud forensic readiness framework for organizations. *Journal of Cloud Computing (Heidelberg, Germany), 8*(1), 11. Advance online publication. DOI: 10.1186/s13677-019-0133-z

Al-Fayad, F. S. (2020). The European Union's GDPR and Its Effect on Data-Driven Marketing Strategies. *International Journal of Marketing Studies, 12*(1), 39. DOI: 10.5539/ijms.v12n1p39

Algarni, A. M., & Thayananthan, V. (2025). Digital health: The cybersecurity for AI-based healthcare communication. *IEEE Access : Practical Innovations, Open Solutions, 13*, 5858–5870. DOI: 10.1109/ACCESS.2025.3526666

Alhayan, F., Alshuhail, A., Ismail, A. O. A., Alrusaini, O., Alahmari, S., Yahya, A. E., Albouq, S. S., & Al Sadig, M. (2025). Enhanced anomaly network intrusion detection using an improved snow ablation optimizer with dimensionality reduction and hybrid deep learning model. *Scientific Reports, 15*(1), 13270. Advance online publication. DOI: 10.1038/s41598-025-97398-1 PMID: 40247081

Al-Issa, Y., Ottom, M. A., & Tamrawi, A. (2019). EHealth Cloud Security Challenges: A survey. *Journal of Healthcare Engineering, 2019*, 1–15. DOI: 10.1155/2019/7516035

Ali, T., Al-Khalidi, M., & Al-Zaidi, R. (2024). Information security risk assessment methods in cloud computing: Comprehensive review. *Journal of Computer Information Systems*, •••, 1–28. DOI: 10.1080/08874417.2024.2329985

Alkhoori, O., Hassan, A., Almansoori, O., Debe, M., Salah, K., Jayaraman, R., Arshad, J., & Rehman, M. H. U. (2021). Design and implementation of CryptoCargo: A blockchainpowered smart shipping container for vaccine distribution. *IEEE Access : Practical Innovations, Open Solutions*, *9*, 9. DOI: 10.1109/ACCESS.2021.3070911

Al-Mhiqani, M. N., Zainal Abidin, Z., Ali, N. S., Hassan, A., Ahmad, R., Yunos, Z., Abdulkareem, K. H., & Yassin, W. (2020). A Review of Insider Threat Detection: Classification, Machine Learning Techniques, Datasets, Open Challenges, and Recommendations. *Applied Sciences (Basel, Switzerland)*, *10*(15), 5208. DOI: 10.3390/app10155208

Al-Muntaser, B., Mohamed, M. A., & Tuama, A. Y. (2023). Real-Time Intrusion Detection of Insider Threats in Industrial Control System Workstations Through File Integrity Monitoring. *International Journal of Advanced Computer Science and Applications*, *14*(6). Advance online publication. DOI: 10.14569/IJACSA.2023.0140636

Alnasser, A., Sun, H., & Jiang, J. (2019). Cyber security challenges and solutions for V2X communications: A survey. *Computer Networks*, *151*, 52–67. DOI: 10.1016/j.comnet.2018.12.018

Al-Ofeishat, H. A., & Alshorman, R. (2023). Build a secure network using segmentation and micro-segmentation techniques. *International Journal of Computing and Digital Systems*, *14*(1), 1–16.

Alotaibi, Y. K., & Federico, F. (2017). The impact of health information technology on patient safety. *Saudi Medical Journal*, *38*(12), 1173–1180. DOI: 10.15537/smj.2017.12.20631 PMID: 29209664

Alshammari, M. M., Alwan, A. A., & Aishaikhli, I. (2016, December). *Data Recovery and Business continuity in Cloud computing: A review of the research literature.* International Journal of Advancements in Computing Technology. https://www.researchgate.net/publication/312166397_Data_recovery_and_business_continuity_in_Cloud_computing_A_Review_of_the_Research_Literature

Alshamrani, A., Myneni, S., & Saddik, B. (2021). Security challenges in telemedicine and remote healthcare. *Sensors (Basel)*, *21*(6), 1965. DOI: 10.3390/s21061965 PMID: 33799616

Alsowail, R. A., & Al-Shehari, T. (2022). Techniques and countermeasures for preventing insider threats. *PeerJ. Computer Science*, *8*(12), e938. DOI: 10.7717/peerj-cs.938 PMID: 35494800

Alturi, V., & Ferraiolo, D. (2025). Role-based access control. In *Encyclopedia of Cryptography, Security and Privacy* (pp. 2124–2127). Springer Nature Switzerland. DOI: 10.1007/978-3-030-71522-9_829

Alzahrani, A. (2020). Coronavirus Social Engineering Attacks: Issues and Recommendations. *International Journal of Advanced Computer Science and Applications, 11*(5). Advance online publication. DOI: 10.14569/IJACSA.2020.0110523

Amah, U., Mart, J., & Oyetoro, A. (2023). *Cloud Security Governance Guidelines.* DOI: 10.14293/PR2199.000062.v1

Amajuoyi, C., Nwobodo, L., & Adegbola, M.Chinazor Prisca AmajuoyiLuther Kington NwobodoMayokun Daniel Adegbola. (2024). Transforming business scalability and operational flexibility with advanced cloud computing technologies. *Computer Science &amp. IT Research Journal, 5*(6), 1469–1487. DOI: 10.51594/csitrj.v5i6.1248

Anand, D., & Khemchandani, V. (2019). Identity and access management systems. *Security and Privacy of Electronic Healthcare Records: Concepts, Paradigms and Solutions*, 61.

Andriole, K. P. (2014). Security of Electronic Medical Information and Patient Privacy: What You Need to Know. *Journal of the American College of Radiology, 11*(12, 12 Pt B), 1212–1216. DOI: 10.1016/j.jacr.2014.09.011 PMID: 25467897

Angle, J. (2022, May). *Healthcare Supply Chain Cybersecurity Risk Management 2*. Cloud Security Alliance. https://www.researchgate.net/publication/360550527_Healthcare_Supply_Chain_Cybersecurity_Risk_Management_2

Anjum, M., Shahab, S., Whangbo, T., & Ahmad, S. (2023). Preventing overloaded dissemination in healthcare applications using NonDelay tolerant dissemination technique. *Heliyon, 9*(8), e18783. DOI: 10.1016/j.heliyon.2023.e18783 PMID: 37576207

Antal, C., Cioara, T., Antal, M., & Anghel, I. (2021). Blockchain platform for COVID-19 vaccine supply management. *IEEE Open Journal of the Computer Society, 2*, 164–178. DOI: 10.1109/OJCS.2021.3067450

Anuradha, R., Vandana, C. P., Singh, S. V., Singh, N., Emad, R., & Nitin, V. (2024, May). Integrating Quantum Computing for Enhanced Image Reconstruction in Medical Diagnostics. In *2024 International Conference on Communication, Computer Sciences and Engineering (IC3SE)* (pp. 1294-1298). IEEE. DOI: 10.1109/IC3SE62002.2024.10593044

Arefin, S. (2024). Strengthening Healthcare data security with AI-powered threat detection. [IJSRM]. *International Journal of Scientific Research and Management*, *12*(10), 1477–1483. DOI: 10.18535/ijsrm/v12i10.ec02

Argaw, S. T., Bempong, N.-E., Eshaya-Chauvin, B., & Flahault, A. (2019). The state of research on cyberattacks against hospitals and available best practice recommendations: A scoping review. *BMC Medical Informatics and Decision Making*, *19*(1), 10. Advance online publication. DOI: 10.1186/s12911-018-0724-5

Arshad, M. W., Murtza, I., & Arshad, M. A. (2023). Applications of quantum computing in health sector. *Journal of Data Science and Intelligent Systems*, *1*(1), 19–24. DOI: 10.47852/bonviewJDSIS3202656

Arute, F., Arya, K., Babbush, R., Bacon, D., Bardin, J. C., Barends, R., & Burkett, B. (2019). Quantum supremacy using a programmable superconducting processor. *Nature*, *574*(7779), 505–510. DOI: 10.1038/s41586-019-1666-5 PMID: 31645734

Arya, R., & Verma, A. (2024). Quantum Computing and Healthcare. *International Journal of Advanced Research in Science. Tongxin Jishu*, *4*(2).

Asan, O., Yu, Z., & Crotty, B. H. (2021). How clinician-patient communication affects trust in health information sources: Temporal Trends from a national cross-sectional survey. *PLoS One*, *16*(2), e0247583. Advance online publication. DOI: 10.1371/journal.pone.0247583

Aslam, N., Zhou, H., Urbach, E. K., Turner, M. J., Walsworth, R. L., Lukin, M. D., & Park, H. (2023). Quantum sensors for biomedical applications. *Nature Reviews. Physics*, *5*(3), 157–169. DOI: 10.1038/s42254-023-00558-3 PMID: 36776813

Atlam, H. F., & Yang, Y. (2025). Enhancing Healthcare Security: A Unified RBAC and ABAC Risk-Aware Access Control Approach. *Future Internet*, *17*(6), 262. DOI: 10.3390/fi17060262

Australian Cyber Security Centre. (2023). *Medibank cyber incident update*. Australian Government. https://www.cyber.gov.au

Avatefipour, O., Al-Sumaiti, A. S., El-Sherbeeny, A. M., Awwad, E. M., Elmeligy, M. A., Mohamed, M. A., & Malik, H. (2019). An intelligent secured framework for cyberattack detection in electric vehicles' CAN bus using machine learning. *IEEE Access : Practical Innovations, Open Solutions*, *7*, 127580–127592. DOI: 10.1109/ACCESS.2019.2937576

Azad, M. A., Abdullah, S., Arshad, J., Lallie, H., & Ahmed, Y. H. (2024). Verify and trust: A multidimensional survey of zero-trust security in the age of IoT. *Internet of Things : Engineering Cyber Physical Human Systems*, *27*, 101227. DOI: 10.1016/j.iot.2024.101227

Babu, P. R., Palaniswamy, B., Reddy, A. G., Odelu, V., & Kim, H. S. (2022). A survey on security challenges and protocols of electric vehicle dynamic charging system. *Security and Privacy*, *5*(3), e210. DOI: 10.1002/spy2.210

Bada, M., & Von Solms, B. (2022). *A Cybersecurity Guide for Using Fitness Devices*. Springer., DOI: 10.1007/978-3-030-94285-4_3

Balasubramani, S., Renjith, P. N., Kavisankar, L., Rajavel, R., Malarvel, M., & Shankar, A. (2025). A Quantum-enhanced Artificial Neural Network Model for Efficient Medical Image Compression. *IEEE Access : Practical Innovations, Open Solutions*.

Banimfreg, B. H. (2023). A comprehensive review and conceptual framework for cloud computing adoption in bioinformatics. *Healthcare Analytics*, *3*, 100190. DOI: 10.1016/j.health.2023.100190

Baniulyte, G., Rogerson, N., & Bowden, J. (2023). Evolution – removing paper and digitising the hospital. *Health and Technology*, *13*(2), 263–271. DOI: 10.1007/s12553-023-00740-8 PMID: 36846741

Baseri, Y., Chouhan, V., Ghorbani, A., & Chow, A. (2025). Evaluation framework for Quantum Security Risk Assessment: A Comprehensive Strategy for Quantum-Safe Transition. *Computers &amp. Computers & Security*, *150*, 104272. DOI: 10.1016/j.cose.2024.104272

Basnet, M., & Ali, M. H. (2021). Exploring cybersecurity issues in 5G enabled electric vehicle charging station with deep learning. *IET Generation, Transmission & Distribution*, *15*(24), 3435–3449. DOI: 10.1049/gtd2.12275

Becker, R., Ziaka, A., Tzortzatou-Nanopoulou, O., Comandè, G., Thorogood, A., Dove, E. S., Molnár-Gábor, F., & Chokoshvili, D. (2024). Purpose definition as a crucial step for determining the legal basis under the GDPR: Implications for scientific research. *Journal of Law and the Biosciences*, *11*(1), lsae001. Advance online publication. DOI: 10.1093/jlb/lsae001 PMID: 38313429

Bent, B., & Dunn, J. P. (2020). Optimizing sampling rate of wrist-worn optical sensors for physiologic monitoring. *Journal of Clinical and Translational Science*, *5*(1), e34. Advance online publication. DOI: 10.1017/cts.2020.526 PMID: 33948257

Bergies, S., Aljohani, T. M., Su, S.-F., & Elsisi, M. (2024). An IoT-based deep-learning architecture to secure automated electric vehicles against cyberattacks and data loss. *IEEE Transactions on Systems, Man, and Cybernetics. Systems*, *54*(9), 5717–5732. Advance online publication. DOI: 10.1109/TSMC.2024.3409314

Bernier, A., Molnár-Gábor, F., & Knoppers, B. M. (2022). The international data governance landscape. *Journal of Law and the Biosciences*, *9*(1), lsac005. Advance online publication. DOI: 10.1093/jlb/lsac005 PMID: 35382430

Bertino, E., & Ghinita, G. (2011). *Towards mechanisms for detection and prevention of data exfiltration by insiders*. 10–19. DOI: 10.1145/1966913.1966916

Biamonte, J., Wittek, P., Pancotti, N., Rebentrost, P., Wiebe, N., & Lloyd, S. (2017). Quantum machine learning. *Nature*, *549*(7671), 195–202. DOI: 10.1038/nature23474 PMID: 28905917

Birnstill, P., Wagner, P. G., Krempel, E., & Beyerer, J. (2018). Identity Management and Protection Motivated by the General Data Protection Regulation of the European Union—A Conceptual Framework Based on State-of-the-Art Software Technologies. *Technologies*, *6*(4), 115. DOI: 10.3390/technologies6040115

Bishop, M., & Gates, C. (2008). *Defining the insider threat*. 1–3. DOI: 10.1145/1413140.1413158

Biswal, S. P., & Kulkarni, M. S. (2021). Implications of GDPR on Emerging Technologies. *Revista Gestão Inovação e Tecnologias*, *11*(4), 4898–4912. DOI: 10.47059/revistageintec.v11i4.2512

Bohn, L., & Schiereck, D. (2022). Regulation of data breach publication: The case of US healthcare and the hitech act. *Journal of Economics and Finance*, *47*(2), 386–399. DOI: 10.1007/s12197-022-09607-6

Bollineni, C., Sharma, M., Hazra, A., Kumari, P., Manipriya, S., & Tomar, A. (2025). IoT for Next-Generation Smart Healthcare: A Comprehensive Survey. *IEEE Internet of Things Journal*, *12*(16), 32616–32639. DOI: 10.1109/JIOT.2025.3570188

Botha, N. N., Segbedzi, C. E., Dumahasi, V. K., Maneen, S., Kodom, R. V., Tsedze, I. S., Akoto, L. A., Atsu, F. S., Lasim, O. U., & Ansah, E. W. (2024). Artificial Intelligence in Healthcare: A scoping review of perceived threats to patient rights and safety. *Archives of Public Health = Archives Belges de Santé Publique*, *82*(1), 188. Advance online publication. DOI: 10.1186/s13690-024-01414-1

Bowman, S. (2013). Impact of electronic health record systems on information integrity: Quality and safety implications. *Perspectives in Health Information Management*, •••, 10. PMID: 24159271

Brakeville, S., & Perepa, B. (2018). *Blockchain basics: Introduction to distributed ledgers*. IBM Developer.

Branley-Bell, D., Sillence, E., & Coventry, L. (2021). *Promoting Cybersecurity Culture Change in Healthcare*. 544–549. DOI: 10.1145/3453892.3461622

Brännvall, R., Linge, H., & Forsgren, H. (2023). *HEIDA: Software Examples for Rapid Introduction of Homomorphic Encryption for Privacy Preservation of Health Data* (Vol. 302). Institut F R Ost Und S Dosteuropaforschung., DOI: 10.3233/SHTI230116

Brenner, M., Weir, A., McCann, M., Doyle, C., Hughes, M., Moen, A., Ingvar, M., Nauwelaerts, K., Turk, E., & McCabe, C. (2023). Development of the key performance indicators for Digital Health Interventions: A scoping review. *Digital Health*, *9*, 20552076231152160. Advance online publication. DOI: 10.1177/20552076231152160

Brown, C. (2005). HIPAA Programs: Design and Implementation. *Information Systems Security : ... International Conference, ICISS ... : Proceedings*, *14*(1), 10–20. DOI: 10.1201/1086/45098.14.1.20050301/87267.3

Buchta, R., Gkoktsis, G., Heine, F., & Kleiner, C. (2024). Advanced persistent threat attack detection systems: A review of approaches, challenges, and Trends. *Digital Threats : Research and Practice*, *5*(4), 1–37. DOI: 10.1145/3696014

Campazas-Vega, A., Crespo-Martínez, I. S., Guerrero-Higueras, Á. M., Álvarez-Aparicio, C., Matellán, V., & Fernández-Llamas, C. (2023). Malicious traffic detection on sampled network flow data with novelty-detection-based models. *Scientific Reports*, *13*(1), 15446. Advance online publication. DOI: 10.1038/s41598-023-42618-9 PMID: 37723267

Cao, H., Phan, H. V., & Silveri, S. (2024). Data breach disclosures and stock price crash risk: Evidence from data breach notification laws. *International Review of Financial Analysis*, *93*, 103164. DOI: 10.1016/j.irfa.2024.103164

Cao, Y., Romero, J., & Aspuru-Guzik, A. (2018). Potential of quantum computing for drug discovery. *IBM Journal of Research and Development*, *62*(6), 6–1. DOI: 10.1147/JRD.2018.2888987

Casino, F., Dasaklis, T. K., & Patsakis, C. (2019). A systematic literature review of blockchain-based applications: Current status, classification and open issues. *Telematics and Informatics*, *36*, 55–81. DOI: 10.1016/j.tele.2018.11.006

Celi, L. A., Dee, E. C., Yao, S., Eber, R., Mitchell, W. G., Moukheiber, L., Schirmer, J., Charpignon, M.-L., Park, J., Paguio, J., Dernoncourt, F., Situ, J., Wawira, J. G., & Cellini, J. (2022). Sources of bias in artificial intelligence that perpetuate healthcare disparities-A global review. *PLOS Digital Health, 1*(3), e0000022. DOI: 10.1371/journal.pdig.0000022 PMID: 36812532

Chakraborty, S., Aich, S., & Kim, H. C. 2019. A secure healthcare system design framework using blockchain technology. Int. Conf. Adv. Commun. Technol. ICACT 260–264., 2019-Febru.DOI: 10.23919/ICACT.2019.8701983

Chandramouli, R. (2023). *A Zero Trust Architecture Model for Access Control in Cloud Native Applications in Multi-Cloud Environments*. National Institute Of Standards Technology., DOI: 10.6028/NIST.SP.800-207A.ipd

Chandramouli, R., Iorga, M., & Chokhani, S. (2013). *Cryptographic Key Management Issues and Challenges in Cloud Services*. National Institute Of Standards Technology., DOI: 10.6028/NIST.IR.7956

Chandrasekaran, S., Agrawal, R., Dutt, V., & Vyas, N. (2023, January). Improved healthcare system with quantum computing. In *2023 International Conference on Artificial Intelligence and Smart Communication (AISC)* (pp. 99–103). IEEE.

Chang, S. E., & Chen, Y. (2020). Blockchain in Health Care Innovation: Literature Review and Case Study From a Business Ecosystem Perspective. *Journal of Medical Internet Research, 22*(8), e19480. DOI: 10.2196/19480 PMID: 32865501

Cheimonidis, P., & Rantos, K. (2023). Dynamic Risk Assessment in cybersecurity: A systematic literature review. *Future Internet, 15*(10), 324. DOI: 10.3390/fi15100324

Chen, L. (2022, February 1). *Paving the runway for standardization of Post-Quantum Cryptography*. CSRC. https://csrc.nist.gov/pubs/journal/2022/02/paving-the-runway-for-standardization-of-pqc/final

Chenais, G., Gil-Jardiné, C., & Lagarde, E. (2022). *Artificial Intelligence in Emergency Medicine: Viewpoint of Current Applications and Foreseeable Opportunities and Challenges (Preprint)*. Jmir. DOI: 10.2196/preprints.40031

Chen, G., Xu, B., Lu, M., & Chen, N.-S. (2018). Exploring blockchain technology and its potential applications for education. *Smart Learn. Environ., 5*(1), 1. DOI: 10.1186/s40561-017-0050-x

Chen, Y., Yang, S., Xu, Z., Ding, S., & Zheng, H. (2018). Blockchain-Based Medical Records Secure Storage and Medical Service Framework. *Journal of Medical Systems, 43*(1), 5. Advance online publication. DOI: 10.1007/s10916-018-1121-4 PMID: 30467604

Chin, M. H., Bruch, J. D., Grogan, C. M., Huang, E. S., Kandula, N. R., Kim, D. D., Peek, M. E., & Pollack, H. A. (2025). How to Fix a Broken Health Care System: Pathways to Maximize Health and Well-being for All. *Diabetes Care*, •••, dci250001. DOI: 10.2337/dci25-0001 PMID: 40542616

Chinnasamy, P., & Deepalakshmi, P. (2021). HCAC-EHR: Hybrid cryptographic access control for secure EHR retrieval in Healthcare Cloud. *Journal of Ambient Intelligence and Humanized Computing*, *13*(2), 1001–1019. DOI: 10.1007/s12652-021-02942-2

Chiregi, M., & Navimipour, N. J. (2018). Cloud computing and trust evaluation: A systematic literature review of the state-of-the-art mechanisms. *Journal of Electrical Systems and Information Technology*, *5*(3), 608–622. DOI: 10.1016/j.jesit.2017.09.001

Choi, Y., Johnson, M. E., & Lehmann, C. U. (2019). Data breaches in the healthcare sector: Trends and implications. *Health Affairs*, *38*(2), 206–212. DOI: 10.1377/hlthaff.2018.05072

Chronicled. (2021). *MediLedger Network*. https://www.mediledger.com

Cohen, I. (2008). Improving Time-Critical Decision Making in Life-Threatening Situations: Observations and Insights. *Decision Analysis*, *5*(2), 100–110. DOI: 10.1287/deca.1080.0111

Collins, R. (2019). Clinician Cognitive Overload and Its Implications for Nurse Leaders. *Nurse Leader*, *18*(1), 44–47. DOI: 10.1016/j.mnl.2019.11.007

Colwill, C. (2009). Human factors in information security: The insider threat – Who can you trust these days? *Information Security Technical Report*, *14*(4), 186–196. DOI: 10.1016/j.istr.2010.04.004

Cook, R. I., & Woods, D. D. (2018). *Operating at the Sharp End: The Complexity of Human Error* (pp. 255–310). Crc. DOI: 10.1201/9780203751725-13

Cooper, J., Williams, H., Hibbert, P., Edwards, A., Butt, A., Wood, F., Parry, G., Smith, P., Sheikh, A., Donaldson, L., & Carson-Stevens, A. (2018). Classification of patient-safety incidents in primary care. *Bulletin of the World Health Organization*, *96*(7), 498–505. DOI: 10.2471/BLT.17.199802

Coventry, L., & Branley, D. (2018). Cybersecurity in healthcare: A narrative review of trends, threats and ways forward. *Maturitas*, *113*, 48–52. DOI: 10.1016/j.maturitas.2018.04.008 PMID: 29903648

Cremer, F., Sheehan, B., Fortmann, M., Kia, A. N., Mullins, M., Murphy, F., & Materne, S. (2022). Cyber risk and cybersecurity: A systematic review of data availability. *The Geneva Papers on Risk and Insurance. Issues and Practice*, *47*(3), 698–736. DOI: 10.1057/s41288-022-00266-6

Cresswell, K., Hernández, A. D., Williams, R., & Sheikh, A. (2022). Key challenges and opportunities for Cloud Technology in health care: Semistructured interview study. *JMIR Human Factors*, *9*(1), e31246. Advance online publication. DOI: 10.2196/31246

Croskerry, P. (2002). Achieving Quality in Clinical Decision Making: Cognitive Strategies and Detection of Bias. *Academic Emergency Medicine*, *9*(11), 1184–1204. DOI: 10.1197/aemj.9.11.1184 PMID: 12414468

Cross, J. L., Choma, M. A., & Onofrey, J. A. (2024). Bias in medical AI: Implications for clinical decision-making. *PLOS Digital Health*, *3*(11), e0000651. DOI: 10.1371/journal.pdig.0000651 PMID: 39509461

Daah, C., Awan, I., Konur, S., & Qureshi, A. (2024). Enhancing Zero Trust Models in the Financial Industry through Blockchain Integration: A Proposed Framework. *Electronics (Basel)*, *13*(5), 865. DOI: 10.3390/electronics13050865

Dankolo, N. M., Radzi, N. H. M., Mustaffa, N. H., Arshad, N. I., Nasser, M., Gabi, D., & Yusuf, M. N. (2025). Optimizing resource allocation for IoT applications in the edge cloud continuum using hybrid metaheuristic algorithms. *Scientific Reports*, *15*(1), 14409. Advance online publication. DOI: 10.1038/s41598-025-97648-2 PMID: 40274877

Das, A., Tariq, A., Batalini, F., Dhara, B., & Banerjee, I. (2024). Exposing vulnerabilities in clinical llms through data poisoning attacks: Case study in breast cancer. *The National Library of Medicine*. DOI: 10.1101/2024.03.20.24304627

Davids, J., Lidströmer, N., & Ashrafian, H. (2022). Artificial intelligence in medicine using quantum computing in the future of healthcare. In *Artificial intelligence in medicine* (pp. 423–446). Springer. DOI: 10.1007/978-3-030-64573-1_338

Davis Iii, K. M., & Ruotsalo, T. (2025). Physiological Data: Challenges for Privacy and Ethics. *Computer*, *58*(1), 33–44. DOI: 10.1109/MC.2024.3404994

Davis, N., Raina, G., & Jagannathan, K. (2020). A framework for end-to-end deep learning-based anomaly detection in transportation networks. *Transportation Research Interdisciplinary Perspectives*, *5*, 100112. DOI: 10.1016/j.trip.2020.100112

Dawson, J. K., Missah, Y. M., Frimpong, T., & Hayfron Acquah, J. B. (2023). Ensuring privacy and confidentiality of cloud data: A comparative analysis of diverse cryptographic solutions based on run time trend. *PLoS One*, *18*(9), e0290831. DOI: 10.1371/journal.pone.0290831 PMID: 37676866

De Aguiar, E. J., Faiçal, B. S., Krishnamachari, B., & Ueyama, J. (2020). A survey of blockchain-based strategies for healthcare. *ACM Computing Surveys*, *53*(2), 1–27. Advance online publication. DOI: 10.1145/3376915

Dehling, T., Gao, F., Schneider, S., & Sunyaev, A. (2015). Exploring the far side of mobile health: Information security and privacy of mobile health apps on iOS and Android. *JMIR mHealth and uHealth*, *3*(1), e8. DOI: 10.2196/mhealth.3672 PMID: 25599627

Del-Real, C., De Busser, E., & van den Berg, B. (2025). A systematic literature review of security and privacy by design principles, norms, and strategies for Digital Technologies. *International Review of Law, Computers &amp. International Review of Law Computers & Technology*, 1–32. DOI: 10.1080/13600869.2025.2457227

Department of Health. (2018). *Lessons learned review of the WannaCry ransomware cyber attack*. UK Government. https://www.gov.uk

Dhiman, P., Hamid, Y., Kaur, A., Saini, N., Nisa, K. U., Gulzar, Y., & Turaev, S. (2024). A Review and Comparative Analysis of Relevant Approaches of Zero Trust Network Model. *Sensors (Basel)*, *24*(4), 1328. DOI: 10.3390/s24041328 PMID: 38400486

Dike, U., & Jackson, V.Uzondu C. DikeVictor M. Jackson. (2024). Telemedicine integration with cloud-based IoT: A literature review approach. *World Journal of Advanced Research and Reviews*, *24*(2), 723–131. DOI: 10.30574/wjarr.2024.24.2.3355

Dou, T., Zheng, Z., Qiu, W., & Ge, C. (2025). A Secure Medical Data Framework Integrating Blockchain and Edge Computing: An Attribute-Based Signcryption Approach. *Sensors (Basel)*, *25*(9), 2859. DOI: 10.3390/s25092859 PMID: 40363296

Drake, R., & Ridder, E. (2022). *Healthcare Cybersecurity Vulnerabilities*. 49–56. DOI: 10.19107/CYBERCON.2022.06

Drinkwater, K., & Saeed, S. (2022, April). *Integrating Cybersecurity and Disaster Recovery: A Unified Approach to Business Continuity*. ResearchGate. https://www.researchgate.net/publication/383268245_Integrating_Cybersecurity_and_Disaster_Recovery_A_Unified_Approach_to_Business_Continuity

Dunbar, P., Keyes, L. M., & Browne, J. P. (2023). Determinants of regulatory compliance in health and Social Care Services: A systematic review using the Consolidated Framework for Implementation Research. *PLoS One*, *18*(4), e0278007. Advance online publication. DOI: 10.1371/journal.pone.0278007

Dunjko, V., & Briegel, H. J. (2018). Machine learning & artificial intelligence in the quantum domain: A review of recent progress. *Reports on Progress in Physics*, *81*(7), 074001. DOI: 10.1088/1361-6633/aab406 PMID: 29504942

Durant, T. J., Knight, E., Nelson, B., Dudgeon, S., Lee, S. J., Walliman, D., Young, H. P., Ohno-Machado, L., & Schulz, W. L. (2024). A primer for quantum computing and its applications to healthcare and biomedical research. *Journal of the American Medical Informatics Association : JAMIA*, *31*(8), 1774–1784. DOI: 10.1093/jamia/ocae149 PMID: 38934288

Ekert, A., & Jozsa, R. (1996). Quantum computation and Shor's factoring algorithm. *Reviews of Modern Physics*, *68*(3), 733–753. DOI: 10.1103/RevModPhys.68.733

Elenberg, F., & Howe Iii, E. G. (2020). Ethical Challenges Posed by Big Data. *Innovations in Clinical Neuroscience*, *17*(10–12), 24–30. PMID: 33898098

Elendu, C., Omeludike, E. K., Oloyede, P. O., Obidigbo, B. T., & Omeludike, J. C. (2024). Legal implications for clinicians in cybersecurity incidents. *Revista de Medicina (São Paulo)*, *103*(39), e39887. DOI: 10.1097/MD.0000000000039887 PMID: 39331908

ElHussini, H., Assi, C., Moussa, B., Atallah, R., & Ghrayeb, A. (2021). A tale of two entities: Contextualizing the security of electric vehicle charging stations on the power grid. *ACM Transactions on the Internet of Things*, *2*(2), 1–21. DOI: 10.1145/3437258

Elkourdi, F., Xiao, L., Yu, Z., Wei, C., & Asan, O. (2024). Exploring Current Practices and Challenges of HIPAA Compliance in Software Engineering: Scoping Review. *IEEE Open Journal of Systems Engineering*, *2*, 94–104. DOI: 10.1109/OJSE.2024.3392691

Elmogazy, H., & Bamasag, O. (2016). Securing Healthcare Records in the Cloud Using Attribute-Based Encryption. *Computer and Information Science*, *9*(4), 60. DOI: 10.5539/cis.v9n4p60

El-Rewini, Z., Sadatsharan, K., Selvaraj, D. F., Plathottam, S. J., & Ranganathan, P. (2020). Cybersecurity challenges in vehicular communications. *Vehicular Communications*, *23*, 100214. DOI: 10.1016/j.vehcom.2019.100214

Elsayed, Z., Abdelgawad, A., & Elsayed, N. (2025). *Cybersecurity and Frequent Cyber Attacks on IoT Devices in Healthcare: Issues and Solutions.* /arxiv.2501.11250DOI: 10.1109/ICMI65310.2025.11141075

Enahoro, Q., Daraojimba, A., Anyanwu, E., Odilibe, I., Ogugua, J., & Akomolafe, O. (2023). The impact of electronic health records on healthcare delivery and patient outcomes: A review. *World Journal of Advanced Research and Reviews, 21*(2), 451–460. DOI: 10.30574/wjarr.2024.21.2.0478

Endalamaw, A., Khatri, R. B., Mengistu, T. S., Erku, D., Wolka, E., Zewdie, A., & Assefa, Y. (2024). A scoping review of continuous quality improvement in healthcare system: Conceptualization, models and tools, barriers and facilitators, and impact. *BMC Health Services Research, 24*(1), 487. Advance online publication. DOI: 10.1186/s12913-024-10828-0

Enescu, F. M., Bizon, N., Stirbu, C., & Ionescu, V. M. 2018. Blockchain technology applied in health the study of blockchain application in the health system (II). In: Proceedings of the 10th International Conference on Electronics, Computers and Artificial Intelligence. ECAI. https://doi.org/DOI: 10.1109/ECAI.2018.8679029

Ermakova, T., Sunyaev, A., Fabian, B., Thiebes, S., & Kornacka, M. (2020). Security and Privacy Requirements for Cloud Computing in Healthcare. *ACM Transactions on Management Information Systems, 11*(2), 1–29. DOI: 10.1145/3386160

Esposito, C., De Santis, A., Tortora, G., Chang, H., & Choo, K.-K. R. (2018). Blockchain: A panacea for healthcare cloud-based data security and privacy? *IEEE Cloud Computing, 5*(1), 31–37. DOI: 10.1109/MCC.2018.011791712

European Commission. (2016). *General Data Protection Regulation (GDPR).* https://eur-lex.europa.eu

Ewoh, P., & Vartiainen, T. (2024). Vulnerability to cyberattacks and sociotechnical solutions for Health Care Systems: Systematic review. *Journal of Medical Internet Research, 26*, e46904. Advance online publication. DOI: 10.2196/46904

Farmer, L., & Lundy, A. (2017). Informed Consent: Ethical and Legal Considerations for Advanced Practice Nurses. *The Journal for Nurse Practitioners, 13*(2), 124–130. DOI: 10.1016/j.nurpra.2016.08.011

Fathullah, M. A., Subbarao, A., & Muthaiyah, S. (2023). A systematic review: Risk Management of cloud computing projects in Healthcare. *International Journal of Management. Finance and Accounting, 4*(2), 83–115. DOI: 10.33093/ijomfa.2023.4.2.5

Fedorowicz, J., & Ray, A. W. (2004). Impact of HIPAA on the integrity of healthcare information. *International Journal of Healthcare Technology and Management*, *6*(2), 142. DOI: 10.1504/IJHTM.2004.004954

Feld, A. D. (2005). The Health Insurance Portability and Accountability Act (HIPAA): Its Broad Effect on Practice. *The American Journal of Gastroenterology*, *100*(7), 1440–1443. DOI: 10.1111/j.1572-0241.2005.50621.x PMID: 15984962

Feng, D., Qin, Y., Feng, W., Li, W., Shang, K., & Ma, H. (2024). Survey of research on confidential computing. *IET Communications*, *18*(9), 535–556. DOI: 10.1049/cmu2.12759

Ferdosi, M., Rezayatmand, R., & Molavi Taleghani, Y. (2020). Risk management in executive levels of healthcare organizations: Insights from a scoping review (2018). *Risk Management and Healthcare Policy*, *13*, 215–243. DOI: 10.2147/RMHP.S231712

Fournaris, A. P., Dimopoulos, C., Lampropoulos, K., & Koufopavlou, O. (2020). Anomaly detection trusted hardware sensors for critical infrastructure legacy devices. *Sensors (Basel)*, *20*(11), 3092. DOI: 10.3390/s20113092 PMID: 32486125

Francis, L. P. (2014). Genomic knowledge sharing: A review of the ethical and legal issues. *Applied & Translational Genomics*, *3*(4), 111–115. DOI: 10.1016/j.atg.2014.09.003 PMID: 27294025

Fu, K., & Blum, J. (2013). Controlling for cybersecurity risks of medical device software. *Communications of the ACM*, *56*(10), 35–37. DOI: 10.1145/2508701

Gabarron, E., Househ, M., Bond, C., Lau, A. Y. S., Mayer, M. A., Hansen, M., Merolli, M., Bamidis, P., & Denecke, K. (2015). Ethical Issues of Social Media Usage in Healthcare. *Yearbook of Medical Informatics*, *10*(1), 137–147. DOI: 10.15265/IY-2015-001 PMID: 26293861

Gao, F., Thiebes, S., & Sunyaev, A. (2018). Rethinking the meaning of cloud computing for Health Care: A taxonomic perspective and future research directions. *Journal of Medical Internet Research*, *20*(7), e10041. Advance online publication. DOI: 10.2196/10041

Garbis, J., & Chapman, J. W. (2021). *What Is Zero Trust?* Apress., DOI: 10.1007/978-1-4842-6702-8_2

Garofalaki, Z., Kosmanos, D., Moschoyiannis, S., Kallergis, D., & Douligeris, C. (2022). Electric vehicle charging: A survey on the security issues and challenges of the open charge point protocol (OCPP). *IEEE Communications Surveys and Tutorials*, *24*(3), 1504–1533. Advance online publication. DOI: 10.1109/COMST.2022.3184448

Georgiou, D., & Lambrinoudakis, C. (2020). Compatibility of a Security Policy for a Cloud-Based Healthcare System with the EU General Data Protection Regulation (GDPR). *Information (Basel), 11*(12), 586. DOI: 10.3390/info11120586

Georgiou, D., & Lambrinoudakis, C. (2021). Data Protection Impact Assessment (DPIA) for Cloud-Based Health Organizations. *Future Internet, 13*(3), 66. DOI: 10.3390/fi13030066

Gholami, A., & Laure, E. (2015). *Security and Privacy of Sensitive Data in Cloud Computing : A Survey of Recent Developments*. 131–150. DOI: 10.5121/csit.2015.51611

Gianfrancesco, M. A., Yazdany, J., Schmajuk, G., & Tamang, S. (2018). Potential Biases in Machine Learning Algorithms Using Electronic Health Record Data. *JAMA Internal Medicine, 178*(11), 1544. DOI: 10.1001/jamainternmed.2018.3763 PMID: 30128552

Gill, S. S., Kumar, A., Singh, H., Singh, M., Kaur, K., Usman, M., & Buyya, R. (2022). Quantum computing: A taxonomy, systematic review and future directions. *Software, Practice & Experience, 52*(1), 66–114. DOI: 10.1002/spe.3039

Giordani, M., Polese, M., Mezzavilla, M., Rangan, S., & Zorzi, M. (2020). Toward 6G networks: Use cases and technologies. *IEEE Communications Magazine, 58*(3), 55–61. DOI: 10.1109/MCOM.001.1900411

Gitonga, C. K. (2025). The impact of quantum computing on cryptographic systems: Urgency of quantum-resistant algorithms and practical applications in cryptography. *European Journal of Information Technologies and Computer Science, 5*(1), 1–10. DOI: 10.24018/compute.2025.5.1.146

Gitonga, N. K., Muketha, G. M., & Kamau, G. (2020). Cloud Data Privacy Preserving Model for Health Information Systems Based on Multi Factor Authentication. [IJRTE]. *International Journal of Recent Technology and Engineering, 9*(3), 360–367. DOI: 10.35940/ijrte.C4458.099320

Glockler, J., Sedlmeir, J., Frank, M., & Fridgen, G. (2023). A systematic review of identity and Access Management Requirements in enterprises and potential contributions of self-sovereign identity. *Business &amp. Business & Information Systems Engineering, 66*(4), 421–440. DOI: 10.1007/s12599-023-00830-x

Goel, A., Goel, A. K., & Kumar, A. (2023). The role of artificial neural network and machine learning in utilizing spatial information. *Spatial Information Research, 31*(3), 275–285. DOI: 10.1007/s41324-022-00494-x

Gonçalves-Ferreira, D., Bacelar-Silva, G. M., Sousa, M., Cruz-Correia, R., Beale, T., Frade, S., & Antunes, L. F. (2018). *OpenEHR and General Data Protection Regulation: Evaluation of Principles and Requirements (Preprint).* Jmir. DOI: 10.2196/preprints.9845

González-Granadillo, G., González-Zarzosa, S., & Diaz, R. (2021). Security Information and Event Management (SIEM): Analysis, trends, and usage in critical infrastructures. *Sensors (Basel), 21*(14), 4759. DOI: 10.3390/s21144759

Goswami, S., & Sharma, S. (2024, March). Artificial intelligence, quantum computing and cloud computing enabled personalized medicine in next generation sequencing bioinformatics. In *2024 IEEE International Conference on Interdisciplinary Approaches in Technology and Management for Social Innovation (IATMSI)* (Vol. 2, pp. 1–5). IEEE. DOI: 10.1109/IATMSI60426.2024.10502533

Griesser, G. (1989). Data protection in health information systems (HIS). *Biomedizinische Technik. Biomedical Engineering. Biomedizinische Technik. Biomedical Engineering, 34*(s1), 16–19. DOI: 10.1515/bmte.1989.34.s1.16 PMID: 2819143

Gruska, J. (1999). *Quantum computing* (Vol. 2005). McGraw-Hill.

Gunia, A. (2023). The role of trust in human-machine interaction: Cognitive science perspective. In *Artificial Intelligence, Management and Trust* (pp. 85-126). Routledge.

Guo, H., & Yu, X. (2022). A survey on blockchain technology and its security. *Blockchain: Research and Applications, 3*(2), 100067.

Gupta, S., Modgil, S., Bhatt, P. C., Jabbour, C. J. C., & Kamble, S. (2023). Quantum computing led innovation for achieving a more sustainable Covid-19 healthcare industry. *Technovation, 120*, 102544. DOI: 10.1016/j.technovation.2022.102544

Gu, X., Sabrina, F., Fan, Z., & Sohail, S. (2023). A review of Privacy Enhancement Methods for Federated Learning in healthcare systems. *International Journal of Environmental Research and Public Health, 20*(15), 6539. DOI: 10.3390/ijerph20156539

Habibzadeh, H., Dinesh, K., Shishvan, O. R., Boggio-Dandry, A., Sharma, G., & Soyata, T. (2019). A survey of healthcare Internet of Things (HIoT): A clinical perspective. *IEEE Internet of Things Journal, 7*(1), 53–71. DOI: 10.1109/JIOT.2019.2946359 PMID: 33748312

Haney, J., Jacobs, J., & Lutters, W. (2021). Cybersecurity Advocates: Force Multipliers in Security Behavior Change. *IEEE Security and Privacy, 19*(4), 54–59. DOI: 10.1109/MSEC.2021.3077405 PMID: 37051374

Haque, R. U., Hasan, A. S. M. T., Daria, A., Rasool, A., Chen, H., Jiang, Q., & Zhang, Y. (2023). A novel secure and distributed architecture for privacy-preserving healthcare system. *Journal of Network and Computer Applications*, *217*, 103696. DOI: 10.1016/j.jnca.2023.103696

Hardjono, T., & Smith, N. (2021). Towards an attestation architecture for blockchain networks. *World Wide Web (Bussum)*, *24*(5), 1587–1615. DOI: 10.1007/s11280-021-00869-4

Hassan, J., Shehzad, D., Habib, U., Aftab, M. U., Ahmad, M., Kuleev, R., & Mazzara, M. (2022). The Rise Of Cloud Computing: Data Protection, Privacy, and open research challenges—a systematic literature review (SLR). *Computational Intelligence and Neuroscience*, *2022*, 1–26. DOI: 10.1155/2022/8303504

Hassan, O. F., Fatai, F. O., Sanusi, M. A., Akinde, A. O., Aderibigbe, O., Onasanya, T., & Odukoya, O. (2024). Enhancing Cybersecurity through Cloud Computing Solutions in the United States. *Intelligent Information Management*, *16*(04), 176–193. DOI: 10.4236/iim.2024.164011

Hatzivasilis, G., Goeke, L., Hildebrandt, T., Ioannidis, S., Spanoudakis, G., Lefthériotis, G., Koshutanski, H., Oikonomou, F., Frati, F., Tsakirakis, G., & Smyrlis, M. (2020). Modern Aspects of Cyber-Security Training and Continuous Adaptation of Programmes to Trainees. *Applied Sciences (Basel, Switzerland)*, *10*(16), 5702. DOI: 10.3390/app10165702

Haufe, K., Dzombeta, S., & Brandis, K. (2014). Proposal for a Security Management in Cloud Computing for Health Care. *TheScientificWorldJournal*, *2014*(6), 1–7. DOI: 10.1155/2014/146970 PMID: 24701137

He, Y., Aliyu, A., Evans, M., & Luo, C. (2021). Health Care Cybersecurity challenges and solutions under the climate of covid-19: Scoping review. *Journal of Medical Internet Research*, *23*(4), e21747. Advance online publication. DOI: 10.2196/21747

He, Y., Maglaras, L., Aliyu, A., & Luo, C. (2022). Healthcare Security Incident Response Strategy - A Proactive Incident Response (IR) procedure. *Security and Communication Networks*, *2022*, 1–10. DOI: 10.1155/2022/2775249

He, Y., Zamani, E. D., Lloyd, S., & Luo, C. (2022). Agile incident response (air): Improving the incident response process in healthcare. *International Journal of Information Management*, *62*, 102435. DOI: 10.1016/j.ijinfomgt.2021.102435

HHS (U.S. Department of Health and Human Services). (2023). *Breach portal: Notice to the Secretary of HHS*. https://ocrportal.hhs.gov

Hijji, M., & Alam, G. (2021). A Multivocal Literature Review on Growing Social Engineering Based Cyber-Attacks/Threats During the COVID-19 Pandemic: Challenges and Prospective Solutions. *IEEE Access : Practical Innovations, Open Solutions*, *9*(3), 7152–7169. DOI: 10.1109/ACCESS.2020.3048839 PMID: 34786300

Hiwale, M., Walambe, R., Potdar, V., & Kotecha, K. (2023). A systematic review of privacy-preserving methods deployed with blockchain and federated learning for the telemedicine. *Healthcare Analytics (New York, N.y.)*, *3*, 100192. DOI: 10.1016/j.health.2023.100192

Hong, J., Song, T. J., Lee, H., & Zaboli, A. (2022). Automated cybersecurity tester for IEC61850-based digital substations. *Energies*, *15*(21), 7833. DOI: 10.3390/en15217833

Horowitz, M., & Grumbling, E. (Eds.). (2019). *Quantum computing: progress and prospects*.

Hughes, A., Shandhi, M. M. H., Master, H., Dunn, J., & Brittain, E. (2023). Wearable Devices in Cardiovascular Medicine. *Circulation Research*, *132*(5), 652–670. DOI: 10.1161/CIRCRESAHA.122.322389 PMID: 36862812

Hummel, P., Braun, M., Tretter, M., & Dabrock, P. (2021). Data sovereignty: A Review. *Big Data &amp. Big Data & Society*, *8*(1), 2053951720982012. Advance online publication. DOI: 10.1177/2053951720982012

Hussain, M. I., Razque, F., He, J., Zardari, Z. A., Sabah, F., Zhu, N., & Hussain, S. (2021). AAAA: SSO and MFA Implementation in Multi-Cloud to Mitigate Rising Threats and Concerns Related to User Metadata. *Applied Sciences (Basel, Switzerland)*, *11*(7), 3012. DOI: 10.3390/app11073012

Hussein, Z., Salama, M. A., & El-Rahman, S. A. (2023). Evolution of blockchain consensus algorithms: A review on the latest milestones of blockchain consensus algorithms. *Cybersecurity*, *6*(1), 30. DOI: 10.1186/s42400-023-00163-y

Ianculescu, M., Constantin, V.- ., Gu atu, A.-M., Petrache, M.-C., Mihăescu, A.-G., Bica, O., & Alexandru, A. (2025). Enhancing Connected Health Ecosystems Through IoT-Enabled Monitoring Technologies: A Case Study of the Monit4Healthy System. *Sensors (Basel)*, *25*(7), 2292. DOI: 10.3390/s25072292 PMID: 40218804

IBM. (2023). *X-Force Threat Intelligence Index 2023*. https://www.ibm.com/reports/threat-intelligence

Imoize, A. L., Balas, V. E., Solanki, V. K., Lee, C. C., & Obaidat, M. S. (Eds.). (2023). *Handbook of Security and Privacy of AI-Enabled Healthcare Systems and Internet of Medical Things* (pp. 1–460). CRC press.

Isibor, E. (2024). Regulation of healthcare data security: Legal obligations in a digital age. *Available at SSRN* 4957244. DOI: 10.2139/ssrn.4957244

Islam, M. S., & Rahman, M. S. (2025). LogStamping: A blockchain-based log auditing approach for large-scale systems. *arXiv Preprint arXiv:2505.17236.*

Islam, R., Bose, R., Roy, S., Khan, A. A., Sutradhar, S., Das, S., Ali, F., & AlZubi, A. A. (2025). Decentralized trust framework for smart cities: A blockchain-enabled cybersecurity and data integrity model. *Scientific Reports*, *15*(1), 23454. DOI: 10.1038/s41598-025-06405-y PMID: 40603417

Islam, R., Weir, C. R., Jones, M., Del Fiol, G., & Samore, M. H. (2015). Understanding complex clinical reasoning in infectious diseases for improving clinical decision support design. *BMC Medical Informatics and Decision Making*, *15*(1), 101. Advance online publication. DOI: 10.1186/s12911-015-0221-z PMID: 26620881

Islam, S., Papastergiou, S., & Silvestri, S. (2022). Cyber threat analysis using natural language processing for a secure healthcare system. *2022 IEEE Symposium on Computers and Communications (ISCC)*, 1–7. DOI: 10.1109/ISCC55528.2022.9912768

Isong, B., Kgote, O., & Abu-Mahfouz, A. (2024). Insights into Modern Intrusion Detection Strategies for Internet of Things Ecosystems. *Electronics (Basel)*, *13*(12), 2370. DOI: 10.3390/electronics13122370

Issaoui, A., Örtensjö, J., & Islam, M. S. (2023). Exploring the General Data Protection Regulation (GDPR) compliance in cloud services: Insights from Swedish public organizations on privacy compliance. *Future Business Journal*, *9*(1), 107. Advance online publication. DOI: 10.1186/s43093-023-00285-2

Jaatun, M. G., Cruzes, D. S., Moe, N. B., Tøndel, I. A., Bernsmed, K., & Haugset, B. (2018). Accountability Requirements in the Cloud Provider Chain. *Symmetry*, *10*(4), 124. DOI: 10.3390/sym10040124

Jackson, N., Woods, J., Watkinson, P., Brent, A., Peto, T. E. A., Walker, A. S., & Eyre, D. W. (2023). The quality of vital signs measurements and value preferences in electronic medical records varies by hospital, specialty, and patient demographics. *Scientific Reports*, *13*(1), 3858. Advance online publication. DOI: 10.1038/s41598-023-30691-z PMID: 36890179

Jafleh, E. A., Alnaqbi, F. A., Almaeeni, H. A., Faqeeh, S., Alzaabi, M. A., & Al Zaman, K. (2024). The Role of Wearable Devices in Chronic Disease Monitoring and Patient Care: A Comprehensive Review. *Cureus*, *16*(9). Advance online publication. DOI: 10.7759/cureus.68921 PMID: 39381470

Jafri, R., & Singh, S. (2022). Blockchain applications for the healthcare sector: Uses beyond Bitcoin. In *Elsevier eBooks* (71–92). DOI: 10.1016/B978-0-323-90615-9.00022-0

Jahankhani, H., Kendzierskyj, S., Jamal, A., & Epiphaniou, G. H. 2019. In: Al-Khateeb(Ed.), Blockchain and Clinical Trial Securing Patient Data (Advanced Sciences and Technologies for Security Applications).

Jain, R. B., & Puri, M. (2020). An approach towards the development of scalable data masking for preserving privacy of sensitive business data. In *Artificial Intelligence and Evolutionary Computations in Engineering Systems* (pp. 733–743). Springer Singapore. DOI: 10.1007/978-981-15-0199-9_63

Jaiswal, S., Bahadur, P. S., Singh, S., & Rajpoot, S. (2023a, September). Progressive Technology of InfraRed Spectroscopy for Characterization of Materials. In Proceedings of the 6th International Conference on Contemporary Computing and Informatics (IC3I). IEEE. DOI: 10.1109/IC3I59117.2023.10397795

Jaiswal, S., Machiraju, M. S., & Kaustubh, M. H. (2023b, November 24–26). Review of novel technology in cochlear implants among special needs children. In Proceedings of the 2023 10th IEEE Uttar Pradesh Section International Conference on Electrical, Electronics and Computer Engineering (UPCON) (pp. 370–374). IEEE. DOI: 10.1109/UPCON59197.2023.10434570

Jaiswal, S., Singh, P., Srivastav, S., Chaudhary, R., & Kumar, A. (2024, November 14–16). Noval technology of nano-robot for promising drug delivery system. In Proceedings of the 2024 7th International Conference on Contemporary Computing and Informatics (IC3I) (pp. 858–863). IEEE. DOI: 10.1109/IC3I61595.2024.10829002

Jaiswal, S., & Khanam, S. Z. (2025). Techno-Economic Analysis of Green Hydrogen Production for Industrial Use. In Mabrouki, J. (Ed.), *Obstacles Facing Hydrogen Green Systems and Green Energy* (pp. 479–506). IGI Global Scientific Publishing., DOI: 10.4018/979-8-3693-8980-5.ch028

Jasim, L. H., Mishra, A., Joshi, S. K., & Sapaev, I. B., DR, P., & Babu, A. N. (2023). Analysing blockchain-based cryptography: Enhancing security, transparency, and practical implementations. *2023 International Conference for Technological Engineering and Its Applications in Sustainable Development (ICTEASD)*, 39–44. DOI: 10.1109/ICTEASD57136.2023.10585016

Jayanthi, P., Rai, B. K., & Muralikrishna, I. (2022). The potential of quantum computing in healthcare. In *Technology road mapping for quantum computing and engineering* (pp. 81–101). IGI Global. DOI: 10.4018/978-1-7998-9183-3.ch006

Jeyaraman, N., Jeyaraman, M., Yadav, S., Ramasubramanian, S., & Balaji, S. (2024). Revolutionizing healthcare: The emerging role of quantum computing in enhancing medical technology and treatment. *Cureus, 16*(8). Advance online publication. DOI: 10.7759/cureus.67486 PMID: 39310567

Jiang, L. (2021). IoT Sensors for Smart Health Devices and Data security in Healthcare. *Journal of Biomedical and Sustainable Healthcare Applications*, 105–112. DOI: 10.53759/0088/JBSHA202101013

Jiang, J., & Bai, G. (2019). Types of Information Compromised in Breaches of Protected Health Information. *Annals of Internal Medicine, 172*(2), 159–160. DOI: 10.7326/M19-1759 PMID: 31546251

Jpc Rodrigues, J., De La Torre, I., Fernández, G., & López-Coronado, M. (2013). Analysis of the Security and Privacy Requirements of Cloud-Based Electronic Health Records Systems. *Journal of Medical Internet Research, 15*(8), e186. DOI: 10.2196/jmir.2494 PMID: 23965254

Kabra, M., C, P. H., & Rao, M. (2022). Design and evaluation of performance-efficient SOC-on-FPGA for cloud-based healthcare applications. *2022 IEEE Nordic Circuits and Systems Conference (NorCAS)*, 1–6. DOI: 10.1109/NorCAS57515.2022.9934217

Kagita, M. K., Thilakarathne, N., Gadekallu, T. R., & Maddikunta, P. K. R. (2022). A review on security and privacy of internet of medical things. *Intelligent internet of things for healthcare and industry*, 171-187.

Kang, M., Park, E., Cho, B. H., & Lee, K.-S. (2018). Recent Patient Health Monitoring Platforms Incorporating Internet of Things-Enabled Smart Devices. *International Neurourology Journal, 22*(4), 313. DOI: 10.5213/inj.1820corr.001 PMID: 30599503

Kaplan, B. (2020). Phi protection under hipaa: An overall analysis. *Kaplan, B.(with appendix by Monteiro, APL)," PHI Protection under HIPAA: An Overall Analysis," LGPD na Saúde (LGPD Applicable to Health), Dallari, AB, Monaco, GFC, ed., São Paulo: Editora Revista dos Tribunais (Thomsom Reuters), 2021*, 61-88.

Kassam, I., Ilkina, D., Kemp, J., Roble, H., Carter-Langford, A., & Shen, N. (2023a). Patient perspectives and preferences for consent in the digital health context: State-of-the-art literature review. *Journal of Medical Internet Research, 25*, e42507. Advance online publication. DOI: 10.2196/42507

Kavousi-Fard, A., Jin, T., Su, W., & Parsa, N. (2020). An effective anomaly detection model for securing communications in electric vehicles. *IEEE Transactions on Industry Applications*. Advance online publication. DOI: 10.1109/TIA.2020

Kedi, W. E., Ejimuda, C., & Ajegbile, M. D. (2024). Cloud computing in healthcare: A comprehensive review of data storage and Analysis Solutions. *World Journal of Advanced Engineering Technology and Sciences, 12*(2), 290–298. DOI: 10.30574/wjaets.2024.12.2.0291

Kerasidou, A., & Kerasidou, C. (2023). Data-driven research and Healthcare: Public Trust, data governance and the NHS. *BMC Medical Ethics, 24*(1), 51. Advance online publication. DOI: 10.1186/s12910-023-00922-z

Khadka, K., & Ullah, A. B. (2025). Human factors in cybersecurity: An interdisciplinary review and framework proposal. *International Journal of Information Security, 24*(3), 119. Advance online publication. DOI: 10.1007/s10207-025-01032-0

Khan, B., Hussain, J., Hanan, A., Qureshi, A., Abdullah, S., Kumar, S., & Fatima, H. (2023). Drawbacks of Artificial Intelligence and Their Potential Solutions in the Healthcare Sector. *Biomedical Materials &amp. Biomedical Materials & Devices, 1*(2), 731–738. DOI: 10.1007/s44174-023-00063-2 PMID: 36785697

Khan, M. M., & Alkhathami, M. (2024). Anomaly detection in IOT-based healthcare: Machine Learning for Enhanced Security. *Scientific Reports, 14*(1), 5872. Advance online publication. DOI: 10.1038/s41598-024-56126-x

Kim, J. W., Moon, S.-M., Jang, B., & Kang, S.-U. (2020). Effective Privacy-Preserving Collection of Health Data from a User's Wearable Device. *Applied Sciences (Basel, Switzerland), 10*(18), 6396. DOI: 10.3390/app10186396

Kim, J., Kim, H., Cho, S., Kang, P., & Park, M. (2019). Insider Threat Detection Based on User Behavior Modeling and Anomaly Detection Algorithms. *Applied Sciences (Basel, Switzerland), 9*(19), 4018. DOI: 10.3390/app9194018

Kim, K., Kim, J. S., Jeong, S., Park, J. H., & Kim, H. K. (2021). Cybersecurity for autonomous vehicles: Review of attacks and defense. *Computers & Security, 103*, 102150. DOI: 10.1016/j.cose.2020.102150

Kim, W., & Choi, J. (2016). Challenges for wearable healthcare services. *International Journal of Web and Grid Services, 12*(4), 407. DOI: 10.1504/IJWGS.2016.080141

Kiseleva, A., Kotzinos, D., & De Hert, P. (2022). Transparency of AI in healthcare as a multilayered system of accountabilities: Between legal requirements and technical limitations. *Frontiers in Artificial Intelligence, 5*, 879603. Advance online publication. DOI: 10.3389/frai.2022.879603

Koczkodaj, , W., Masiak, J., F Zabrodskii, P., Strzałka, D., & Mazurek, M. (2019). Massive Health Record Breaches Evidenced by the Office for Civil Rights Data. *Iranian Journal of Public Health, 48*(2). Advance online publication. DOI: 10.18502/ijph.v48i2.826 PMID: 31205882

Kombe, C., Ally, M., & Sam, A. (2018). A review on healthcare information systems and consensus protocols in blockchain technology. *Int. J. Adv. Technol. Eng. Explor., 5*(49), 473–483. DOI: 10.19101/IJATEE.2018.547023

Koonin, L. M., Hoots, B., Tsang, C. A., Leroy, Z., Farris, K., Jolly, B., Antall, P., McCabe, B., Zelis, C. B. R., Tong, I., & Harris, A. M. (2020). Trends in the use of telehealth during the emergence of the COVID-19 pandemic—United States, January–March 2020. *MMWR. Morbidity and Mortality Weekly Report, 69*(43), 1595–1599. DOI: 10.15585/mmwr.mm6943a3 PMID: 33119561

Kop, M., Slijpen, S., Liu, K., Lee, J.H., Albrecht, C., & Cohen, I.G. (2024). How Quantum Technologies May Be Integrated Into Healthcare, What Regulators Should Consider. *What Regulators Should Consider (December 05, 2024).*

Kotsias, J., Ahmad, A., & Scheepers, R. (2022). Adopting and integrating cyber-threat Intelligence in a commercial organisation. *European Journal of Information Systems, 32*(1), 35–51. DOI: 10.1080/0960085X.2022.2088414

Kritikos, K., Papageorgiou, N., & Tsamoura, E. (2021). A systematic review of API security threats in healthcare applications. *Computer Standards & Interfaces, 75*, 103513. DOI: 10.1016/j.csi.2021.103513

Krotsiani, M., Spanoudakis, G., & Kloukinas, C. (2015). Monitoring-based certification of Cloud Service Security. *Lecture Notes in Computer Science, 9415*, 644–659. DOI: 10.1007/978-3-319-26148-5_44

Kruse, C. S., Frederick, B., Jacobson, T., & Monticone, D. K. (2017). Cybersecurity in healthcare: A systematic review of modern threats and trends. *Technology and Health Care, 25*(1), 1–10. DOI: 10.3233/THC-161263 PMID: 27689562

Kumar, G., Yadav, S., Mukherjee, A., Hassija, V., & Guizani, M. (2024). Recent advances in quantum computing for drug discovery and development. *IEEE Access : Practical Innovations, Open Solutions, 12*, 64491–64509. DOI: 10.1109/ACCESS.2024.3376408

Kuo, A. M.-H. (2011). Opportunities and Challenges of Cloud Computing to Improve Health Care Services. *Journal of Medical Internet Research, 13*(3), e67. DOI: 10.2196/jmir.1867 PMID: 21937354

Lamptey, M., & Zhou, G. (2020). Survey of Data Confidentiality and Privacy in the Cloud Computing Environment. *Computer Engineering and Intelligent Systems, 11*(5). Advance online publication. DOI: 10.7176/CEIS/11-5-03

LaPierre, R. (2021). *Introduction to quantum computing*. Springer Nature. DOI: 10.1007/978-3-030-69318-3

Lee, T.-F., Chang, I.-P., & Su, G.-J. (2023). Compliance with hipaa and gdpr in certificateless-based authenticated key agreement using extended chaotic maps. *Electronics (Basel), 12*(5), 1108. DOI: 10.3390/electronics12051108

Li, D. M., Parikh, S., & Costa, A. (2025). A critical look into artificial intelligence and healthcare disparities. *Frontiers in Artificial Intelligence, 8*, 1545869. Advance online publication. DOI: 10.3389/frai.2025.1545869 PMID: 40115119

Li, E., Clarke, J., Ashrafian, H., Darzi, A., & Neves, A. L. (2022). The impact of electronic health record interoperability on safety and quality of care in high-income countries: Systematic Review. *Journal of Medical Internet Research, 24*(9), e38144. Advance online publication. DOI: 10.2196/38144

Lieneck, C., McLauchlan, M., & Phillips, S. (2023). Healthcare cybersecurity ethical concerns during the COVID-19 Global Pandemic: A Rapid Review. *Healthcare (Basel), 11*(22), 2983. DOI: 10.3390/healthcare11222983

Linkov, I., & Kott, A. (2019). Fundamental concepts of cyber resilience: Introduction and overview. In *Cyber resilience of systems and networks* (pp. 1–25). Springer. DOI: 10.1007/978-3-319-77492-3_1

Lin, Y. D., Wang, Z. Y., Lin, P. C., Nguyen, V. L., Hwang, R. H., & Lai, Y. C. (2022). Multi-datasource machine learning in intrusion detection: Packet flows, system logs and host statistics. *Journal of Information Security and Applications, 68*, 103248. DOI: 10.1016/j.jisa.2022.103248

Liu, G., Xie, H., Wang, W., & Huang, H. (2024). A secure and efficient electronic medical record data sharing scheme based on blockchain and proxy re-encryption. *Journal of Cloud Computing (Heidelberg, Germany), 13*(1), 44. Advance online publication. DOI: 10.1186/s13677-024-00608-w

Liu, N., & Chen, S. (2022). The Protection Mechanism of Personal Health Information in the Digital Economy Environment. *Journal of Environmental and Public Health, 2022*(10), 1–17. DOI: 10.1155/2022/2314468 PMID: 35733982

Liu, S., Chen, B., Zourntos, T., Kundur, D., & Butler-Purry, K. (2014). A coordinated multi-switch attack for cascading failures in smart grid. *IEEE Transactions on Smart Grid, 5*(3), 1183–1195. DOI: 10.1109/TSG.2014.2302476

Liu, X., Shah, R., Shandilya, A., Shah, M., & Pandya, A. (2024). A systematic study on integrating blockchain in healthcare for electronic health record management and tracking medical supplies. *Journal of Cleaner Production*, *447*, 141371. DOI: 10.1016/j.jclepro.2024.141371

Liu, Y.-K., & Moody, D. (2024). Post-quantum cryptography and the Quantum Future of Cybersecurity. *Physical Review Applied*, *21*(4), 040501. Advance online publication. DOI: 10.1103/PhysRevApplied.21.040501

Li, Y., Wang, Y., Wu, M., & Li, H. (2019). Replay attack and defense of electric vehicle charging on GB/T 27930-2015 communication protocol. *Journal of Computer and Communications*, *7*(12), 20–30. DOI: 10.4236/jcc.2019.712003

Lopes, , A. P., & Gondim, P. R. L. (2020). Mutual Authentication Protocol for D2D Communications in a Cloud-Based E-Health System. *Sensors (Basel)*, *20*(7), 2072. DOI: 10.3390/s20072072 PMID: 32272675

Lorenzini, G., Shaw, D. M., & Elger, B. S. (2022). It takes a pirate to know one: Ethical hackers for healthcare cybersecurity. *BMC Medical Ethics*, *23*(1), 131. Advance online publication. DOI: 10.1186/s12910-022-00872-y PMID: 36494715

Loyka, K., Zhou, H., & Khatri, S. P. (2018). *A Homomorphic Encryption Scheme Based on Affine Transforms*. 51–56. DOI: 10.1145/3194554.3194585

Macedo, E. L. C., De Rezende, J. F., Delicato, F. C., De Oliveira, E. A. R., Silva, F. H., Mello, R. R., Franca, F. M. G., & De Moraes, L. F. M. (2019). On the security aspects of Internet of Things: A systematic literature review. *Journal of Communications and Networks (Seoul)*, *21*(5), 444–457. DOI: 10.1109/JCN.2019.000048

Machal, M. L. (2023). *An Overview About Connected Medical Devices and Their Risks*. Institut F R Ost Und S Dosteuropaforschung., DOI: 10.3233/SHTI230438

Mackey, T. K., & Nayyar, G. (2017). A review of existing and emerging digital technologies to combat the global trade in fake medicines. *Expert Opinion on Drug Safety*, *16*(5), 587–602. DOI: 10.1080/14740338.2017.1313227 PMID: 28349715

Madanian, S., Airehrour, D., Subasinghage, M., Chinbat, T., Yongchareon, S., & Hassandoust, F. (2024). Health IoT Threats: Survey of Risks and Vulnerabilities. *Future Internet*, *16*(11), 389. DOI: 10.3390/fi16110389

Mahboubi, A., Luong, K., Aboutorab, H., Bui, H. T., Jarrad, G., Bahutair, M., Camtepe, S., Pogrebna, G., Ahmed, E., Barry, B., & Gately, H. (2024). Evolving techniques in cyber threat hunting: A systematic review. *Journal of Network and Computer Applications*, *232*, 104004. DOI: 10.1016/j.jnca.2024.104004

Maksuti, S., Bicaku, A., Zsilak, M., Ivkic, I., Péceli, B., Singler, G., Kovács, K., Tauber, M., & Delsing, J. (2021). Automated and secure onboarding for system of systems. *IEEE Access : Practical Innovations, Open Solutions*, *9*, 111095–111113. DOI: 10.1109/ACCESS.2021.3102280

Malina, L., Dzurenda, P., Ricci, S., Hajny, J., Srivastava, G., Matulevičius, R., Affia, A.-A. O., Laurent, M., Sultan, N. H., & Tang, Q. (2021). Post-quantum era privacy protection for intelligent infrastructures. *IEEE Access : Practical Innovations, Open Solutions*, *9*, 36038–36077. DOI: 10.1109/ACCESS.2021.3062201

Mamdiwar, S. D., & Srinivasan, K. (2021). Recent Advances on IoT-Assisted Wearable Sensor Systems for Healthcare Monitoring. *Biosensors (Basel)*, *11*(10), 372. DOI: 10.3390/bios11100372 PMID: 34677328

Mandarino, V., Pappalardo, G., & Tramontana, E. (2024). A Blockchain-Based Electronic Health Record (EHR) System for Edge Computing Enhancing Security and Cost Efficiency. *Computers*, *13*(6), 132. DOI: 10.3390/computers13060132

Marengo, A., & Santamato, V. (2025). Quantum algorithms and complexity in healthcare applications: A systematic review with machine learning-optimized analysis. *Frontiers of Computer Science*, *7*, 1584114. Advance online publication. DOI: 10.3389/fcomp.2025.1584114

Marko, J. G. O., Neagu, C. D., & Anand, P. B. (2025). Examining inclusivity: the use of AI and diverse populations in health and social care: a systematic review. *BMC Medical Informatics and Decision Making*, *25*(1), 57. Advance online publication. DOI: 10.1186/s12911-025-02884-1 PMID: 39910518

Maronese, M., Destri, C., & Prati, E. (2022). Quantum activation functions for quantum neural networks. *Quantum Information Processing*, *21*(4), 128. DOI: 10.1007/s11128-022-03466-0

Martin, G., Ghafur, S., Kinross, J., Hankin, C., & Darzi, A. (2017). WannaCry—A year on. *BMJ (Clinical Research Ed.)*, *361*, k2381. DOI: 10.1136/bmj.k2381 PMID: 29866711

Mayer, R. C., & Mayer, B. M. (2024). Towards interdisciplinary scholarship in trust: the needs, some leads, and a seed. In *A Research Agenda for Trust* (pp. 1–10). Edward Elgar Publishing. DOI: 10.4337/9781802200942.00008

McCallen, J., Schmardebeck, R., Shipman, J. E., & Whited, R. L. (2022). Evidence on the 2020 exemption of low-revenue issuers from the internal control audit requirement. *Available at SSRN* 3420787.

McLeod, A., & Dolezel, D. (2018). Cyber-analytics: Modeling factors associated with healthcare data breaches. *Decision Support Systems*, *108*, 57–68. DOI: 10.1016/j.dss.2018.02.007

Mehrtak, M., SeyedAlinaghi, S. A., MohsseniPour, M., Noori, T., Karimi, A., Shamsabadi, A., Heydari, M., Barzegary, A., Mirzapour, P., Soleymanzadeh, M., Vahedi, F., Mehraeen, E., & Dadras, O. (2021). Security challenges and solutions using healthcare cloud computing. *Journal of Medicine and Life*, *14*(4), 448–461. DOI: 10.25122/jml-2021-0100

Memon, M., Wagner, S. R., Pedersen, C. F., Beevi, F. H. A., & Hansen, F. O. (2014). Ambient assisted living healthcare frameworks, platforms, standards, and quality attributes. *Sensors (Basel)*, *14*(3), 4312–4341. DOI: 10.3390/s140304312 PMID: 24599192

Mennella, C., Maniscalco, U., De Pietro, G., & Esposito, M. (2024). Ethical and regulatory challenges of AI technologies in healthcare: A narrative review. *Heliyon*, *10*(4), e26297. DOI: 10.1016/j.heliyon.2024.e26297 PMID: 38384518

Mensah, F. (2024). Zero trust architecture: A comprehensive review of principles, implementation strategies, and future directions in enterprise cybersecurity. [IJAIRI]. *International Journal of Academic and Industrial Research Innovations*, *10*, 339–346.

Merlec, M. M., Lee, Y. K., Hong, S.-P., & In, H. P. (2021). A smart contract-based dynamic consent management system for personal data usage under GDPR. *Sensors (Basel)*, *21*(23), 7994. DOI: 10.3390/s21237994 PMID: 34883997

Mishra, A. K., Govil, M. C., Pilli, E. S., & Bijalwan, A. (2022). Digital Forensic Investigation of healthcare data in cloud computing environment. *Journal of Healthcare Engineering*, *2022*, 1–11. DOI: 10.1155/2022/9709101

Mittelstadt, B. (2019). The Ethics of Biomedical 'Big Data' Analytics. *Philosophy &amp. Philosophy & Technology*, *32*(1), 17–21. DOI: 10.1007/s13347-019-00344-z

Mittelstadt, B. D., & Floridi, L. (2015). The Ethics of Big Data: Current and Foreseeable Issues in Biomedical Contexts. *Science and Engineering Ethics*, *22*(2), 303–341. DOI: 10.1007/s11948-015-9652-2 PMID: 26002496

Mohamed, N. (2025). Artificial Intelligence and machine learning in cybersecurity: A deep dive into state-of-the-art techniques and future paradigms. *Knowledge and Information Systems*, *67*(8), 6969–7055. Advance online publication. DOI: 10.1007/s10115-025-02429-y

Mone, V., & Shakhlo, F. (2023). Health Data on the Go: Navigating Privacy Concerns with Wearable Technologies. *Legal Information Management, 23*(3), 179–188. DOI: 10.1017/S1472669623000427

Montesinos, L., Checa Rifá, P., Rifá Fabregat, M., Maldonado-Romo, J., Capacci, S., Maccaro, A., & Piaggio, D. (2024). Sustainability across the medical device lifecycle: A scoping review. *Sustainability (Basel), 16*(4), 1433. DOI: 10.3390/su16041433

Morić, Z., Dakić, V., & Regvart, D. (2025). Advancing Cybersecurity with honeypots and deception strategies. *Informatics (MDPI), 12*(1), 14. DOI: 10.3390/informatics12010014

Morita, P. P., Kaur, J., & Miranda, P. A. (2024a). Enhancing public health research: A viewpoint report on the transition to secure, cloud-based systems. *Frontiers in Public Health, 11*, 1270450. Advance online publication. DOI: 10.3389/fpubh.2023.1270450

Mukta, R., Paik, H., Lu, Q., & Kanhere, S. S. (2022). A survey of data minimisation techniques in blockchain-based healthcare. *Computer Networks, 205*, 108766. DOI: 10.1016/j.comnet.2022.108766

Munjal, K., & Bhatia, R. (2022). A systematic review of homomorphic encryption and its contributions in healthcare industry. *Complex &amp. Complex & Intelligent Systems, 9*(4), 3759–3786. DOI: 10.1007/s40747-022-00756-z

Musamih, A., Jayaraman, R., Salah, K., Hasan, H. R., Yaqoob, I., & Al-Hammadi, Y. (2021b). Blockchain-based solution for distribution and delivery of COVID-19 vaccines. *IEEE Access : Practical Innovations, Open Solutions, 9*, 71372–71387. DOI: 10.1109/ACCESS.2021.3079197 PMID: 34812393

Musamih, A., Salah, K., Jayaraman, R., Arshad, J., Debe, M., Al-Hammadi, Y., & Ellahham, S. (2021a). A Blockchain-Based approach for drug traceability in healthcare supply chain. *IEEE Access : Practical Innovations, Open Solutions, 9*, 9728–9743. DOI: 10.1109/ACCESS.2021.3049920

Musamih, A., Salah, K., Jayaraman, R., Yaqoob, I., Al-Hammadi, Y., & Antony, J. (2022). Blockchain-based solution for COVID-19 vaccine waste reduction. *Journal of Cleaner Production, 372*(August), 133619. DOI: 10.1016/j.jclepro.2022.133619 PMID: 35999948

Mysore, N. R. (2022). Healthcare System 4.0 Driven by Quantum Computing and Its Use Cases: A COVID-19 Perspective. In *Artificial Intelligence, Machine Learning and Blockchain in Quantum Satellite, Drone and Network* (pp. 107–126). CRC Press.

Nabil, S. S., Alam Pran, M. S., Al Haque, A. A., Chakraborty, N. R., Chowdhury, M. J. M., & Ferdous, M. S. (2022). Blockchain-based COVID vaccination registration and monitoring. *Blockchain Res. Appl.*, *3*(4), 100092. Advance online publication. DOI: 10.1016/j.bcra.2022.100092

Nadji, B. (2024). Data security, integrity, and protection. In *Data, Security, and Trust in Smart Cities* (pp. 59–83). Springer Nature Switzerland. DOI: 10.1007/978-3-031-61117-9_4

Nasir, M., Siddiqui, K., & Ahmed, S. (2025). Ethical-legal implications of AI-powered healthcare in critical perspective. *Frontiers in Artificial Intelligence*, *8*, 1619463. Advance online publication. DOI: 10.3389/frai.2025.1619463 PMID: 40673212

Natarajan, M., Bharathi, A., Varun, C. S., & Selvarajan, S. (2025). Quantum secure patient login credential system using blockchain for electronic health record sharing framework. *Scientific Reports*, *15*(1), 4023. Advance online publication. DOI: 10.1038/s41598-025-86658-9 PMID: 39894869

Nazer, L. H., Ma, H., Mathur, P., Khanna, A. K., Zatarah, R., Moukheiber, L., Moukheiber, M., Moukheiber, D., Hicklen, R. S., Waldrip, S., & Ke, J. X. C. (2023). Bias in artificial intelligence algorithms and recommendations for mitigation. *PLOS Digital Health*, *2*(6), e0000278. DOI: 10.1371/journal.pdig.0000278 PMID: 37347721

Neaimeh, M., & Andersen, P. B. (2020). Mind the gap—Open communication protocols for vehicle grid integration. *Energy Informatics*, *3*(1), 1–17. DOI: 10.1186/s42162-020-0103-1

Neisse, R., Fovino, I. N., & Steri, G. (2018). *Blockchain-based Identity Management and Data Usage Control (Extended Abstract)*. Springer., DOI: 10.1007/978-3-319-92925-5_15

O'Sullivan, E., & Schofield, S. (2018). Cognitive Bias in Clinical Medicine. *Journal of the Royal College of Physicians of Edinburgh*, *48*(3), 225–232. DOI: 10.4997/jrcpe.2018.306 PMID: 30191910

OAIC (Office of the Australian Information Commissioner). (2022). *Notifiable Data Breaches Report: January–June 2022*. https://www.oaic.gov.au

Odeh, A., Abdelfattah, E., & Salameh, W. (2024). Privacy-Preserving Data Sharing in Telehealth Services. *Applied Sciences (Basel, Switzerland)*, *14*(23), 10808. DOI: 10.3390/app142310808

Office for Civil Rights (OCR). (2016). *Anthem pays OCR $16 million in record HIPAA settlement*. U.S. Department of Health and Human Services. https://www.hhs.gov

Olateju, O. O., Olaniyi, O. O., Oladoyinbo, T. O., Okon, S. U., Salami, A. A., & Igwenagu, U. T. I. (2024). Combating the Challenges of False Positives in AI-Driven Anomaly Detection Systems and Enhancing Data Security in the Cloud. *Asian Journal of Research in Computer Science*, *17*(6), 264–292. DOI: 10.9734/ajrcos/2024/v17i6472

Ollitrault, P. J., Miessen, A., & Tavernelli, I. (2021). Molecular quantum dynamics: A quantum computing perspective. *Accounts of Chemical Research*, *54*(23), 4229–4238. DOI: 10.1021/acs.accounts.1c00514 PMID: 34787398

Oluoha, O. M., Odeshina, A., Reis, O., Okpeke, F., Attipoe, V., & Orieno, O. H. (2022). A Unified Framework for Risk-Based Access Control and Identity Management in Compliance-Critical Environments.

Omar, I. A., Jayaraman, R., Debe, M. S., Salah, K., Yaqoob, I., & Omar, M. (2021). Automating procurement contracts in the healthcare supply chain using blockchain smart contracts. *IEEE Access : Practical Innovations, Open Solutions*, *9*, 37397–37409. DOI: 10.1109/ACCESS.2021.3062471

Omotosho, A., Emuoyibofarhe, J., & Meinel, C. (2017). Ensuring patients' privacy in a cryptographic-based-electronic health records using bio-cryptography. *International Journal of Electronic Healthcare*, *9*(4), 227. DOI: 10.1504/IJEH.2017.085800

Ovabor, K., Atkison, T., Benedict, J., Fabusoro, A., & Sule-Odu, I. (2024). AI-driven threat intelligence for real-time cybersecurity: Frameworks, tools, and future directions. *Open Access Research Journal of Science and Technology*, *12*(2), 040–048. DOI: 10.53022/oarjst.2024.12.2.0135

Ozair, F. F., Jamshed, N., Sharma, A., & Aggarwal, P. (2015). Ethical issues in electronic health records: A general overview. *Perspectives in Clinical Research*, *6*(2), 73–76. DOI: 10.4103/2229-3485.153997 PMID: 25878950

Padmapriya, S. T., & Parthasarathy, S. (2023). Ethical Data Collection for Medical Image Analysis: A Structured Approach. *Asian Bioethics Review*, *16*(1), 95–108. DOI: 10.1007/s41649-023-00250-9 PMID: 37361687

Pakela, J. M., Tseng, H. H., Matuszak, M. M., Ten Haken, R. K., McShan, D. L., & El Naqa, I. (2020). Quantum-inspired algorithm for radiotherapy planning optimization. *Medical Physics*, *47*(1), 5–18. DOI: 10.1002/mp.13840 PMID: 31574176

Pal, S., Bhattacharya, M., Lee, S. S., & Chakraborty, C. (2024). Quantum computing in the next-generation computational biology landscape: From protein folding to molecular dynamics. *Molecular Biotechnology*, *66*(2), 163–178. DOI: 10.1007/s12033-023-00765-4 PMID: 37244882

Panch, T., Mattie, H., & Atun, R. (2019). Artificial intelligence and algorithmic bias: Implications for health systems. *Journal of Global Health*, *9*(2), 010318. Advance online publication. DOI: 10.7189/jogh.09.020318 PMID: 31788229

Pascarella, G., Rossi, M., Montella, E., Capasso, A., De Feo, G., Botti, G., Nardone, A., Montuori, P., Triassi, M., D'Auria, S., & Morabito, A. (2021). Risk analysis in healthcare organizations: Methodological Framework and critical variables. *Risk Management and Healthcare Policy*, *14*, 2897–2911. DOI: 10.2147/RMHP.S309098

Pattanaik, P. K., Gupta, S., Pani, A. K., Himanshu, U., & Pappas, I. O. (2024). Impact of inter and intra organizational factors in healthcare digitalization: A Conditional Mediation Analysis. *Information Systems Frontiers*. Advance online publication. DOI: 10.1007/s10796-024-10522-w

Paul, B., & Rao, M. (2022). Zero-Trust Model for Smart Manufacturing Industry. *Applied Sciences (Basel, Switzerland)*, *13*(1), 221. DOI: 10.3390/app13010221

Peltier, T. R. (2006). Social Engineering: Concepts and Solutions. *Information Systems Security : ... International Conference, ICISS ... : Proceedings*, *15*(5), 13–21. DOI: 10.1201/1086.1065898X/46353.15.4.20060901/95427.3

Perets, O., Stagno, E., Yehuda, E. B., Mcnichol, M., Anthony Celi, L., Rappoport, N., & Dorotic, M. (2024). Inherent Bias in Electronic Health Records: A Scoping Review of Sources of Bias. In medRxiv *: the preprint server for health sciences*. Cold Spring Harbor Laboratory. DOI: 10.1101/2024.04.09.24305594

Perry, H., Tsai, E. M., Perusse, K., Herschorn, S. D., & Watson, E. J. (2022). Breast Imaging During a Cyberattack and Global Pandemic: What We Did to Pick Up the Pieces. *Seminars in Ultrasound. Seminars in Ultrasound, CT, and MR*, *44*(1), 18–22. DOI: 10.1053/j.sult.2022.10.001 PMID: 36792269

Peterson, C., & Watzlaf, V. (2015). Telerehabilitation Store and Forward Applications: A Review of Applications and Privacy Considerations in Physical and Occupational Therapy Practice. *International Journal of Telerehabilitation*, *6*(2), 75–84. DOI: 10.5195/ijt.2014.6161 PMID: 25945231

Phyo, A. H., Furnell, S. M., & Portilla, F. (2004). *A Framework for Role-Based Monitoring of Insider Misuse*. Kluwer Academic., DOI: 10.1007/1-4020-8145-6_4

Pietrzykowski, T., & Smilowska, K. (2021). The reality of informed consent: Empirical studies on patient comprehension—systematic review. *Trials*, *22*(1), 57. Advance online publication. DOI: 10.1186/s13063-020-04969-w

Podder, P., Mondal, M. R. H., Bharati, S., & Paul, P. K. (2020). Review on the Security Threats of Internet of Things. *International Journal of Computer Applications*, *176*(41), 37–45. DOI: 10.5120/ijca2020920548

Pöhn, D., & Hillmann, P. (2021). *Reference Service Model for Federated Identity Management*. Springer., DOI: 10.1007/978-3-030-79186-5_13

Pokharel, B. P., Paudel, S., Kshetri, N., & Sharma, S. R. (2025). blockHealthSecure: Integrating Blockchain and Cybersecurity in Post-Pandemic Healthcare Systems. *Information (Basel)*, *16*(2), 133. DOI: 10.3390/info16020133

Ponemon Institute. (2022). *The cost of a data breach report 2022*. IBM Security. https://www.ibm.com/security/data-breach

Popoola, O., Rodrigues, M. A., Marchang, J., Shenfield, A., Ikpehai, A., & Popoola, J. (2024). An optimized hybrid encryption framework for smart home healthcare: Ensuring data confidentiality and security. *Internet of Things : Engineering Cyber Physical Human Systems*, *27*, 101314. DOI: 10.1016/j.iot.2024.101314

Portela, D., Almeida, R., Nogueira-Leite, D., & Cruz-Correia, R. (2022). *Economic Impact of a Hospital Cyberattack in a National Health System: Descriptive Case Study (Preprint)*. Jmir. DOI: 10.2196/preprints.41738

Prashanth Joshi, A., Han, M., & Wang, Y. (2018). A survey on security and privacy issues of blockchain technology. *Mathematical Foundations of Computing*, *1*(2), 121–147. DOI: 10.3934/mfc.2018007

Price, W. N.II, & Cohen, I. G. (2019). Privacy in the age of medical big data. *Nature Medicine*, *25*(1), 37–43. DOI: 10.1038/s41591-018-0272-7 PMID: 30617331

Pulipeti, S., & Kumar, A. (2023). Secure quantum computing for healthcare sector: A short analysis. *Security and Privacy*, *6*(5), e293. DOI: 10.1002/spy2.293

Pu, X., Jiang, R., Song, Z., Liang, Z., & Yang, L. (2024). A medical big data access control model based on smart contracts and risk in the blockchain environment. *Frontiers in Public Health*, *12*, 1358184. DOI: 10.3389/fpubh.2024.1358184 PMID: 38605878

Qayyum, A. (2023). Quantum computing for healthcare: A review. *Authorea Preprints*.

Radanliev, P. (2024). Artificial Intelligence and Quantum Cryptography. *Journal of Analytical Science and Technology*, *15*(1), 4. Advance online publication. DOI: 10.1186/s40543-024-00416-6

Radanliev, P., De Roure, D., Nurse, J. R. C., Nicolescu, R., Huth, M., Cannady, S., & Montalvo, R. M. (2020). Cyber risk at the edge: Current and future trends on cyber risk analytics and artificial intelligence in the industrial internet of things and industry 4.0 supply chains. *Cybersecurity*, *3*(13), 13. Advance online publication. DOI: 10.1186/s42400-020-00052-8

Raghupathi, W., Saharia, A., & Raghupathi, V. (2023). Analyzing Health Data Breaches: A Visual Analytics Approach. *AppliedMath*, *3*(1), 175–199. DOI: 10.3390/appliedmath3010011

Raikwar, M., Mazumdar, S., Ruj, S., Sen Gupta, S., Chattopadhyay, A., & Lam, K. Y. 2018.A blockchain framework for insurance processes. In: 2018 9th IFIP International Conference On New Technologies, Mobility And Security, NTMS 2018 - Proceedings,vol. 2018, pp. 1–4. https://doi.org/DOI: 10.1109/NTMS.2018.8328731

Ramesh, D., Sharma, R. P., & Edla, D. R. (2020). HHDSSC: Harnessing healthcare data security in cloud using ciphertext policy attribute-based encryption. *International Journal of Information and Computer Security*, *13*(3/4), 322. DOI: 10.1504/IJICS.2020.109480

Ramezanpour, K., & Jagannath, J. (2022). Intelligent zero trust architecture for 5G/6G networks: Principles, challenges, and the role of machine learning in the context of O-RAN. *Computer Networks*, *217*, 109358. DOI: 10.1016/j.comnct.2022.109358

Rana, M. M. (2017). Attack resilient wireless sensor networks for smart electric vehicles. *IEEE Sensors Letters*, *1*(2), 1–4. DOI: 10.1109/LSENS.2017.2690907

Rashmi, R. V., & Karthikeyan, A. (2018, March). Secure boot of embedded applications-a review. In *2018 Second International Conference on Electronics, Communication and Aerospace Technology (ICECA)* (pp. 291-298). IEEE.

Rathore, R. S., Hewage, C., Kaiwartya, O., & Lloret, J. (2022). In-vehicle communication cyber security: Challenges and solutions. *Sensors (Basel)*, *22*(17), 6679. DOI: 10.3390/s22176679

Rauf, A., Shaikh, R. A., & Shah, A. (2022). Trust Modelling and management for IoT healthcare. *International Journal of Wireless and Microwave Technologies*, *12*(5), 21–35. DOI: 10.5815/ijwmt.2022.05.03

Reale, C., Andreae, M. H., Sushereba, C., Banerjee, A., Militello, L. G., Slagle, J., Weinger, M. B., Anders, S., Mcivor, W. R., Gaba, D. M., Salwei, M. E., Torsher, L. C., & Burden, A. (2023). Decision-Making During High-Risk Events: A Systematic Literature Review. *Journal of Cognitive Engineering and Decision Making*, *17*(2), 188–212. DOI: 10.1177/15553434221147415 PMID: 37823061

Reddy, R. P. (2025). Zero Trust Architectures in Modern Enterprises: Principles, Implementation Challenges, and Best Practices. *International Journal of Computer Trends and Technology*, *73*(6), 48–57. DOI: 10.14445/22312803/IJCTT-V73I6P107

Reddy, S., Cooper, P., Allan, S., & Coghlan, S. (2019). A governance model for the application of AI in health care. *Journal of the American Medical Informatics Association : JAMIA*, *27*(3), 491–497. DOI: 10.1093/jamia/ocz192 PMID: 31682262

Regueiro, C., Seco, I., Gutiérrez-Agüero, I., Urquizu, B., & Mansell, J. (2021). A blockchain-based audit trail mechanism: Design and implementation. *Algorithms*, *14*(12), 341. DOI: 10.3390/a14120341

Reis, O., Abrahams, T., Ehimuan, B., Olorunsogo, T., Eneh, N., & Anyanwu, A. (2024). PRIVACY LAW CHALLENGES IN THE DIGITAL AGE: A GLOBAL REVIEW OF LEGISLATION AND ENFORCEMENT. *International Journal of Applied Research in Social Sciences*, *6*(1), 73–88. DOI: 10.51594/ijarss.v6i1.733

Rengamani, H., Upadhyaya, S., Kumaraguru, P., & Rao, H. R. (2010). *Protecting senior citizens from cyber security attacks in the e-health scenario.* 1–4. DOI: 10.1145/1852666.1852759

Rhayha, R., El Ouali Lalami, A., El Malki, H., Merabti, A., El Hilaly, J., Mahla, T., Bahli, B., & Alaoui Ismaili, A. (2025). Factors influencing clinician performance post-electronic health record implementation: An empirical analysis in Moroccan hospitals. *BMC Health Services Research*, *25*(1), 324. Advance online publication. DOI: 10.1186/s12913-025-12438-w PMID: 40016779

Ribeiro De Mello, E., Silva Wangham, M., Da Silva, C. E., Cavalcanti Da Silva, G., De Chaves, S. A., Bristot Loli, S., & Bristot Loli, B. (2020). Multi-factor authentication for shibboleth identity providers. *Journal of Internet Services and Applications*, *11*(1), 8. Advance online publication. DOI: 10.1186/s13174-020-00128-1

Richter, S., & Ammenwerth, E. (2023). IT risk management for medical devices in hospital IT networks: A catalogue of measures and indicators. *BMJ Health & Care Informatics*, *30*(1), e100639. DOI: 10.1136/bmjhci-2022-100639 PMID: 36724909

Rieffel, E., & Polak, W. (2000). An introduction to quantum computing for non-physicists. *ACM Computing Surveys*, *32*(3), 300–335. DOI: 10.1145/367701.367709

Rigaud, M., Buekers, J., Bessems, J., Basagaña, X., Mathy, S., Nieuwenhuijsen, M., & Slama, R. (2024). The methodology of Quantitative Risk Assessment Studies. *Environmental Health : A Global Access Science Source*, *23*(1), 13. Advance online publication. DOI: 10.1186/s12940-023-01039-x

Robinson, T., Harkin, J., & Shukla, P. (2021). Hardware acceleration of genomics data analysis: Challenges and opportunities. *Bioinformatics (Oxford, England), 37*(13), 1785–1795. DOI: 10.1093/bioinformatics/btab017 PMID: 34037688

Rocchiccioli, J. (2003). Health Insurance Portability and Accountability Act: Administrative Simplification to Understand the Revised Proposed Privacy Standards—A Policy Update. *The Journal of the Association of Nurses in AIDS Care: JANAC, 14*(2), 63–66. DOI: 10.1177/1055329002251000 PMID: 12698767

Rockwern, B., Johnson, D., & Snyder Sulmasy, L. (2021). Health Information Privacy, protection, and use in the expanding digital health ecosystem: A position paper of the American College of Physicians. *Annals of Internal Medicine, 174*(7), 994–998. DOI: 10.7326/M20-7639

Rogers, J., Someya, T., & Malliaras, G. (2018). Biomedical devices go wild. *Science Advances, 4*(9), eaav1889. Advance online publication. DOI: 10.1126/sciadv.aav1889 PMID: 30255157

Ronanki, D., & Karneddi, H. (2023). Electric vehicle charging infrastructure: Review, cyber security considerations, potential impacts, countermeasures and future trends. *IEEE Journal of Emerging and Selected Topics in Power Electronics.* Advance online publication. DOI: 10.1109/JESTPE.2023

Rony, M. K. K., Akter, F., Tushar, H., Johra, F. T., Numan, S. M., Akter, K., Mondal, S., Parvin, M. R., Uddin, M. J., Das, M., Debnath, M., & Begum, J. (2024). Nurses' perspectives on privacy and ethical concerns regarding artificial intelligence adoption in healthcare. *Heliyon, 10*(17), e36702. DOI: 10.1016/j.heliyon.2024.e36702 PMID: 39281626

Roopa, M. S., & Venugopal, K. R. (2025). Digital twins for cyber-physical healthcare systems: Architecture, requirements, systematic analysis, and future prospects. *IEEE Access : Practical Innovations, Open Solutions, 13*, 44963–44996. DOI: 10.1109/ACCESS.2025.3547991

Rose, S., Borchert, O., Mitchell, S., & Connelly, S. (2020). *Zero Trust Architecture (SP 800-207).* National Institute of Standards and Technology. https://doi.org/DOI: 10.6028/NIST.SP.800-207

Rose, S., Borchert, O., Mitchell, S., & Connelly, S. (2020). *Zero Trust Architecture. National Institute of Standards and Technology (NIST), Special Publication 800-207.*

Roy Sarkar, K. (2010). Assessing insider threats to information security using technical, behavioural and organisational measures. *Information Security Technical Report, 15*(3), 112–133. DOI: 10.1016/j.istr.2010.11.002

Rutherford, A., Walden, A., Noblin, A., Gabriel, M. H., & Cortelyou-Ward, K. (2018). Data breach locations, types, and associated characteristics among US hospitals. *The American Journal of Managed Care*, *24*(2), 78–84. PMID: 29461854

S, M., & K R, J. (2025). Blockchain-enabled federated learning with edge analytics for secure and efficient electronic health records management. *Scientific Reports*, *15*(1). DOI: 10.1038/s41598-025-12225-x

SaberiKamarposhti, M., Ng, K.-W., Chua, F.-F., Abdullah, J., Yadollahi, M., Moradi, M., & Ahmadpour, S.SaberiKamarposhti. (2024). Post-quantum Healthcare: A roadmap for cybersecurity resilience in medical data. *Heliyon*, *10*(10), e31406. Advance online publication. DOI: 10.1016/j.heliyon.2024.e31406

Sachdeva, S., Bhatia, S., Al Harrasi, A., Shah, Y. A., Anwer, M., Philip, A. K., Shah, S. F. A., Khan, A., & Ahsan Halim, S. (2024). Unraveling the role of Cloud Computing in health care system and biomedical sciences. *Heliyon*, *10*(7), e29044. Advance online publication. DOI: 10.1016/j.heliyon.2024.e29044

Saeed, S., Suayyid, S. A., Al-Ghamdi, M. S., Al-Muhaisen, H., & Almuhaideb, A. M. (2023). A systematic literature review on Cyber Threat Intelligence for Organizational Cybersecurity Resilience. *Sensors (Basel)*, *23*(16), 7273. DOI: 10.3390/s23167273

Salahdine, F., & Kaabouch, N. (2019). Social Engineering Attacks: A Survey. *Future Internet*, *11*(4), 89. DOI: 10.3390/fi11040089

Salem, A. H., Azzam, S. M., Emam, O. E., & Abohany, A. A. (2024). Advancing cybersecurity: A comprehensive review of AI-Driven Detection Techniques. *Journal of Big Data*, *11*(1), 105. Advance online publication. DOI: 10.1186/s40537-024-00957-y

Salim, D. T., Singh, M. M., & Keikhosrokiani, P. (2023). A systematic literature review for APT detection and Effective Cyber Situational Awareness (ECSA) conceptual model. *Heliyon*, *9*(7), e17156. Advance online publication. DOI: 10.1016/j.heliyon.2023.e17156

Sanghvi, A., & Markel, T. (2021, June). Cybersecurity for electric vehicle fast-charging infrastructure. In *2021 IEEE Transportation Electrification Conference & Expo (ITEC)* (pp. 573–576). IEEE. DOI: 10.1109/ITEC51675.2021.9490069

Sanghvi, A., Markel, T., Granda, S., Nagarajan, A., & Jun, M. (2021). *Identification and testing of electric vehicle fast charger cybersecurity mitigations* (No. NREL/TP-5R00-80799). National Renewable Energy Laboratory. DOI: 10.2172/1786046

Santos, P., Abreu, R., Reis, M. J., Serôdio, C., & Branco, F. (2025). A systematic review of Cyber Threat Intelligence: The effectiveness of technologies, strategies, and collaborations in Combating modern threats. *Sensors (Basel)*, *25*(14), 4272. DOI: 10.3390/s25144272

Sarkar, S., Choudhary, G., Shandilya, S. K., Hussain, A., & Kim, H. (2022). Security of zero trust networks in cloud computing: A comparative review. *Sustainability (Basel)*, *14*(18), 11213. DOI: 10.3390/su141811213

Sarker, I. H. (2024). Introduction to AI-driven cybersecurity and threat intelligence. In *AI-driven cybersecurity and threat intelligence: Cyber automation, intelligent decision-making and explainability* (pp. 3–19). Springer Nature Switzerland. DOI: 10.1007/978-3-031-54497-2_1

Scheibner, J., Raisaro, J. L., Troncoso-Pastoriza, J. R., Ienca, M., Fellay, J., Vayena, E., & Hubaux, J.-P. (2021). Revolutionizing medical data sharing using advanced privacy-enhancing technologies: Technical, legal, and ethical synthesis. *Journal of Medical Internet Research*, *23*(2), e25120. Advance online publication. DOI: 10.2196/25120

Seh, A. H., Zarour, M., Alenezi, M., Sarkar, A. K., Agrawal, A., Kumar, R., & Ahmad Khan, R. (2020). Healthcare Data Breaches: Insights and Implications. *Health Care*, *8*(2), 133. DOI: 10.3390/healthcare8020133 PMID: 32414183

Semantha, F. H., Azam, S., Yeo, K. C., & Shanmugam, B. (2020). A systematic literature review on privacy by design in the healthcare sector. *Electronics (Basel)*, *9*(3), 452. DOI: 10.3390/electronics9030452

Sergiu, E. (2020). Insider threats and thermal stress in the working environment. *Scientific Bulletin of Naval Academy*, *23*(1), 271–276. DOI: 10.21279/1454-864X-20-I1-038

Seth, D., Najana, M., & Ranjan, P. (2024). Compliance and Regulatory Challenges in Cloud Computing: A Sector-Wise Analysis. *International Journal of Global Innovations and Solutions (IJGIS)*. DOI: 10.21428/e90189c8.68b5dea5

Seth, M., Jalo, H., Högstedt, Å., Medin, O., Sjöqvist, B. A., & Candefjord, S. (2025). Technologies for interoperable internet of medical things platforms to manage medical emergencies in home and Prehospital Care: Scoping Review. *Journal of Medical Internet Research*, *27*, e54470. Advance online publication. DOI: 10.2196/54470

Sevin, A., & Osman Mohammed, A. A. (2024). Comparative Study of Blockchain Hashing Algorithms with a Proposal for HashLEA. *Applied Sciences (Basel, Switzerland)*, *14*(24), 11967. DOI: 10.3390/app142411967

Shahnaz, A., Qamar, U., & Khalid, A. (2019). Using blockchain for electronic health records. *IEEE Access : Practical Innovations, Open Solutions*, *7*, 147782–147795. DOI: 10.1109/ACCESS.2019.2946373

Shaikh, J. A., Wang, C., Muhammad, W. U. S., Arshad, M., Owais, M., Alnashwan, R. O., Chelloug, S. A., & Muthanna, M. S. A. (2024). RCLNet: An effective anomaly-based intrusion detection for securing the IoMT system. *Frontiers in Digital Health*, *6*, 1467241. Advance online publication. DOI: 10.3389/fdgth.2024.1467241 PMID: 39421756

Shaikh, J. A., Wang, C., Sima, M. W. U., Arshad, M., Owais, M., Hassan, D. S. M., Alkanhel, R., & Muthanna, M. S. A. (2025). A deep Reinforcement learning-based robust Intrusion Detection System for securing IoMT Healthcare Networks. *Frontiers in Medicine*, *12*, 1524286. Advance online publication. DOI: 10.3389/fmed.2025.1524286 PMID: 40309737

Shamszare, H., & Choudhury, A. (2023). Clinicians' Perceptions of Artificial Intelligence: Focus on Workload, Risk, Trust, Clinical Decision Making, and Clinical Integration. *Health Care*, *11*(16), 2308. DOI: 10.3390/healthcare11162308 PMID: 37628506

Sharma, S., & Ali, I. (2025). IEC 61850 communication-enabled cost optimisation for electric vehicle integration in microgrids. *International Journal of Ambient Energy*, *46*(1), 2516065. Advance online publication. DOI: 10.1080/01430750.2025.2516065

Sheikh, N., Pawar, M., & Lawrence, V. (2021). Zero Trust Using Network Micro Segmentation. *IEEE INFOCOM 2021 - IEEE Conference on Computer Communications Workshops (INFOCOM WKSHPS)*, 1–6. DOI: 10.1109/INFOCOMWKSHPS51825.2021.9484645

Shemshi, V., & Jakimovski, B. (2025). Extended Model for Efficient Federated Identity Management with Dynamic Levels of Assurance Across eIDAS, REFEDS, and Kantara Frameworks for Educational Institutions. *Information (Basel)*, *16*(5), 385. DOI: 10.3390/info16050385

Shin, H., Ryu, K., Kim, J.-Y., & Lee, S. (2024). Application of privacy protection technology to Healthcare Big Data. *Digital Health*, *10*, 20552076241282242. Advance online publication. DOI: 10.1177/20552076241282242

Shojaei, P., Vlahu-Gjorgievska, E., & Chow, Y.-W. (2024). Security and privacy of technologies in Health Information Systems: A systematic literature review. *Computers*, *13*(2), 41. DOI: 10.3390/computers13020041

Siddiqi, M. A., Doerr, C., & Strydis, C. (2020). IMDfence: Architecting a Secure Protocol for Implantable Medical Devices. *IEEE Access : Practical Innovations, Open Solutions*, *8*, 147948–147964. DOI: 10.1109/ACCESS.2020.3015686

Sills, M., Ranade, P., & Mittal, S. (2020). Cybersecurity threat intelligence augmentation and embedding improvement - A healthcare USECASE. *2020 IEEE International Conference on Intelligence and Security Informatics (ISI)*, 1–6. DOI: 10.1109/ISI49825.2020.9280482

Singapore Ministry of Health. (2018). *SingHealth cyberattack—Public report.* https://www.moh.gov.sg

Singh, Y., Jaiswal, S., & Kumar, V. (2024). A Comprehensive Literature Review on Privacy, Security, and Data Management in Healthcare. *2024 2nd International Conference on Disruptive Technologies (ICDT)*, 220–224.

Singh, C., Thakkar, R., & Warraich, J. (2023). IAM identity access management—Importance in maintaining security systems within organizations. *European Journal of Engineering and Technology Research*, *8*(4), 30–38. DOI: 10.24018/ejeng.2023.8.4.3074

Skopik, F., & Pahi, T. (2020). Under false flag: Using technical artifacts for cyber attack attribution. *Cybersecurity*, *3*(1), 8. DOI: 10.1186/s42400-020-00048-4

Solve.Care. (2021). *Solve.Care Platform Overview*. https://solve.care

Sookhak, M., Jabbarpour, M. R., Safa, N. S., & Yu, F. R. (2021). Blockchain and smart contract for access control in healthcare: A survey, issues and challenges, and open issues. *Journal of Network and Computer Applications*, *178*, 102950. DOI: 10.1016/j.jnca.2020.102950

Sowmya, T., & Mary Anita, E. A. (2023). A comprehensive review of AI based intrusion detection system. *Measurement. Sensors*, *28*, 100827. DOI: 10.1016/j.measen.2023.100827

Srivastava, D., Budhiraja, V., Srivastava, A., & Verma, M. (2025). A systematic review of applications, challenges, data collection and academic research in healthcare using IoT. *Transforming Healthcare: Mode, Technologies, and Implementation*, 181.

Stavrou, E., & Piki, A. (2024). Cultivating self-efficacy to empower professionals' re-up skilling in cybersecurity. *Information &amp. Information and Computer Security*, *32*(4), 523–541. DOI: 10.1108/ICS-02-2024-0038

Stern, A. D., Gordon, W. J., Landman, A. B., & Kramer, D. B. (2019). Cybersecurity features of digital medical devices: An analysis of FDA product summaries. *BMJ Open*, *9*(6), e025374. DOI: 10.1136/bmjopen-2018-025374 PMID: 31256020

Stewart, J., & Dawson, M. (2018). How the modification of personality traits leave one vulnerable to manipulation in social engineering. *International Journal of Information Privacy. Security and Integrity*, *3*(3), 187. DOI: 10.1504/IJIPSI.2018.10013213

Subudhi, S. (2024). Effectiveness of AI/ML in SOAR (security automation and orchestration) platforms. [IJSR]. *International Journal of Science and Research (Raipur, India)*, *13*(8), 201–206. DOI: 10.21275/MR24802085215

Suleski, T., Ahmed, M., Yang, W., & Wang, E. (2023). A review of multi-factor authentication in the Internet of Healthcare Things. *Digital Health*, *9*, 205520762311771. DOI: 10.1177/20552076231177144 PMID: 37252257

Sulmasy, L. S., Horwitch, C. A., & López, A. M. (2017). Ethical Implications of the Electronic Health Record: In the Service of the Patient. *Journal of General Internal Medicine*, *32*(8), 935–939. DOI: 10.1007/s11606-017-4030-1 PMID: 28321550

Syed, R. (2018). Enterprise reputation threats on social media: A case of data breach framing. *The Journal of Strategic Information Systems*, *28*(3), 257–274. DOI: 10.1016/j.jsis.2018.12.001

Tabassum, M., Mahmood, S., Bukhari, A., Alshemaimri, B., Daud, A., & Khalique, F. (2024). Anomaly-based threat detection in Smart Health Using Machine Learning. *BMC Medical Informatics and Decision Making*, *24*(1), 347. Advance online publication. DOI: 10.1186/s12911-024-02760-4

Tahir, N. U. A., Alshara, M. A., Javed, Y., Cao, Y., Rashid, U., Ahmad, N., & Hadi, H. J. (2024). Blockchain-Based Healthcare Records Management Framework: Enhancing Security, Privacy, and Interoperability. *Technologies*, *12*(9), 168. DOI: 10.3390/technologies12090168

Tahmasebi, M. (2024). Beyond defense: Proactive approaches to disaster recovery and threat intelligence in modern enterprises. *Journal of Information Security*, *15*(2), 106–133. DOI: 10.4236/jis.2024.152008

Tall, A., Wang, J., & Han, D. (2016). *Survey of data intensive computing technologies application to to security log data management*. 268–273. DOI: 10.1145/3006299.3006336

Tanimura, J. K., & Wehrly, E. W. (2015). The Market Value and Reputational Effects from Lost Confidential Information. *International Journal of Financial Management*, *5*(4). Advance online publication. DOI: 10.21863/ijfm/2015.5.4.020

Tao, Q., Liu, S., Zhang, J., Jiang, J., Jin, Z., Huang, Y., Liu, X., Lin, S., Zeng, X., Li, X., Tao, G., & Chen, H. (2023). Clinical applications of smart wearable sensors. *iScience*, *26*(9), 107485. DOI: 10.1016/j.isci.2023.107485 PMID: 37636055

Taylor, R. A., Sangal, R. B., Smith, M. E., Haimovich, A. D., Rodman, A., Iscoe, M. S., Pavuluri, S. K., Rose, C., Janke, A. T., Wright, D. S., Socrates, V., & Declan, A. (2024). Leveraging artificial intelligence to reduce diagnostic errors in emergency medicine: Challenges, opportunities, and future directions. *Academic Emergency Medicine*, *32*(3), 327–339. DOI: 10.1111/acem.15066 PMID: 39676165

Thapa, C., & Camtepe, S. (2020a). Precision health data: Requirements, challenges and existing techniques for data security and privacy. *Computers in Biology and Medicine*, *129*, 104130. DOI: 10.1016/j.compbiomed.2020.104130 PMID: 33271399

Theodoropoulos, T., Rosa, L., Benzaid, C., Gray, P., Marin, E., Makris, A., Cordeiro, L., Diego, F., Sorokin, P., Girolamo, M. D., Barone, P., Taleb, T., & Tserpes, K. (2023). Security in cloud-native services: A survey. *Journal of Cybersecurity and Privacy*, *3*(4), 758–793. DOI: 10.3390/jcp3040034

Theodos, K., & Sittig, S. (2020, December 7). *Health Information Privacy Laws in the digital age: HIPAA doesn't apply*. Perspectives in health information management. https://pmc.ncbi.nlm.nih.gov/articles/PMC7883355/

Tikkinen-Piri, C., Rohunen, A., & Markkula, J. (2018). EU General Data Protection Regulation: Changes and implications for personal data collecting companies. *Computer Law & Security Review*, *34*(1), 134–153. DOI: 10.1016/j.clsr.2017.05.015

Tong, Y., Li, P., Sun, J., & Chow, S. S. M. (2013, October 1). *Towards auditable cloud-assisted access of encrypted health data*. DOI: 10.1109/CNS.2013.6682769

Touchie, C., Kinnear, B., Schumacher, D., Caretta-Weyer, H., Hamstra, S. J., Hart, D., Gruppen, L., Ross, S., Warm, E., & Ten Cate, O. (2021). On the validity of summative entrustment decisions. *Medical Teacher*, *43*(7), 780–787. DOI: 10.1080/0142159X.2021.1925642 PMID: 34020576

Tseng, J. H., Liao, Y. C., Chong, B., & Liao, S. W. (2018). Governance on the drug supply chain via gcoin blockchain. *International Journal of Environmental Research and Public Health*, *15*(6), 1055. Advance online publication. DOI: 10.3390/ijerph15061055 PMID: 29882861

Tsiostas, D., Chouliaras, N., Douligeris, C., Kittes, G., Maglaras, L., Vlachos, V., & Kantzavelou, I. (2020). *The Insider Threat: Reasons, Effects and Mitigation Techniques*. 340–345. DOI: 10.1145/3437120.3437336

Udendhran, R. (2017). *A hybrid approach to enhance data security in cloud storage.* 1–6. DOI: 10.1145/3018896.3025138

Udroiu, A.-M., Dumitrache, M., & Sandu, I. (2022). Improving the cybersecurity of medical systems by applying the NIST framework. *2022 14th International Conference on Electronics, Computers and Artificial Intelligence (ECAI)*, 1–7. DOI: 10.1109/ECAI54874.2022.9847498

Ur Rasool, R., Ahmad, H. F., Rafique, W., Qayyum, A., Qadir, J., & Anwar, Z. (2023). Quantum computing for healthcare: A review. *Future Internet, 15*(3), 94. DOI: 10.3390/fi15030094

Uygun Ilikhan, S., Özer, M., Tanberkan, H., & Bozkurt, V. (2024). How to mitigate the risks of deployment of artificial intelligence in medicine? *Turkish Journal of Medical Sciences, 54*(3), 483–492. DOI: 10.55730/1300-0144.5814 PMID: 39050000

Vashishth, T. K., Sharma, V., Sharma, K. K., Kumar, B., Chaudhary, S., & Panwar, R. (2025). Securing the cloud: Strategies for protecting sensitive patient data in cloud-based Healthcare Recommender Systems. *Healthcare Recommender Systems*, 185–220. DOI: 10.1007/978-3-031-80056-6_9

Vayena, E., Brownstein, J. S., Dzenowagis, J., & Sheikh, A. (2017). Policy implications of big data in the health sector. *Bulletin of the World Health Organization, 96*(1), 66–68. DOI: 10.2471/BLT.17.197426 PMID: 29403102

Veeraballi, V. R. (2025). Implementing the NIST risk management framework in cloud environments: A comprehensive approach. *INTERNATIONAL JOURNAL OF COMPUTER ENGINEERING AND TECHNOLOGY, 16*(1), 3655–3670. DOI: 10.34218/IJCET_16_01_252

Venkatesha, S., Reddy, K. R., & Chandavarkar, B. R. (2021). Social Engineering Attacks During the COVID-19 Pandemic. *SN Computer Science, 2*(2), 78. Advance online publication. DOI: 10.1007/s42979-020-00443-1 PMID: 33585823

Verizon. (2023). *Data Breach Investigations Report (DBIR).* https://www.verizon.com/business/resources/reports/dbir/

Vickrey, B. G., Samuels, M. A., & Ropper, A. H. (2010). How neurologists think: A cognitive psychology perspective on missed diagnoses. *Annals of Neurology, 67*(4), 425–433. DOI: 10.1002/ana.21907 PMID: 20437577

Vitorino, J., Praça, I., & Maia, E. (2023). SoK: Realistic adversarial attacks and defenses for intelligent network intrusion detection. *Computers &amp. Computers & Security, 134*, 103433. DOI: 10.1016/j.cose.2023.103433

Voss, W. G. (2019). Cross-border data flows, the GDPR, and data governance. *Wash. Int'l LJ*, *29*, 485.

Vukotich, G. (2023). Healthcare and cybersecurity: Taking a Zero trust approach. *Health Services Insights*, *16*, 11786329231187826. Advance online publication. DOI: 10.1177/11786329231187826

Wang, C., Song, R., & Liu, Z. (2020). Simulation of vehicle network communication security based on random geometry and data mining. *IEEE Access : Practical Innovations, Open Solutions*, *8*, 69389–69400. DOI: 10.1109/ACCESS.2020.2986338

Wang, H., Wang, Y., Cao, Z., Li, Z., & Xiong, G. (2019). *An Overview of Blockchain Security Analysis* (Vol. 970). Springer Singapore., DOI: 10.1007/978-981-13-6621-5_5

Wang, Y., Zhao, Z., Qi, B., Cheng, Y., Tang, K., & Li, B. (2024). Vulnerability analysis of an electric vehicle fleet for car-sharing service under cyber attacks. *Sustainable Energy. Grids and Networks*, *37*, 101207. DOI: 10.1016/j.segan.2024.101207

Wang, Z., Yu, X., Xue, P., Qu, Y., & Ju, L. (2023). Research on medical security system based on Zero trust. *Sensors (Basel)*, *23*(7), 3774. DOI: 10.3390/s23073774

Wani, T. A., Mendoza, A., & Gray, K. (2020). Hospital bring-your-own-device security challenges and solutions: Systematic review of Gray Literature. *JMIR mHealth and uHealth*, *8*(6), e18175. Advance online publication. DOI: 10.2196/18175

Wan, J., O'Grady, M., Cao, N., Li, M., & Al-Awlaqi, A A H. (2018). M., Gu, X., & Wang, J. (2018). Wearable IoT enabled real-time health monitoring system. *EURASIP Journal on Wireless Communications and Networking*, (1). Advance online publication. DOI: 10.1186/s13638-018-1308-x

Wasserman, L., & Wasserman, Y. (2022). Hospital cybersecurity risks and gaps: Review (for the non-cyber professional). *Frontiers in Digital Health*, *4*(Suppl 6), 862221. Advance online publication. DOI: 10.3389/fdgth.2022.862221 PMID: 36033634

Weinberg, A. I., & Cohen, K. (2024). Zero trust implementation in the emerging technologies era: A survey. *Complex Engineering Systems*, *4*(3). Advance online publication. DOI: 10.20517/ces.2024.41

Weng, S., Li, Y., & Ding, X. (2020). Resilient distributed coordination of plug-in electric vehicles charging under cyber-attack. *Electronics (Basel)*, *9*(5), 770. DOI: 10.3390/electronics9050770

Wheatley, M. C. (2024). Quantum Shifts: The Societal Implications of Quantum Computing on Security, Privacy, and the Economy. *Journal of Computational Science, 1*, 100002.

Williams, P. A., & Woodward, A. J. (2015). Cybersecurity vulnerabilities in medical devices: a complex environment and multifaceted problem. *Medical Devices: Evidence and Research*, 305-316.

Williams, M. S., Taylor, C. O., Walton, N. A., Goehringer, S. R., Aronson, S., Freimuth, R. R., Rasmussen, L. V., Hall, E. S., Prows, C. A., Chung, W. K., Fedotov, A., Nestor, J., Weng, C., Rowley, R. K., Wiesner, G. L., Jarvik, G. P., & Del Fiol, G. (2019). Genomic Information for Clinicians in the Electronic Health Record: Lessons Learned From the Clinical Genome Resource Project and the Electronic Medical Records and Genomics Network. *Frontiers in Genetics, 10*(146), 1059. DOI: 10.3389/fgene.2019.01059 PMID: 31737042

Williams, P., & Woodward, A. (2015). Cybersecurity vulnerabilities in medical devices: A complex environment and multifaceted problem. *Medical Devices (Auckland, N.Z.), 8*(10), 305. DOI: 10.2147/MDER.S50048 PMID: 26229513

Wu, C. M., Schulz, E., Speekenbrink, M., & Pleskac, T. J. (2022). Time pressure changes how people explore and respond to uncertainty. *Scientific Reports, 12*(1), 4122. Advance online publication. DOI: 10.1038/s41598-022-07901-1 PMID: 35260717

Wutthikarn, R., & Hui, Y. G. 2018. Prototype of blockchain in dental care service application based on hyperledger composer in hyperledger fabric framework, 2018. In: International Computer Science and Engineering Conference, *22nd*. ICSEC. . Jul. 2018.DOI: 10.1109/ICSEC.2018.8712639

Xia, L., Cao, Z., & Zhao, Y. (2024). Paradigm transformation of global health data regulation: Challenges in governance and human rights protection of cross-border data flows. *Risk Management and Healthcare Policy, 17*, 3291–3304. DOI: 10.2147/RMHP.S450082

Xiang, D., & Cai, W. (2021). Privacy protection and secondary use of health data: Strategies and methods. *BioMed Research International, 2021*(1). DOI: 10.1155/2021/6967166

Xu, J. (2024). The current status and promotional strategies for Cloud Migration of Hospital Information Systems in China: Strengths, weaknesses, opportunities, and threats analysis. *JMIR Medical Informatics, 12*, e52080. Advance online publication. DOI: 10.2196/52080

Xu, J., Glicksberg, B. S., Su, C., Walker, P., Bian, J., & Wang, F. (2020). Federated Learning for Healthcare Informatics. *Journal of Healthcare Informatics Research, 5*(1), 1–19. DOI: 10.1007/s41666-020-00082-4

Xu, S., Rogers, J. A., Ghaffari, R., Walter, J. R., & Kim, J. (2022). Translational gaps and opportunities for medical wearables in digital health. *Science Translational Medicine, 14*(666), eabn6036. Advance online publication. DOI: 10.1126/scitranslmed.abn6036 PMID: 36223451

Yadav, A., Kumar, A., & Singh, V. (2023). Open-source intelligence: A comprehensive review of the current state, applications and future perspectives in Cyber Security. *Artificial Intelligence Review, 56*(11), 12407–12438. DOI: 10.1007/s10462-023-10454-y

Yang, B., Guo, L., Li, F., Ye, J., & Song, W. (2019, June). Impact analysis of data integrity attacks on power electronics and electric drives. In *2019 IEEE Transportation Electrification Conference and Expo (ITEC)* (pp. 1–6). IEEE. DOI: 10.1109/ITEC.2019.8790574

Yazdi, M., Zarei, E., Adumene, S., & Beheshti, A. (2024). Navigating the power of Artificial Intelligence in Risk Management: A comparative analysis. *Safety (Basel, Switzerland), 10*(2), 42. DOI: 10.3390/safety10020042

Ye, J., Guo, L., Yang, B., Li, F., Du, L., Guan, L., & Song, W. (2020). Cyber-physical security of powertrain systems in modern electric vehicles: Vulnerabilities, challenges and future visions. *IEEE Journal of Emerging and Selected Topics in Power Electronics, 9*(4), 4639–4657. DOI: 10.1109/JESTPE.2020.3045667

Yeng, P. K., Fauzi, M. A., Sun, L., & Yang, B. (2022). Assessing the Legal Aspects of Information Security Requirements for Health Care in 3 Countries: Scoping Review and Framework Development. *JMIR Human Factors, 9*(2), e30050. DOI: 10.2196/30050 PMID: 35612891

Yeole, A., & Kalbande, D. R. (2021). *Ensuring Security and Privacy in IoT for Healthcare Applications*. 299–314. DOI: 10.1002/9781119711308.ch11

Yimam, D., & Fernandez, E. B. (2016). A survey of compliance issues in cloud computing. *Journal of Internet Services and Applications, 7*(1), 5. Advance online publication. DOI: 10.1186/s13174-016-0046-8

Yle News. (2020). *Vastaamo data breach: Finnish psychotherapy scandal deepens*. https://yle.fi/news

Yogi, M. K., MangaDevi, A., & Mundru, Y. (2025). Heartbeat Hackers: Protecting Privacy in the IoMT Age. *Convergence of Internet of Medical Things (IoMT) and Generative AI*, 133-170.

Young, D. L., Goodie, A. S., Hall, D. B., & Wu, E. (2012). Decision making under time pressure, modeled in a prospect theory framework. *Organizational Behavior and Human Decision Processes, 118*(2), 179–188. DOI: 10.1016/j.obhdp.2012.03.005 PMID: 22711977

Zandesh, Z. (2024). Privacy, Security, and Legal Issues in the Health Cloud: Structured Review for Taxonomy Development. *JMIR Formative Research*, *8*(1), e38372. DOI: 10.2196/38372 PMID: 38345858

Zeydan, E., Arslan, S. S., & Liyanage, M. (2024). Managing distributed machine learning lifecycle for healthcare data in the cloud. *IEEE Access : Practical Innovations, Open Solutions*, *12*, 115750–115774. DOI: 10.1109/ACCESS.2024.3443520

Zhang, P., Schmidt, D. C., White, J., & Lenz, G. (2018). Blockchain technology use cases in healthcare. In *Advances in computers*,1–41. https://doi.org/DOI: 10.1016/bs.adcom.2018.03.006

Zhang, G., Yang, Z., & Liu, W. (2022a). Blockchain-based privacy preserving e-health system for healthcare data in cloud. *Computer Networks*, *203*, 108586. DOI: 10.1016/j.comnet.2021.108586

Zhu, L., Wu, Y., Gai, K., & Choo, K. K. R. (2019). Controllable and trustworthy blockchain-based cloud data management. *Future Generation Computer Systems*, *91*, 527–535. DOI: 10.1016/j.future.2018.09.019

Ziwei, H., Dongni, Z., Man, Z., Yixin, D., Shuanghui, Z., Chao, Y., & Chunfeng, C. (2024). The applications of internet of things in smart healthcare sectors: A bibliometric and deep study. *Heliyon*, *10*(3), e25392. DOI: 10.1016/j.heliyon.2024.e25392 PMID: 38356528

Zlatolas, L. N., Welzer, T., & Lhotska, L. (2024). Data breaches in Healthcare: Security Mechanisms for attack mitigation. *Cluster Computing*, *27*(7), 8639–8654. DOI: 10.1007/s10586-024-04507-2

Zobaed, S. M., & Amini Salehi, M. (2025). Confidential Computing Across Edge-To-Cloud for Machine Learning: A Survey Study. *Software, Practice & Experience*, *55*(5), 896–924. DOI: 10.1002/spe.3398

Zoppi, T., Bondavalli, A., Capecchi, T., & Ceccarelli, A. (2021). Unsupervised Anomaly Detectors to Detect Intrusions in the Current Threat Landscape. *ACM/IMS Transactions on Data Science*, *2*(2), 1–26. DOI: 10.1145/3441140

Zwitter, A. (2014). Big Data ethics. *Big Data &amp. Big Data & Society*, *1*(2), 205395171455925. DOI: 10.1177/2053951714559253

About the Contributors

Chin-Shiuh Shieh is a distinguished academic and researcher in the field of electronic engineering and computer science, currently serving as a Professor in the Department of Electronic Engineering at National Kaohsiung University of Science and Technology (NKUST), Taiwan. He received his Ph.D. in Computer Science and Engineering from the National Sun Yat-sen University, Taiwan, and has since dedicated his career to pioneering research and teaching in areas including computer networking, wireless communication, information security, computational intelligence, embedded systems, and medical informatics. With a career spanning several decades, Professor Shieh has made significant contributions to both academia and industry. In the past five years alone, he has authored or co-authored 28 journal papers, of which 24 are indexed in SCI (Science Citation Index), and 80 conference papers, encompassing 26 international and 54 domestic conferences. His editorial acumen is evident in his role as editor for two international academic conference proceedings. Professor Shieh has been actively engaged in various research initiatives, participating in 10 Ministry of Science and Technology (MOST) projects, leading five of them. He has also been involved in three Ministry of Education projects, one of which he led, and a campus research project. Furthermore, his strong industry collaboration is reflected in 10 industry-academia cooperation projects, eight of which he led. He has also contributed to one technology transfer authorization. As a recognized figure in the global research community, Professor Shieh is affiliated with four professional societies, and serves as a reviewer for 106 academic journals. He has participated as a committee member for 21 journals and 175 international conferences, underscoring his influence and expertise in his fields of specialization. Among his recent notable publications is the 2024 SCI-indexed paper titled "Open-set recognition in unknown DDoS attacks detection with reciprocal points learning" published in IEEE Access, which highlights his innovative work in cybersecurity and artificial intelligence. He has also played key editorial roles in conferences such as the International Conference on Genetic and Evolutionary Computing (ICGEC) and Intelligent Information Hiding and Multimedia Signal Processing (IIHMSP). His work has earned multiple accolades including Best Paper Awards and Excellent Paper Awards in international conferences. He has co-developed cutting-edge methods in machine learning, optimization algorithms, and adversarial defense mechanisms, particularly in the domain of cybersecurity threats such as DDoS attacks. His academic journey, prolific publication record, leadership in research projects, and commitment to interdisciplinary collaboration have established him as a leading voice in advancing electronic engineering and computing sciences in Taiwan and beyond.

Pawan Kumar Goel is a seasoned academician, researcher, and institutional leader with over two decades of rich experience in the field of Computer Science and Engineering. Presently serving as an Associate Professor in the Department of Computer Science & Engineering at Raj Kumar Goel Institute of Technology, Ghaziabad (affiliated to Dr. A.P.J. Abdul Kalam Technical University, Lucknow), Dr. Goel has made significant contributions to teaching, research, innovation, and academic administration. His academic journey is marked by a relentless pursuit of excellence, supported by strong educational credentials that include a Ph.D. in Computer Science Engineering, M.Tech in Computer Science & Engineering, and an MBA in Human Resource Management. He is also UGC-NET qualified in Computer Science and Applications and has cleared GATE multiple times. He earned his B.Tech in Information Technology with distinction. His impressive academic qualifications are complemented by numerous certifications from premier institutes in cutting-edge fields like AI, Blockchain, Cloud Computing, Cybersecurity, Quantum Computing, and more. Over his professional career, Dr. Goel has held several key academic and administrative positions. Throughout his journey, he has consistently demonstrated leadership in institutional development, curriculum innovation, accreditation processes (NAAC and NBA), and faculty mentoring. Dr. Goel is a prolific writer and editor, having authored and edited numerous books with globally reputed academic publishers such as IGI Global, Bentham Science, and Scientific International Publishing House. Some of his notable titles include Strategies for E-Commerce Data Security, Cloud Computing and IoT Strategies for Industry 5.0 Innovation, and Improving Security, Privacy, and Trust in Cloud Computing. He has authored over 50 book chapters in diverse areas such as AI for mental health, blockchain for social media, AI-based security for communication networks, and ethical considerations in cybersecurity and artificial emotional intelligence. His scholarly work is widely published in Scopus and UGC-indexed journals, and he has presented at leading IEEE international conferences such as IC3SE, ICDT, ICCSP, and AECE. Dr. Goel's research interests are interdisciplinary, encompassing cloud and edge computing, AI and machine learning, cybersecurity,

IoT, wireless sensor networks, and blockchain technology. He has also filed several patents, including designs and systems for smart agricultural drones, IoT health monitoring devices, and blockchain-integrated IoT data management systems. His technological innovations reflect his commitment to solving real-world problems through applied research. Dr. Goel has received multiple awards and accolades for his academic and professional excellence. He was honored with the International Achiever Award 2023 for Distinguished Teaching by Gyan Uday Foundation and the Educator of the Year Award 2022 by Namaste India Council of Educators. He has also been recognized for his role in quality assurance and curriculum development by institutions like Quantum University and IIMT Greater Noida. In addition, he has received appreciation for his contributions as a reviewer and advisor at various international conferences and journals. An active contributor to professional and academic communities, Dr. Goel holds memberships in a wide range of reputed organizations including IEEE, ACM, CSI, IAENG, IACSIT, IFERP, CSTA, and SCIEI. He serves as an editorial and review board member for several international journals such as IJRAR, IJCSIS, JITE, and IJSCE. He is also the Institutional Ambassador for IFERP and serves as the Single Point of Contact (SPOC) for Infosys Campus Connect Program, further strengthening academia-industry collaboration. As a committed educator and academic facilitator, Dr. Goel has organized and coordinated several faculty development programs (FDPs), seminars, and workshops. He has played key roles in AICTE-sponsored FDPs, including being the Co-Coordinator of the ATAL FDP on Quantum Machine Learning in January 2025. He also serves as the Local Coordinator for the Remote Center of NITTTR Chandigarh, enabling the conduction of numerous FDPs and STCs through ICT mode. His organizational acumen and passion for innovation have enabled the successful execution of national-level events and knowledge dissemination platforms. Dr. Goel continues to actively participate in continuous learning and professional development, having completed numerous AICTE-ATAL FDPs in areas such as Cybersecurity in AI, Deep Learning, Quantum Computing, and Ethical AI. He has also successfully completed various NPTEL MOOCs on subjects including Blockchain Architecture, Data Science, Privacy and Security in Online Social Media, and NBA Accreditation processes. An enthusiastic academic with a strong foundation in pedagogy and research, Dr. Goel teaches core computer science courses such as Programming in C, Data Structures, Computer Networks, Database Management Systems, Cloud Computing, and Cybersecurity. His teaching philosophy emphasizes conceptual clarity, problem-solving, and the integration of emerging technologies into the curriculum. Dr. Goel's personal qualities—leadership, optimism, perseverance, and hard work—have earned him admiration among his peers and students alike. His multifaceted contributions to academia, research, and innovation position him as a thought leader and change-maker in the Indian higher education landscape. He continues to inspire generations of learners and researchers, contributing significantly to the digital and technological transformation of the education ecosystem.

Mong-Fong Horng received his B.S., Ms. and Ph.D degrees from National Chiao Tung University and National Cheng Kung University, Taiwan in 1989, 1991 and 2003, respectively. He now is a jointly-appointed professor with the department of Electronics Engineering at National Kaohsiung University of Science and Technology, and Kaohsiung Medical University, Taiwan. He served as the president of Taiwanese Association of Consumer Electronics (TACE), Chair of Tainan Chapter, IEEE Signal Processing Society. His research interest includes Internet of Things, machine learning, computer networks and medical informatics and related industrial cooperation.

***

Nathaniel Akande is a renowned Information Analyst with over 8 years of experience in threat intelligence, incident response, vulnerability management, Quality Assurance, Governance, Risk, and Compliance (GRC). He holds an MBA, an M.Sc. in Cybersecurity, and is a Certified ISO 27001 Lead Implementer. Adept at implementing data governance, identity and access management, and aligning operations with standards like GDPR, ISO 27001, and NIST, Nathaniel has led enterprise projects involving data governance and AI risk management. He is a conference speaker and has authored and reviewed several articles. He is recognized for his strong analytical skills, technical acumen, and proactive approach to security operations and compliance.

Shalini Jaiswal has more than 17 years' experience in academics and research and is the author of more than 65 scientific publications in Scopus\SCI\UGC and other reputed journal\Conference. Dr. Shalini Jaiswal received her D.Phil degree in Organic Chemistry from University of Allahabad, Allahabad India, in 2009. Dr. Shalini Jaiswal has14 month experience as a project fellow on UGC sponsored project entitled Green synthesis of multi- target nucleosides as a potential anti-viral agent. Her research interest includes different area of Chemistry, Nanotechnology, AI, Biotechnology and Environmental science. She is a Life Member of the Indian science congress association. She has reviewed more than 50 papers of various reputed journal and conferences. She is Editorial board member and Reviewer of various reputed journals like TPI (International Journal), IJATES, International journal of advance research, Advanced Scientific Research, IJEEE, Asian Journal of Research in Chemistry (AJRC) etc.Dr. Shalini Jaiswal Worked as

Moderator in TOKYO SUMMIT-II (2020) and TOKYO SUMMIT-III (2021), Turkey (2022,2023,2024)

Deepti Khurge is currently an Associate Professor in the Department of Electronics and Telecommunication Engineering at Pimpri Chinchwad College of Engineering (PCCoE), Pune, India. She has over 18 year of academic experience and has guided various undergraduate, postgraduate, and doctoral research projects. She holds a Ph.D. in Electronics Engineering from RTM Nagpur University (2019) and an M.Tech and B.E. in Electronics. Her research interests include VLSI Design, FPGA-based System Design, Quantum Computing, and Digital System Design using Verilog and VHDL. She has published over 18 journal papers, more than 20 conference papers, and has contributed 3 book chapters. She also holds 4 granted patents and 5 copyrights. Dr. Khurge has been actively involved in roles such as Autonomy Coordinator, Technical Program Chair for ICCUBEA 2024, BoS member, Ph.D. co-guide, and reviewer. She has participated in various international FDPs, including DAAD ProGRANT, and has certifications in Quantum Computing, AVR Programming, and Innovation Ambassador Training. Her work integrates academia-industry collaboration and promotes student research in VLSI, Semiconductor Design, FPGA Systems.

Swati Sharma received the B.Eng. degree in Electrical Engineering from Maharishi Dayanand University, Rohtak, India and the M.Eng. degree in Control and Instrumentation from Delhi Technological University, Delhi, India and Completed her Doctor of Philosophy at Faculty of Electrical Engineering in Jamia Millia Islamia, New Delhi, India. Her research interests include renewable energy, metaheuristic algorithms, smart grids, battery chargers, demand response, power distribution protection, artificial intelligence, cybersecurity.

Yaduvir Singh is a distinguished academician and researcher with over 19 years of experience in teaching undergraduate and postgraduate students. Currently serving as an Assistant Professor in the Department of Computer Science and Engineering (AI) at NIET, Greater Noida, he brings a wealth of expertise in emerging fields such as Blockchain Technology, Artificial Intelligence, and Data Science.He has authored more than 20 research papers in esteemed national and international journals and is a frequent contributor and organizer of national-level workshops on AI, Blockchain, and Entrepreneurship. A lifetime member of MISTE and affiliated with MIAENG, MIFERP, MCSTA, and MIRED, Prof. Singh continues to be an inspiring figure in academia, driven by his passion for learning and innovation in teaching.

Indumathi Srinivasan's career spans healthcare, consulting, and technology sectors, delivering impactful results at Smiligence, HCL Technologies, Sodexo

India, Juran Academy, and Apollo Hospitals. Her expertise in SQL, Tableau, Power BI, JIRA, and Confluence enables her to develop data-driven strategies for business optimization. Her academic background includes an MBA in Health Service Management, a Bachelor's in Microbiology, and a Post Graduate Diploma in Strategic Digital Marketing. At SIMATS University, her Ph.D. research in Healthcare Management focuses on EHR Data Quality Management, examining data integrity and interoperability to improve clinical decision-making accuracy. As a certified Lean Six Sigma practitioner from ASQ and Indian Statistical Institute, she has trained professionals in process optimization. Indumathi combines analytical skills with technology expertise to advance business intelligence and healthcare informatics.

A. K. Subramani Professor at Saveetha School of Management, Saveetha Institute of Medical and Technical Sciences, Chennai, Dr. Subramani AK brings 18 years of teaching experience to the classroom. Holding a Ph.D. in Business Administration from Manonmaniam Sundaranar University, Tirunelveli, Dr. Subramani A K has contributed significantly to the field with 70 articles published in international journals, including 28 in Scopus indexed journals, 4 in Anna University Annexure journals, and 2 in national journals.

Index

A

B

C

D

E

G

H

I

M

O

P

Q

R

S

T

V

Z

www.ingramcontent.com/pod-product-compliance
Lightning Source LLC
LaVergne TN
LVHW080903300926
849162LV00003B/539